Antioxidants in Human Health and Disease

Antioxidants in Human Health and Disease

Edited by Nina Pegg

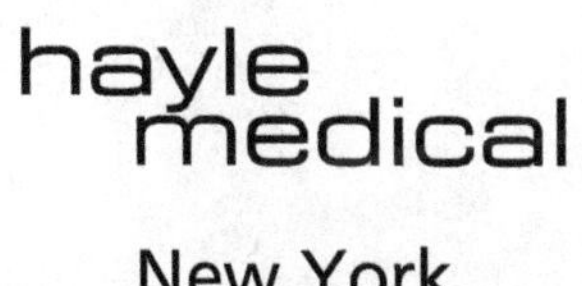

New York

Hayle Medical,
750 Third Avenue, 9th Floor,
New York, NY 10017, USA

Visit us on the World Wide Web at:
www.haylemedical.com

ISBN: 978-1-63241-831-9

Cataloging-in-Publication Data

Antioxidants in human health and disease / edited by Nina Pegg.
p. cm.
Includes bibliographical references and index.
ISBN 978-1-63241-831-9
1. Antioxidants. 2. Health. 3. Healing. 4. Antioxidants--Health aspects.
5. Antioxidants--Therapeutic use. I. Pegg, Nina.

RB170 .A583 2020
613.286--dc23

Table of Contents

Preface

Living organisms require oxygen for survival, but it is also a highly reactive molecule that can damage organisms by producing reactive oxygen species. Oxidation is the chemical reaction that produces free radicals and thereby leads to chain reactions with the potential to damage the cells of organisms. Antioxidants inhibit oxidation. Ascorbic acid or thiols are antioxidants that can terminate these chain reactions. Organisms have a complex system of antioxidant metabolites and enzymes that work in tandem to prevent oxidative damage to DNA, proteins and lipids. However, reactive oxygen species have useful cellular functions as well, such as redox signaling. Antioxidant systems therefore do not remove oxidants completely but keep them at an optimum level. The role of oxidative stress in degenerative diseases, such as diabetes, kidney disease, neurological disorders, obesity, cancer and aging is understood. This makes antioxidant dietary supplements a potential strategy to overcome these conditions. This book provides comprehensive insights into antioxidants and their role in human health and disease. It will also provide interesting topics for research, which interested readers can take up. With state-of-the-art inputs by acclaimed experts of this field, this book targets students and professionals.

Various studies have approached the subject by analyzing it with a single perspective, but the present book provides diverse methodologies and techniques to address this field. This book contains theories and applications needed for understanding the subject from different perspectives. The aim is to keep the readers informed about the progresses in the field; therefore, the contributions were carefully examined to compile novel researches by specialists from across the globe.

Indeed, the job of the editor is the most crucial and challenging in compiling all chapters into a single book. In the end, I would extend my sincere thanks to the chapter authors for their profound work. I am also thankful for the support provided by my family and colleagues during the compilation of this book.

Editor

1

Lipid Peroxidation-Derived Aldehydes, 4-Hydroxynonenal and Malondialdehyde in Aging-Related Disorders

Giuseppina Barrera [1,*], Stefania Pizzimenti [1], Martina Daga [1], Chiara Dianzani [2], Alessia Arcaro [3], Giovanni Paolo Cetrangolo [3], Giulio Giordano [4], Marie Angele Cucci [1], Maria Graf [4] and Fabrizio Gentile [3]

[1] Dipartimento di Scienze Cliniche e Biologiche, Università di Torino, 10124 Turin, Italy; stefania.pizzimenti@unito.it (S.P.); martina.daga@unito.it (M.D.); marieangele.cucci@unito.it (M.A.C.)
[2] Dipartimento di Scienze e Tecnologia del Farmaco, Università di Torino, 10124 Turin, Italy; chiara.dianzani@unito.it
[3] Dipartimento di Medicina e Scienze della Salute "V. Tiberio", Università del Molise, 86100 Campobasso, Italy; alessia.arcaro@unimol.it (A.A.); gianpaolo.cet@tiscali.it (G.P.C.); gentilefabrizio@unimol.it (F.G.)
[4] Presidio Ospedaliero "A. Cardarelli", Azienda Sanitaria Regione Molise, 86100 Campobasso, Italy; giuliogiordano@hotmail.com (G.G.); mariagraf@tiscali.it (M.G.)
* Correspondence: giuseppina.barrera@unito.it

Abstract: Among the various mechanisms involved in aging, it was proposed long ago that a prominent role is played by oxidative stress. A major way by which the latter can provoke structural damage to biological macromolecules, such as DNA, lipids, and proteins, is by fueling the peroxidation of membrane lipids, leading to the production of several reactive aldehydes. Lipid peroxidation-derived aldehydes can not only modify biological macromolecules, by forming covalent electrophilic addition products with them, but also act as second messengers of oxidative stress, having relatively extended lifespans. Their effects might be further enhanced with aging, as their concentrations in cells and biological fluids increase with age. Since the involvement and the role of lipid peroxidation-derived aldehydes, particularly of 4-hydroxynonenal (HNE), in neurodegenerations, inflammation, and cancer, has been discussed in several excellent recent reviews, in the present one we focus on the involvement of reactive aldehydes in other age-related disorders: osteopenia, sarcopenia, immunosenescence and myelodysplastic syndromes. In these aging-related disorders, characterized by increases of oxidative stress, both HNE and malondialdehyde (MDA) play important pathogenic roles. These aldehydes, and HNE in particular, can form adducts with circulating or cellular proteins of critical functional importance, such as the proteins involved in apoptosis in muscle cells, thus leading to their functional decay and acceleration of their molecular turnover and functionality. We suggest that a major fraction of the toxic effects observed in age-related disorders could depend on the formation of aldehyde-protein adducts. New redox proteomic approaches, pinpointing the modifications of distinct cell proteins by the aldehydes generated in the course of oxidative stress, should be extended to these age-associated disorders, to pave the way to targeted therapeutic strategies, aiming to alleviate the burden of morbidity and mortality associated with these disturbances.

Keywords: aldehydes; osteopenia; sarcopenia; myelodysplastic syndromes; immunosenescence

1. Introduction

In recent years, increased life expectancy due to an improved quality of life and decline in mortality rates, is leading to a society in which the aging population is growing more rapidly than the entire population. Life expectancy is projected to increase in industrialized countries. In 2016, 27.3 million very old adults were living in the European Union, and in the UK, 2.4% of the population (1.6 million) were aged 85 and over [1]. It has been calculated that there is more than a 50% probability that, by 2030, female life expectancy will exceed the 90-year barrier, a level that was deemed unattainable at the turn of the 21st century [2]. The functional disturbances appearing in old age are referred to as the "aging process", which entails changes in body composition, imbalances in energy production and use, homeostatic dysregulation, neurodegeneration and loss of neuroplasticity [3]. The scientific community has formulated over 300 theories to explain the driving forces behind aging [4], but none has proven, so far, to be universally applicable. The free radical theory of aging has gained widespread acceptance, thus becoming one of the leading explanations of the aging process at the molecular level. It is commonly believed that the aging process is related to an imbalance favoring pro-oxidant over antioxidant molecules and a consequent increase of oxidative stress [5]. Oxidative stress entails elevated intracellular levels of reactive oxygen species (ROS), which can cause damage to proteins, lipids, and DNA. The mitochondria are the primary sources of intracellular ROS (~1–5%), due to the electron leakage primarily resulting from the electron transport chain [6]. Indeed, mitochondrial dysfunction has long been considered a major contributor to aging and age-related diseases. In elderly subjects, mitochondria are characterized by functional impairment, such as lowered oxidative capacity, reduced oxidative phosphorylation, decreased adenosine triphosphate production, significantly increased ROS generation, and diminished antioxidant defense [7]. Depending on their concentration in the cells, ROS are either physiological signals essential for cell life or toxic species which damage cell structure and functions. In particular, ROS cause the oxidation of polyunsaturated fatty acids in membrane lipid bilayers, leading eventually to the formation of aldehydes, which have been considered as toxic messengers of oxidative stress, able to propagate and amplify oxidative injury [8].

Among the aldehydes produced by lipid peroxidation (LPO), malonaldehyde (MDA) and 4-hydroxynonenal (HNE) have gained most attention, since MDA is produced at high levels during LPO, so that it is commonly used as a measure of oxidative stress, and HNE has been shown to be endowed with the highest biological activity. The production, metabolism, and signaling mechanisms of two main omega-6 fatty acids lipid peroxidation products, MDA and HNE, have been extensively studied and reported in an excellent review [9]. Briefly, MDA and HNE originate from the peroxidation of polyunsaturated fatty acids. LPO can be described generally as a process under which oxidant, free radical or non-radical chemical species attack lipids containing carbon–carbon double bond(s). This process involves hydrogen abstraction from a carbon atom and oxygen insertion, resulting in the formation of peroxyl radicals and lipid hydroperoxides, as illustrated in Figure 1.

Since aldehydes have high chemical reactivities, mammals have evolved a full set of enzymes converting them into less reactive chemical species and contributing to the control of their intracellular concentrations, which reflect the steady-state between the rates of formation by LPO and catabolism into less reactive compounds. Once formed, MDA and HNE can be reduced to alcohols by aldo-keto reductases or alcohol dehydrogenases, or can be oxidized to acids by aldehyde dehydrogenases [10]. Moreover, HNE, which is the most reactive among aldehydes, easily reacts with low-molecular-weight compounds, such as glutathione. This reaction can occur spontaneously or can be catalyzed by glutathione-S-transferases [10]. HNE and MDA are able to affect several signaling processes. Most of these effects depend on their ability to bind covalently to proteins and DNA.

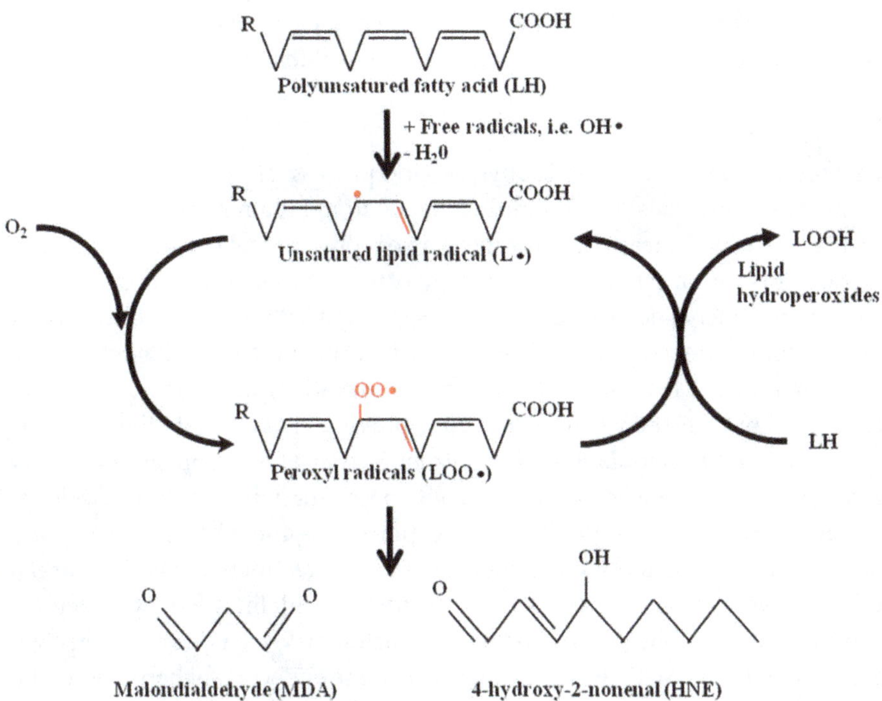

Figure 1. Malondialdehyde (MDA) and 4-hydroxynonenal (HNE) formation from polyunsaturated fatty acids.

Aldehyde–Protein Adduct in Human Disease

LPO-derived aldehydes easily react with proteins, generating a wide variety of intra- and inter-molecular covalent adducts. Depending on their structural features, they can form Schiff bases and/or Michael adducts with the free amine group of lysine, the imidazoline group of histidine, the guanidine group of arginine and the thiol group of cysteine [11]. HNE can affect cell functions, through its ability to form adducts with proteins involved in signal transduction and gene expression, including receptors, kinases, phosphatases and transcription factors [11]. MDA can form protein adducts by specifically modifying the lysyl residues of proteins [12], and modified autologous biomolecules can generate neoepitopes from self epitopes, capable of inducing undesired innate and adaptive immune responses, including atherosclerosis [13]. HNE adducts can accumulate progressively in the vascular system, leading to cellular dysfunctions and tissue damaging effects, which are involved in the progression of atherosclerosis. Moreover, HNE, by forming HNE-apoB adducts, contributes to the atherogenicity of oxidized low-density lipoproteins (LDL), leading to the formation of foam cells [14]. The presence of HNE-protein adducts has been detected in inflammation-related diseases, such as alcoholic liver disorders and chronic alcoholic pancreatitis, in which the increased formation of HNE-protein adducts was evidenced in acinar cells adjacent to the interlobular connective tissue [15]. Moreover, HNE-protein adducts have been detected in brain tissues and body fluids in several neurodegenerative diseases, such as Alzheimer's disease, Huntington disease, Parkinson's disease, amyotrophic lateral sclerosis, and Down syndrome [10].

The involvement of MDA and HNE in age-related diseases has been supported by the observations that the concentrations of MDA and HNE, in human erythrocytes and blood plasma, increased during the aging process [16]. The role of reactive aldehydes in age-related pathologies, such as atherosclerosis [13], neurodegenerations [17], inflammation, and cancer [10] has been discussed by many excellent reviews. Other age-related disorders, such as osteopenia/osteoporosis, sarcopenia, immunosenescence and myelodysplastic syndromes have received less attention. In this review, we focus our attention on to recent advances in the role of LPO-derived aldehydes and aldehyde-protein adducts in these age-related disorders, all of which are characterized by increases of oxidative stress and consequent increases in the generation of LPO-derived aldehydes.

2. Osteopenia/Osteoporosis

Bone remodeling is a highly dynamic physiological process: osteoblasts (bone-forming cells) and osteoclasts (bone-resorbing cells) work simultaneously to maintain bone density and strength [18]. During aging, bone density decreases and the measure of bone mineral density is commonly employed to evaluate whether or not a patient is affected by osteopenia or osteoporosis. Osteopenia is the thinning of bone mass. Such a decrease in bone mass is not usually "severe", but is considered a very serious risk factor for the development of osteoporosis. Osteoporosis is characterized by profound losses of skeletal mass, coupled with architectural deterioration, which increase bone fragility and susceptibility to fractures. Several recent papers have provided insights into the current prevalence of osteoporosis in specific older populations. The current National Osteoporosis Foundation guidelines for the USA, coupled with the most recently available population data from the National Health and Nutrition Survey, show that the eligibility for osteoporosis treatment increases exponentially with age; roughly 10% of both men and women meet criteria for treatment at age 50 years, whereas 48% of men and 79% of women over 80 years meet treatment guidelines [19]. Current treatments for osteoporosis, which increase bone density and reduce fracture risk, include anti-resorptive medications (bisphosphonates and denosumab), which primarily increase endocortical bone and cortical thickness, and anabolic medications (teriparatide and abaloparatide), which increase the periosteal and endosteal perimeters, without causing large changes in cortical thickness [20].

Increases of ROS levels have been observed consistently in osteopenia and osteoporosis. In aging people, the number and activity of individual osteoblasts decrease and osteoblast apoptosis increases, in association with oxidative stress-induced osteoporosis [21]. Some studies explored the relationships between the use of antioxidants and bone metabolism. Indeed, a marked decrease in plasma antioxidants was found in aged or osteoporotic rats and in aged or osteoporotic women [22–24]. The loss of antioxidant capacity leads to accelerated bone loss through the activation of a tumor necrosis factor alpha (TNF-α)-dependent signalling pathway [25]. In turn, the administration of antioxidants such as vitamin C, E, N-acetyl-cysteine and linoleic acid, had beneficial effects in individuals with osteoporosis [26].

Osteoblast apoptosis was induced by oxidative stress through the activation of the c-Jun N-terminal kinase (JNK) pathway [27] and the NF-kB pathway [28]. In unstimulated cells, NF-κB proteins are sequestered in the cytoplasm because of their association with IκB (inhibitor of κ light gene enhancer in B cells) proteins. Phosphorylation and degradation of IκB disrupt this association and allow the translocation of NF-κB proteins into the nucleus. ROS induce the oxidation of critical cysteines and enhance the activity of several cytoplasmic kinases, which promote IκB phosphorylation and degradation, including IκB kinase and the PKC family of serine/threonine kinases [29]. Additionally, ROS-induced modifications control key steps in the nuclear phase of the NF-κB program, including recruitment of coactivators, chromatin remodeling, and DNA binding. The activation of NF-kB in osteoblastic cells increased the phosphorylation of p66 (shc) protein, which amplified mitochondrial ROS generation and stimulated apoptosis [29]. The increase of ROS in osteoblastic MC3T3-E1 cells induced phosphorylation of MAPKs (mitogen-activated protein kinases), which subsequently triggered the intrinsic apoptosis pathway. Moreover, the advanced oxidation protein products induced osteoblast apoptosis in aged Sprague–Dawley rats [30].

The NF-κB pathway is involved in osteoclast activity, as well. Indeed, ROS stimulated osteoclast differentiation and activity through activation of the NF-κB pathway, and these effects were reversed upon NF-κB suppression [31].

Other than by the direct actions mentioned above, ROS can affect bone turnover by enhancing the production of LPO-derived reactive intermediates, thereby causing protein damage and inflammatory responses [32]. In vitro experiments have proved that HNE, the most biologically active aldehyde produced by LPO, can induce intense oxidative stress, inflammatory reactions, and apoptosis in osteoblasts, via the induction of protein phosphatase 2A activity, which has earned a reputation as a mediator of oxidative stress-induced apoptosis in these cells [21]. The role of LPO-derived aldehydes in osteoblast apoptosis is also supported by studies on aldehyde dehydrogenases (ALDH), a family of enzymes involved in aldehyde degradation [33]. ALDH inhibition by disulfiram resulted in bone loss in rats [34]. Additional confirmation of the role of ALDH activity in osteoporosis comes from the results obtained with transgenic mice expressing the Aldh2*2 (Aldh2*2 Tg) dominant-negative form of ALDH2. These transgenic mice exhibited severe osteoporosis, indicating that ALDH2 regulates physiological bone homeostasis. Moreover, the Aldh2*2 transgene or treatment with acetaldehyde induced the accumulation of HNE and the expression of peroxysome proliferator-activated receptor γ (PPAR-γ) a transcription factor that promotes adipogenesis and inhibits osteoblastogenesis [35]. On the contrary, the activation of ALDH2 by *N*-(1,3-benzodioxol-5-ylmethyl)-2,6-dichlorobenzamide (alda-1) had an osteogenic effect, involving increased production of bone morphogenetic protein-2 by osteoblasts [36]. Taken together, these experimental data seem to delineate a role for the products of LPO in the induction of osteoporosis. However, the measurements of MDA as an indicator of LPO in post-menopausal osteoporotic women gave conflicting results. One study disclosed significant increases in plasma MDA concentrations in post-menopausal osteoporotic women, compared with control subjects [37], whereas another one failed to detect changes of MDA concentrations between osteoporotic and non-osteoporotic post-menopausal women [38]. Thus, further studies are needed to precisely define the role played by LPO-derived aldehydes and to validate the possible inclusion of targeted therapies aimed to reducing the effects of reactive aldehydes in the development and progression of age-related osteopenia/osteoporosis.

3. Sarcopenia

Sarcopenia is a geriatric syndrome characterized by a progressive and generalized loss of skeletal muscle mass, together with low muscle strength and/or poor physical performance in the elderly [39]. A recent study in Brazilians aged 60 years or older demonstrated that the overall prevalence of sarcopenia in older Brazilians was 17.0%. Sensitivity analysis showed rates of 20.0% in women and 12.0% in men [40]. In order to counteract the age-related muscle decline several interventions have been explored, including protein supplementation, testosterone replacement in men, estrogen replacement in women, growth hormone replacement, and treatment with vitamin D. To date, adequate protein intake and physical exercise are the most promising interventions aiming to prevent and/or delay the decline of muscle mass [41].

Oxidative stress and inflammation are implicated in the pathogenesis of sarcopenia [42]. It has been suggested that an increase of oxidative stress might activate apoptosis, leading to the loss of skeletal muscle fibers, thus contributing to the progression of sarcopenia [43]. Skeletal muscle tissue is unique, with respect to apoptosis, because muscle cells are one of the three cell types, along with osteoclasts and cytotrophoblasts, that are multinucleated [44]. The process by which nuclei are eliminated from multinucleated muscle fibers appears to be similar to apoptosis, since it involves chromatin condensation and DNA fragmentation. Moreover, it has been suggested that oxidative stress and the consequent mitochondrial genotoxic damage might play a causal role in the numerical loss of muscle fibers with aging [45].

Deregulation of redox homeostasis has emerged in recent years as a common pathogenetic mechanism and potential therapeutic target in collagen VI-related congenital muscular dystrophies, and in Duchenne muscular dystrophy, as well as in other more prevalent processes, such as age-related muscle loss [46]. Moreover, sarcopenia can be associated with obesity. This association is defined as sarcopenic obesity and represents a chronic condition, whose increase in prevalence has been related to parallel increases in the mean age of the population, the prevalence of obesity, and the changes in lifestyle during the last several decades [47]. In obese individuals, adipose tissue secretes both bioactive molecules, called "adipokines", and ROS, which might represent the mechanistic link between obesity and its associated metabolic complications, including sarcopenia [48].

The aging of human skeletal muscle cells is marked by a progressive functional decline of mitochondria, resulting in the accumulation of ROS [43]. *Sod1*$^{-}$/$^{-}$ mice lack the superoxide dismutase [Cu-Zn] 1 (CuZnSOD1) enzyme and undergo accelerated sarcopenia, i.e., display the characteristics of aging muscle in an accelerated manner. In *Sod1*$^{-}$/$^{-}$ mice, muscle loss was accompanied by a progressive decline of mitochondrial function, with an increased mitochondrial generation of ROS and faster induction of mitochondrial-mediated apoptosis and loss of myonuclei. *Sod1*$^{-}$/$^{-}$ mice also exhibited a strikingly increased number of dysfunctional mitochondria near neuromuscular junctions [49]. Increased ROS production is a necessary response to exercise of a sufficient intensity [50]. ROS and RNS (reactive nitrogen species, such as NO and the peroxynitrite anion) play important roles in the function of skeletal muscle, as they may mediate muscle adaptive responses, e.g., to physical exercise [51], by facilitating glucose uptake or inducing mitochondrial biogenesis [52,53]. However, during extended disuse periods, redox imbalance contributes to deleterious muscle remodeling via myonuclear apoptosis and atrophy, with the mediation of a redox-sensitive transcriptional regulator, NF-κB [54,55]. ROS can stimulate the production of TNF-α and IL-1β, through the activation of NF-κB-mediated pathways [56]. Systemic inflammation, impaired responses to stressors, and weakened regenerative capacity are all associated with sarcopenia. In Wistar rats, aging (40 weeks) was accompanied by reduced mitochondrial respiratory chain complex activities in saponin-skinned soleus muscle fibers, increased production of ROS and decreased transcription of the genes encoding mitochondrial superoxide dismutase 2 (*SOD2*), PPAR-γ coactivator-1β (*PGC-1β*) and sirtuin 1, in comparison with young (16 weeks) rats. Chronic intake of polyphenols normalized V_{max}, decreased ROS production and enhanced *SOD2* and *PGC-1β* expression, in comparison with age-matched untreated rats [57].

Notably, sarcopenia is also accompanied by fat infiltration in the skeletal muscle, which can not only affect muscle quality and functional performance [58], but might render muscle tissue prone to oxidative stress-induced LPO. In disease processes marked by increased ROS production, novel 2,4-dinitrophenylhydrazine (DNPH)-reactive carbonyl groups in proteins, susceptible to spectrometric or antibody-mediated detection, might be either produced by the direct metal-catalyzed oxidation of aminoacyl side chains or introduced by stable adduct formation via the reaction of the latter with reducing sugars or reactive carbonyl species, including MDA and HNE. Age-related increases in protein carbonyl levels were detected in skeletal muscle by derivatization with DNPH, followed by fluorescent anti-DNPH antibodies, in descending ranking order, in the extracellular space, subsarcolemmal mitochondria, intermyofibrillar mitochondria and cytoplasm [59]. By the use of quantitative proteomics, a number of mitochondrial proteins susceptible to carbonylation in a muscle type-dependent (slow- vs. fast-twitch) and age-dependent manner were identified in Fischer 344 rat skeletal muscle. Fast-twitch muscle revealed twice as many carbonylated mitochondrial proteins than slow-twitch muscle, with 22 proteins showing significant changes (mostly increases) in carbonylation state with age. Ingenuity pathway analysis revealed that these proteins belonged to functional classes and pathways known to be impaired in muscle aging, including cellular function and maintenance, fatty acid metabolism and citric acid cycle. Although proof was not provided that carbonylation was responsible for any functional changes, these data delineated a catalog of protein targets deserving investigation, because of their potential implication in muscle aging [60]. In the gastrocnemius muscle of male C57B1/6 mice, a distinct increase of HNE adducts was noticed, upon the progression of age from 5 to 25 months. This was accompanied by increased expression of inducible nitric oxide synthase, decreased expression of G6PDH, activation of JNK, caspase 2, caspase 9, and inactivation of BCL-2, through phosphorylation at Ser70 [61]. Other observations have been collected in transgenic mice expressing a dominant-negative form of ALDH2 (ALDH2*2 Tg mice), which indicate a role of HNE as an inducer of apoptosis. Mice, in whose muscles ALDH activity was selectively attenuated, exhibited small body size, muscle atrophy, decreased fat content, osteopenia, and kyphosis, accompanied by increased muscular HNE levels [62].

Oxidative stress, in sarcopenic patients, can lead to increased LPO production. The mechanistic importance of apoptosis in the loss of muscle cells in age-related sarcopenia and the involvement of LPO-derived aldehydes in this process are supported by several studies. The abundance of protein carbonyl adducts was determined within skeletal muscle sarcoplasmic, myofibrillar, and mitochondrial protein subfractions from musculus *vastus lateralis* biopsies, using immunoblotting techniques, in two groups of 16 old males ("old" and "old sarcopenic") [63]. Concentrations of cytoprotective proteins (e.g., heat shock proteins, αβ-crystallin) were also assayed. Aging was associated with increased mitochondrial (but not myofibrillar or sarcoplasmic) protein carbonyl adducts, independent of (stage-I) sarcopenia. Mitochondrial protein carbonyl abundance negatively correlated with muscle strength, but not muscle mass. According to this study, mitochondrial protein carbonylation increased moderately with age, and this increase might impact upon skeletal muscle function, but was not a hallmark of sarcopenia, per se. It should be considered, though, that the subjects under study were affected by low-grade (stage-I) sarcopenia [63].

A recent study, conducted with an urban Spanish cohort of elderly people (≥70 years), demonstrated a significant increase of MDA and HNE in blood samples of sarcopenic subjects, with respect to sarcopenia-exempt control subjects [64]. Notably, among several parameters examined in this study, only MDA and HNE levels were significantly associated with sarcopenia. These observations have been confirmed by studies demonstrating the presence of plasma MDA/HNE protein adducts in sarcopenic patients [65]. Interestingly, proteomic analysis of muscle extracts from adult and aged post-menopausal women demonstrated that ALDH2 and AKR1A1 were up-regulated in aged women, suggesting that the scavenging of reactive aldehyde products in skeletal muscle cells of the elderly was enhanced [66]. These results may be interpreted as a demonstration of the existence of a mechanism of adaptation of muscle cells to increased oxidative stress and to the consequently increased production of LPO-derived aldehydes.

Taken together, these results support a pathogenic link between oxidative stress, LPO-derived aldehydes, aldehyde-protein adducts and age-related sarcopenia in humans.

4. Immunosenescence

Immunosenescence takes a relevant part in the aging phenotype, and there is growing consensus on the idea that it might result from a progressive imbalance, favoring inflammatory over anti-inflammatory mechanisms, which some authors define as "inflammaging". According to this view, continuing antigenic stimulation in the course of life, with accompanying oxidative stress, steadily leads, as enzymatic and non-enzymatic antioxidant defences fade off with age, to an up-regulation of inflammatory responses and a remodeling of immune responses, as revealed by the increased serum levels of pro-inflammatory cytokines, such as IL-6 and TNF-α, and a loss of efficacy of adaptive responses. Pro-inflammatory cytokines stimulate further the generation of ROS and cytotoxic LPO products.

As already well documented in other tissues and organ systems, accumulation of ROS and LPO products might cause significant damage to cell lipids, nucleic acids and crucial cell proteins also in cells of the immune system. This pro-inflammatory condition negatively affects the overall chances for good health, self-sufficiency and extended survival of the elderly and is a hallmark of the so-called "fragility" of the elderly [67,68]. Moreover, the remodeling of immunity strongly contributes to a number of age-associated diseases (infectious diseases, autoimmunity, cancer, metabolic, vascular and neurodegenerative diseases). Immunosenescence is best revealed by the changes in the modulation of survival of T cells, which become more resistant to damage-induced apoptosis. As a consequence, CD28-senescent T cells increase in number (with effector/memory cells, most of the CD8+ CD45RO+ CD25+ phenotype, prevailing over naïve cells), dysfunctional cells accumulate, and the immunological space in lymphoid tissues is reduced. Increased activation-induced cell death (AICD), in response to TNF-α, causes a progressive depletion of lymphoid niches, particularly of the naïve T cell compartment. At the same time, the generation of immunocompetent T cells in thymus declines with age [68–72].

The age-dependent shortening of DNA telomeres, which is associated with increased mortality in individuals over 65 years of age, contributes to the reduction of the potential for clonal expansion and differentiation of naïve T cells, which is revealed by the dramatic decay of T-cell-receptor excision circles (TREC). The overall outcome is a reduction in the repertoire of clonal antigenic specificities, which is reflected in a decreased ability to enact recall immune responses to formerly encountered antigens (e.g., cytomegalovirus, CMV) and to mount adaptive responses to novel antigenic stimuli, combined with an increased tendency to autoimmunity [68–72]. The inversion of the CD4+/CD8+ cell number ratio, the increased fraction of effector-memory cells and the seropositivity for CMV identify an immune risk phenotype in elderly patients [73]. Reduced B cell function with age reflects the decreases both of CD19+ cell number and of T helper-mediated cooperation with B cell responses. Age-associated changes in innate immunity include reductions of antigen uptake by DCs, phagocytosis and production of lymphocyte-derived chemotactic factor by macrophages, FCγRIII (CD16)-stimulated production of superoxide anion by neutrophils, and IFN-γ secretion and expression of activating NKp receptors by NK cells.

Thymus involution is associated with a drastic reduction in organ volume and replacement of functional cortical and medullary areas with adipose tissue. This process, which starts early in life, is almost complete by the age of 40–50 years. Increasing formation of lipid-laden cells with aging has also been observed in lympho-hematopoietic organs, including the thymus [74,75]. Age-related thymic involution appears to reflect the compound effects of increased rates of thymocyte death in the thymus and decreased thymic differentiation and output of T cells. The former might result from intrathymic inflammation and lipotoxicity, the latter from the failure of stromal cell-dependent thymocyte maturation and survival (Figure 2) [76].

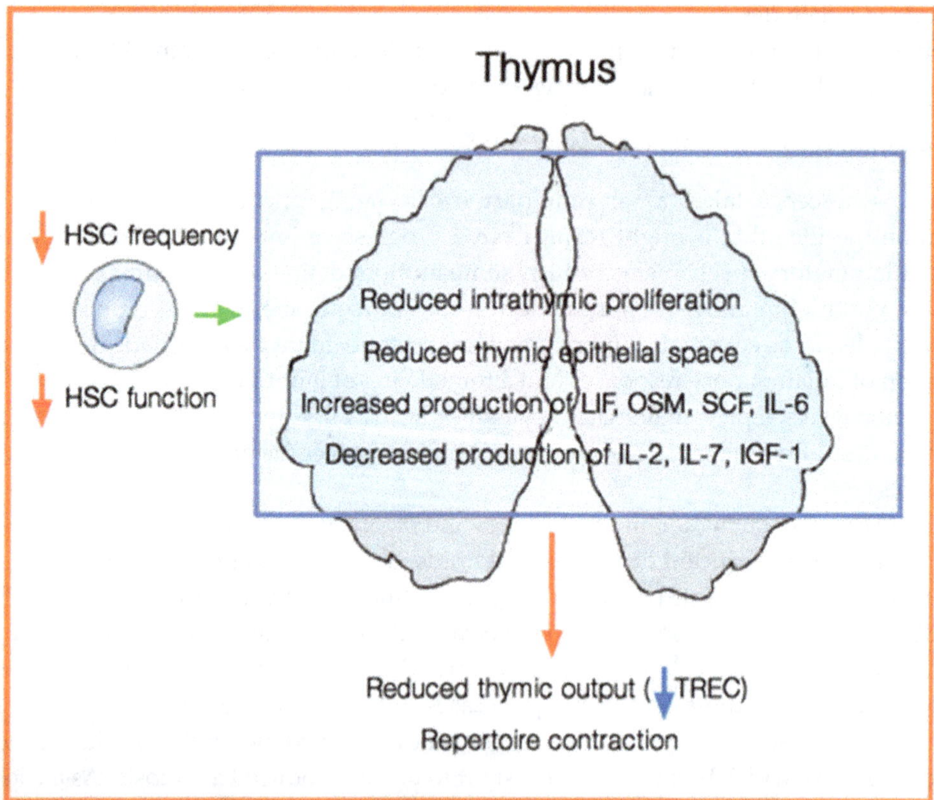

Figure 2. Main aspects of thymic involution. The decrease of hematopoietic cells causes a decrease of production of T cells from the thymus. HSC: hematopoietic stem cells; LIF: leukemia- inhibitory factor; OSM: Oncostatin M; SCF: stem cell factor; IL-2: interleukin 2; IL-6 interleukin 6; IL-7: interleukin 7; IGF-1: insulin-like growth factor 1; TREC: T cell receptor excision circles (modified from [68]).

The levels of pro-inflammatory chemokines (MIP-1α, MIP-1β, RANTES) secreted by activated DC, macrophages and endothelial cells and recognized by CCR5 increase in the aging thymus, just like intrathymic lipid-laden multilocular and adipose cells (LLC), whose number is inversely related with thymic function [76]. It was suggested that LLC derive from CCR5-expressing, perithymic and perivascular preadipocytes, migrating into the aging thymus [77]. They produce pro-inflammatory cytokines (LIF, Oncostatin M, IL-6, TNF-α), thus creating a pro-oxidative, cytotoxic intrathymic *milieu*, which might favor thymocyte death [77]. The age-related alterations of lipid metabolism and redox balance were studied in mouse thymus and isolated thymocytes. An evaluation of the lipidomics profile of the whole thymus, between the ages of 4 weeks (young age) and 18 months (old age), revealed increased amounts of triacylglycerides, cholesterol, HNE, sulfatide ceramide and ganglioside GD1a in the aged thymus. Increased levels of cholesterol esters and HNE adducts were also found in isolated thymocytes from elder mice, compared with younger individuals. Increased levels of TNF-α and increased expression of CD204, a scavenger receptor of oxidized LDL, were detected in the thymic parenchyma of older individuals, as compared to younger ones. GH reduced thymic levels of TNF-α and HNE and increased the number of thymocytes, in accordance with several observations that indicated growth hormone as a powerful immunomodulating agent, stimulating thymopoiesis and limiting the number of adipocytes and fat locules in rodent and human thymus [74]. The levels of MDA and protein carbonyls (PC), as well as of oxidized and reduced glutathione and the activities of several antioxidant enzymes were measured in peripheral blood lymphocytes from 100 individuals, equally subdivided into groups of ages varying from 11–20 to 51–60 years. This study evidenced distinct, steady increases in MDA and PC levels with age, and decreasing glutathione levels and antioxidant enzyme activities, documenting a progressive redox imbalance with aging [78]. When rats subjected to ovariectomy, which undergo premature aging of the immune system, were subjected to dietary supplementation with polyphenolic antioxidants (soybean and green tea polyphenols), beneficial effects were observed on several parameters of the immune function (macrophage phagocytosis, chemotaxis and ROS production; lymphocyte mitogenic responses; NK activity) and redox balance (catalase and glutathione peroxidase activity, oxidized versus reduced glutathione ratio, MDA levels) of peritoneal leukocytes [60].

5. Myelodysplastic Syndromes

Myelodysplastic syndromes (MDS) include a heterogeneous range of stem cell disorders characterized by peripheral cytopenias and increased risk of progression to acute myeloid leukemia. The incidence of MDS increases markedly with age. It is conservatively estimated that >10,000 new cases of MDS occur in the United States annually [79]. In MDS, next-generation sequencing allowed the identification of molecular mutations in nearly 90% of the patients. Consequently, molecular mutation markers were integrated into current classification systems. The growing insights into molecular aspects of the pathogenesis of MDS may help to predict the possible evolution towards leukemia [80].

Most MDS patients have anemia and many develop transfusion dependence and iron overload (IOL). IOL is considered a negative independent prognostic factor, associated with a higher risk of leukemic transformation and shorter survival [81]. Serologic and molecular markers of oxidative stress have been evidenced in many patients with MDS [82], with the concentration of the LPO product MDA being significantly increased in patients with MDS and IOL, compared with IOL-exempt patients and control subjects. Moreover, both plasma nitrite and MDA concentrations were positively correlated with the ferritin levels, suggesting a relationship between IOL and the increased production of ROS in MDS [83]. In regard, it has to be noticed that the impact of iron on the redox balance of cells and body fluids is strictly dependent on transferrin saturation (TSAT). In the presence of normal TSAT, the M1 polarization of macrophages is decreased and the production of pro-inflammatory cytokines, ROS and LPO products are inhibited [84]. Conversely, patients with IOL and high TSAT show higher O_2% saturation levels than patients at the time of diagnosis and normal controls. Antioxidant systems, with the exception of SOD, exhibit significant activity changes in IOL patients, compared with controls.

Moreover, iron chelation treatment with deferoxamine has also been shown to reduce cytopenia in patients with MDS. In a study of 11 patients with MDS who were receiving deferoxamine for up to 60 months, increases in platelet and neutrophil counts were observed in 64% and 78% of patients, respectively [85]. Furthermore, mitochondrial dysfunction has been detected only in IOL cases, but not in control subjects [86]. High-level ROS production in MDS can be responsible for genotoxic damage to nuclear and mitochondrial DNA, resulting in genomic instability, which contributes to disease progression and leukemia onset [87,88].

Even though the role of ROS in MDS is well established, the role played by LPO products in the disease and its progression has not been completely assessed. It was suggested that the loss of ALDHs, which are mainly responsible for the metabolism of reactive aldehydes, might lead to the alteration of various cell processes, which may foster MDS progression to leukemic transformation [89]. Recent data indicate that ALDH1A1-defective cell lines, as well as primary leukemic cells, are sensitive to the treatment with drugs that directly or indirectly generate toxic ALDH substrates, including HNE. On the contrary, normal HSCs are relatively resistant to these compounds, suggesting that LPO-derived aldehydes could selectively kill ALDH1A1-defective leukemic cells [90]. According to these observations, in human lymphoid leukemic CDM-NKR cells, high concentrations of HNE caused significant cytotoxic effects on DNA synthesis and mitochondrial activity, whereas no significant toxicity of HNE was detected in normal hematopoietic precursor cells [91]. In addition, murine erythroleukemia (MEL) cells from HNE-treated mice exhibit a higher degree of differentiation, in comparison with dimethyl sulfoxide-treated MEL cells. These findings indicate that HNE, at concentrations physiologically detected in many normal tissues and in plasma, induces MEL cell differentiation, by modulating the expression of specific genes [92].

However, the role of HNE and other reactive aldehydes in the development of leukemia is controversial. The ALDH1A1 and ALDH3A1 isoforms are important for the metabolism of reactive aldehydes and ROS, and are expressed at high levels in HSCs. Indeed, the loss of these two isoforms resulted in a variety of effects on HSC biology, such as increased DNA damage and increased rates of leukemic transformation [93]. On the other hand, ALDH activity in human leukemic cells also mediates resistance to a number of drugs [94], and high levels of ALDH activity are predictors of poor therapeutic outcomes [95]. These conclusions are supported by the identification, by the in silico screening of the Gene Expression Omnibus database, using the *PTL* gene signature as a template, of 2 new agents, celastrol and HNE, which were able to eradicate acute myeloid leukemia (AML) at the bulk, progenitor, and stem cell level [96].

Serologic and molecular markers of oxidative stress in patients with MDS include increased concentrations of the LPO product MDA and the presence of oxidized bases in CD34+ cells. Potential mechanisms of oxidative stress include mitochondrial dysfunction via IOL and mitochondrial DNA mutation, systemic inflammation, and bone marrow stromal defects [82]. MDA levels in plasma correlated moderately with serum ferritin and free iron levels and were significantly higher in MDS patients with iron overload, when compared to healthy blood donors, once more emphasizing the role of oxidative stress in the development of MDS [97]. Moreover, a cytoprotective effect was reported of erythropoietin on the plasma membrane of erythroid cells in MDS, which was closely reminiscent of effects detected in certain conditions of impaired glucose metabolism, which were associated with increased LPO-dependent cell stress in the elderly [98]. The selective cytotoxic activities exhibited by LPO products towards transformed hematopoietic cells might be partly responsible for the effectiveness of hypomethylating drugs, widely employed in the chemotherapy of AML and MDS. In fact, the use of these chemotherapeutic agents is associated with the generation of enormous amounts of ROS. Antioxidant supplementation in these patients must be approached with caution, because of the high probability that it might result in significant reductions of the therapeutic efficacy of hypomethylating drugs, whose cytotoxic effect is probably mediated by plasma MDA concentrations, which increase significantly during the 14-day post-chemotherapy period [99].

In conclusion, it appears that the overall effects of LPO products within the context of MDS are strictly dependent on their concentrations, the degree of inflammation and the disease phase. Physiological HNE and MDA concentrations in an early phase of MDS, with low-grade inflammation and normal iron concentrations, seem to favor blast apoptosis and normal hematopoietic cell differentiation in bone marrow niches, whereas high HNE and MDA concentrations in later phases of MDS, with high-grade inflammation and higher than normal iron levels, might favor normal cell death and awry maturation of bone marrow cells [99].

6. Conclusions

From the overall body of evidence presented, the pathogenic involvement of oxidative stress and lipid peroxidation appears to be firmly grounded in all of the senile pathological and dysfunctional conditions examined in this review. In turn, increases in the production of ROS and reactive aldehydes from lipid peroxidation concur to induce apoptosis, which has been observed during aging in osteoblasts, muscle cells, thymocytes and hematopoietic cells. The use of antioxidants as an adjuvant therapy to counteract ROS increases in these disorders gave interesting results [26,87,100,101]. However, the efficacy of antioxidants in reducing the concentrations of aldehydes and/or protein-aldehyde adducts in blood or in tissues has not yet been measured. It is our conception that osteoporosis/osteopenia, sarcopenia, immunosenescence and myelodysplastic syndromes may all represent concurring expressions of the age-related decay of molecular turnover and repair capabilities in post-mitotic cells, altogether expressing themselves as the progressive multiorgan/multisystem failure of senescence. A few systematic redox proteomic approaches, pinpointing the modifications of distinct cell proteins with LPO products generated in the course of oxidative stress, have been conducted to date, mostly in the skeletal muscle of rodents. It is warranted that studies of this kind be extended to the other organ systems undergoing age-associated decay, and be complemented by functional studies as well. We anticipate that continuing investigation in this field may pave the way, in the end, to targeted therapeutic strategies aiming to alleviate the burden of morbidity and mortality associated with these disturbances.

Author Contributions: G.B. and F.G. wrote the paper, S.P., M.D., C.D., A.A, G.P.C., G.G., M.A.C. and M.G. were involved in the previous work on these topics in our group and/or substantively revised it.

Funding: This work was supported by the University of Turin and the Department of Clinical and Biological Sciences (Local Funds ex-60%).

Conflicts of Interest: The authors declare no conflict of interest.

Abbreviations

ALDH	aldehyde dehydrogenase
AML	acute myeloid leukemia
apoB	apolipoprotein B
CMV	cytomegalovirus
DNPH	dinitrophenylhydrazine
HNE	4-hydroxynonenal
HSC	hematopoietic stem cell
IkB	inihibitor of κ light gene enhancer in B cells
IGF-1	insulin-like growth factor 1
IOL	iron overload
JNK	c-jun N-terminal kinase
LDL	low-density lipoprotein
LIF	leukemia-inhibitory factor
LLC	lipid-laden multilocular and adipose cell
LPO	lipid peroxidation
MAPK	mitogen-activated protein kinase
MDA	malondialdehyde

MDS	myelodysplastic syndromes
MEL	murine erythroleukemia
NK-κB	nuclear factor of κ light gene enhancer in B cells
OSM	oncostatin M
PC	protein carbonyl
PPAR-γ	peroxysome proliferator-activated receptor γ
SCF	stem cell factor
TNF-α	tumor necrosis factor alpha
TREC	T-cell receptor excision circle
TSAT	transferrin saturation

References

1. Granic, A.; Mendonça, N.; Hill, T.R.; Jagger, C.; Stevenson, E.J.; Mathers, J.C.; Sayer, A.A. Nutrition in the Very Old. *Nutrients* **2018**, *10*, 269. [CrossRef] [PubMed]
2. Kontis, V.; Bennett, J.E.; Mathers, C.D.; Li, G.; Foreman, K.; Ezzati, M. Future life expectancy in 35 industrialised countries: Projections with a Bayesian model ensemble. *Lancet* **2017**, *389*, 1323–1335. [CrossRef]
3. Bektas, A.; Schurman, S.H.; Sen, R.; Ferrucci, L. Aging, inflammation and the environment. *Exp. Gerontol.* **2018**, *105*, 10–18. [CrossRef] [PubMed]
4. Vina, J.; Borras, C.; Miquel, J. Theories of ageing. *IUBMB Life* **2007**, *59*, 249–254. [CrossRef] [PubMed]
5. Sohal, R.S.; Orr, W.C. The redox stress hypothesis of aging. *Free Radic. Biol. Med.* **2012**, *52*, 539–555. [CrossRef] [PubMed]
6. Boveris, A.; Chance, B. The mitochondrial generation of hydrogen peroxide. General properties and effect of hyperbaric oxygen. *Biochem. J.* **1973**, *134*, 707–716. [CrossRef] [PubMed]
7. Chistiakov, D.A.; Sobenin, I.A.; Revin, V.V.; Orekhov, A.N.; Bobryshev, Y.V. Mitochondrial aging and age-related dysfunction of mitochondria. *BioMed. Res. Int.* **2014**, *2014*, 238463. [CrossRef] [PubMed]
8. Esterbauer, H.; Schaur, R.J.; Zollner, H. Chemistry and Biochemistry of 4-hydroxynonenal, malonaldehyde and related aldehydes. *Free Radic. Biol. Med.* **1991**, *11*, 81–128. [CrossRef]
9. Ayala, A.; Muñoz, M.F.; Argüelles, S. Lipid peroxidation: Production, metabolism, and signaling mechanisms of malondialdehyde and 4-hydroxy-2-nonenal. *Oxid. Med. Cell. Longev.* **2014**, *2014*, 360438. [CrossRef] [PubMed]
10. Barrera, G.; Pizzimenti, S.; Ciamporcero, E.S.; Daga, M.; Ullio, C.; Arcaro, A.; Cetrangolo, G.P.; Ferretti, C.; Dianzani, C.; Lepore, A.; et al. Role of 4-hydroxynonenal-protein adducts in human diseases. *Antioxid. Redox Signal.* **2015**, *22*, 1681–1702. [CrossRef] [PubMed]
11. Domingues, R.M.; Domingues, P.; Melo, T.; Pérez-Sala, D.; Reis, A.; Spickett, C.M. Lipoxidation adducts with peptides and proteins: Deleterious modifications or signaling mechanisms? *J. Proteom.* **2013**, *92*, 110–131. [CrossRef] [PubMed]
12. Esterbauer, H.; Zollern, H. Methods for determination of aldehydic lipid peroxidation products. *Free Radic. Biol. Med.* **1989**, *7*, 197–203. [CrossRef]
13. Papac-Milicevic, N.; Busch, C.J.; Binder, C.J. Malondialdehyde Epitopes as Targets of Immunity and the Implications for Atherosclerosis. *Adv. Immunol.* **2016**, *131*, 1–59. [CrossRef] [PubMed]
14. Nègre-Salvayre, A.; Garoby-Salom, S.; Swiader, A.; Rouahi, M.; Pucelle, M.; Salvayre, R. Proatherogenic effects of 4-hydroxynonenal. *Free Radic. Biol. Med.* **2017**, *111*, 127–139. [CrossRef] [PubMed]
15. Casini, A.; Galli, A.; Pignalosa, P.; Frulloni, L.; Grappone, C.; Milani, S.; Pederzoli, P.; Cavallini, G.; Surrenti, C. Collagen type I synthesized by pancreatic periacinar stellate cells (PSC) co-localizes with lipid peroxidation-derived aldehydes in chronic alcoholic pancreatitis. *J. Pathol.* **2000**, *192*, 81–89. [CrossRef]
16. Gil, L.; Siems, W.; Mazurek, B.; Gross, J.; Schroeder, P.; Voss, P.; Grune, T. Age-associated analysis of oxidative stress parameters in human plasma and erythrocytes. *Free Radic. Res.* **2006**, *40*, 495–505. [CrossRef] [PubMed]
17. Sultana, R.; Perluigi, M.; Allan Butterfield, D. Lipid peroxidation triggers neurodegeneration: A redox proteomics view into the Alzheimer disease brain. *Free Radic. Biol. Med.* **2013**, *62*, 157–169. [CrossRef] [PubMed]
18. Manolagas, S.C. Birth and death of bone cells: Basic regulatory mechanisms and implications for the pathogenesis and treatment of osteoporosis. *Endocr. Rev.* **2000**, *2*, 115–137. [CrossRef]

19. Dawson-Hughes, B.; Looker, A.C.; Tosteson, A.N.; Johansson, H.; Kanis, J.A.; Melton, L.J., III. The potential impact of the National Osteoporosis Foundation guidance on treatment eligibility in the USA: An update in NHANES 2005–2008. *Osteoporos. Int.* **2012**, *23*, 811–820. [CrossRef] [PubMed]
20. Choksi, P.; Jepsen, K.J.; Clines, G.A. The challenges of diagnosing osteoporosis and the limitations of currently available tools. *Clin. Diabetes Endocrinol.* **2018**, *4*, 12. [CrossRef] [PubMed]
21. Huang, C.X.; Lv, B.; Wang, Y. Protein Phosphatase 2A Mediates Oxidative Stress Induced Apoptosis in Osteoblasts. *Mediat. Inflamm.* **2015**, *2015*, 804260. [CrossRef] [PubMed]
22. Sendur, O.F.; Turan, Y.; Tastaban, E.; Serter, M. Antioxidant status in patients with osteoporosis: A controlled study. *Joint Bone Spine* **2009**, *76*, 514–518. [CrossRef] [PubMed]
23. Almeida, M.; Han, L.; Martin-Millan, M.; Plotkin, L.I.; Stewart, S.A.; Roberson, P.K.; Kousteni, S.; O'Brien, C.A.; Bellido, T.; Parfitt, A.M.; et al. Skeletal involution by age-associated oxidative stress and its acceleration by loss of sex steroids. *J. Biol. Chem.* **2007**, *282*, 27285–27297. [CrossRef] [PubMed]
24. Maggio, D.; Barabani, M.; Pierandrei, M.; Polidori, M.C.; Catani, M.; Mecocci, P.; Senin, U.; Pacifici, R.; Cherubini, A. Marked decrease in plasma antioxidants in aged osteoporotic women: Results of a cross-sectional study. *J. Clin. Endocrinol. Metab.* **2003**, *88*, 1523–1527. [CrossRef] [PubMed]
25. Lean, J.M.; Jagger, C.J.; Kirstein, B.; Fuller, K.; Chambers, T.J. Hydrogen peroxide is essential for estrogen-deficiency bone loss and osteoclast formation. *Endocrinology* **2005**, *146*, 728–735. [CrossRef] [PubMed]
26. Domazetovic, V.; Marcucci, G.; Iantomasi, T.; Brandi, M.L.; Vincenzini, M.T. Oxidative stress in bone remodeling: Role of antioxidants. *Clin. Cases Miner. Bone Metab.* **2017**, *14*, 209–216. [CrossRef] [PubMed]
27. Li, X.; Han, Y.; Guan, Y.; Zhang, L.; Bai, C.; Li, Y. Aluminum induces osteoblast apoptosis through the oxidative stress-mediated JNK signaling pathway. *Biol. Trace Elem. Res.* **2012**, *150*, 502–508. [CrossRef] [PubMed]
28. Pantano, C.; Reynaert, N.L.; van der Vliet, A.; Janssen-Heininger, Y.M. Redox-sensitive kinases of the nuclear factor-κB signaling pathway. *Antioxid. Redox Signal.* **2006**, *8*, 1791–1806. [CrossRef] [PubMed]
29. Almeida, M.; Han, L.; Ambrogini, E.; Bartell, S.M.; Manolagas, S.C. Oxidative stress stimulates apoptosis and activates NF-κB in osteoblastic cells via a PKCβ/p66shc signaling cascade: Counter regulation by estrogens or androgens. *Mol. Endocrinol.* **2010**, *24*, 2030–2037. [CrossRef] [PubMed]
30. Zhu, S.Y.; Zhuang, J.S.; Wu, Q.; Liu, Z.Y.; Liao, C.R.; Luo, S.G.; Chen, J.T.; Zhong, Z.M. Advanced oxidation protein products induce pre-osteoblast apoptosis through a nicotinamide adenine dinucleotide phosphate oxidase-dependent, mitogen-activated protein kinases-mediated intrinsic apoptosis pathway. *Aging Cell* **2018**, e12764. [CrossRef] [PubMed]
31. Wang, X.; Chen, B.; Sun, J.; Jiang, Y.; Zhang, H.; Zhang, P.; Fei, B.; Xu, Y. Iron-induced oxidative stress stimulates osteoclast differentiation via NF-κB signaling pathway in mouse model. *Metabolism* **2018**, *83*, 167–176. [CrossRef] [PubMed]
32. Rachner, T.D.; Khosla, S.; Hofbauer, L.C. Osteoporosis: Now and the future. *Lancet* **2011**, *377*, 1276–1287. [CrossRef]
33. Muzio, G.; Maggiora, M.; Paiuzzi, E.; Oraldi, M.; Canuto, R.A. Aldehyde dehydrogenases and cell proliferation. *Free Radic. Biol. Med.* **2012**, *52*, 735–746. [CrossRef] [PubMed]
34. Mittal, M.; Khan, K.; Pal, S.; Porwal, K.; China, S.P.; Barbhuyan, T.K.; Baghel, K.S.; Rawat, T.; Sanyal, S.; Bhadauria, S.; et al. The thiocarbamate disulphide drug, disulfiram induces osteopenia in rats by inhibition of osteoblast function due to suppression of acetaldehyde dehydrogenase activity. *Toxicol. Sci.* **2014**, *139*, 257–270. [CrossRef] [PubMed]
35. Hoshi, H.; Hao, W.; Fujita, Y.; Funayama, A.; Miyauchi, Y.; Hashimoto, K.; Miyamoto, K.; Iwasaki, R.; Sato, Y.; Kobayashi, T.; et al. Aldehyde-stress resulting from Aldh2 mutation promotes osteoporosis due to impaired osteoblastogenesis. *J. Bone Miner. Res.* **2012**, *27*, 2015–2023. [CrossRef] [PubMed]
36. Mittal, M.; Pal, S.; China, S.P.; Porwal, K.; Dev, K.; Shrivastava, R.; Raju, K.S.; Rashid, M.; Trivedi, A.K.; Sanyal, S.; et al. Pharmacological activation of aldehyde dehydrogenase 2 promotes osteoblast differentiation via bone morphogenetic protein-2 and induces bone anabolic effect. *Toxicol. Appl. Pharmacol.* **2017**, *316*, 63–73. [CrossRef] [PubMed]
37. Akpolat, V.; Bilgin, H.M.; Celik, M.Y.; Erdemoglu, M.; Isik, B. An evaluation of nitric oxide, folate, homocysteine levels and lipid peroxidation in postmenopausal osteoporosis. *Adv. Clin. Exp. Med.* **2013**, *22*, 403–409. [PubMed]

38. Wu, Q.; Zhong, Z.M.; Pan, Y.; Zeng, J.H.; Zheng, S.; Zhu, S.Y.; Chen, J.T. Advanced Oxidation Protein Products as a Novel Marker of Oxidative Stress in Postmenopausal Osteoporosis. *Med. Sci. Monit.* **2015**, *21*, 2428–2432. [CrossRef] [PubMed]
39. Cruz-Jentoft, J.P.; Baeyens, J.M.; Bauer, Y.; Boirie, T.; Cederholm, F.; Landi, F.C.; Martin, J.P.; Michel, Y.; Rolland, S.M.; Schneider, E.; et al. European consensus on definition and diagnosis: Report of the European Working Group on Sarcopenia in Older People. *Age Ageing* **2010**, *39*, 412–423. [CrossRef] [PubMed]
40. Diz, J.B.; Leopoldino, A.A.; Moreira, B.S.; Henschke, N.; Dias, R.C.; Pereira, L.S.; Oliveira, V.C. Prevalence of sarcopenia in older Brazilians: A systematic review and meta-analysis. *Geriatr. Gerontol. Int.* **2017**, *17*, 5–16. [CrossRef] [PubMed]
41. Zanandrea, V.; Giua, R.; Costanzo, L.; Vellas, B.; Zamboni, M.; Cesari, M. Interventions against sarcopenia in older persons. *Curr. Pharm. Des.* **2014**, *20*, 5983–6006. [PubMed]
42. Marzetti, E.; Calvani, R.; Bernabei, R.; Leeuwenburgh, C. Apoptosis in skeletal myocytes: A potential target for interventions against sarcopenia and physical frailty—A mini-review. *Gerontology* **2012**, *58*, 99–106. [CrossRef] [PubMed]
43. Buonocore, D.; Rucci, S.; Vandoni, M.; Negro, M.; Marzatico, F. Oxidative system in aged skeletal muscle. *Muscles Ligaments Tendons J.* **2011**, *1*, 85–90. [PubMed]
44. Dupont-Versteegden, E.E. Apoptosis in muscle atrophy: Relevance to sarcopenia. *Exp. Gerontol.* **2005**, *40*, 473–481. [CrossRef] [PubMed]
45. Aiken, J.; Bua, E.; Cao, Z.; Lopez, M.; Wanagat, J.; McKenzie, D.; McKiernan, S. Mitochondrial DNA deletion mutations and sarcopenia. *Ann. N. Y. Acad. Sci.* **2002**, *959*, 412–423. [CrossRef] [PubMed]
46. Moulin, M.; Ferreiro, A. Muscle redox disturbances and oxidative stress as pathomechanisms and therapeutic targets in early-onset myopathies. *Semin. Cell Dev. Biol.* **2017**, *64*, 213–223. [CrossRef] [PubMed]
47. Polyzos, S.A.; Margioris, A.N. Sarcopenic obesity. *Hormones* **2018**. [CrossRef] [PubMed]
48. Lefranc, C.; Friederich-Persson, M.; Palacios-Ramirez, R.; Nguyen Dinh Cat, A. Mitochondrial oxidative stress in obesity: Role of the mineralocorticoid receptor. *J. Endocrinol.* **2018**, *238*, R143–R159. [CrossRef] [PubMed]
49. Jang, Y.C.; Lustgarten, M.S.; Liu, Y.; Muller, F.L.; Bhattacharya, A.; Liang, H.; Salmon, A.B.; Brooks, S.V.; Larkin, L.; Hayworth, C.R.; et al. Increased superoxide in vivo accelerates age-associated muscle atrophy through mitochondrial dysfunction and neuromuscular junciton degeneration. *FASEB J.* **2010**, *24*, 1376–1390. [CrossRef] [PubMed]
50. Vollaard, N.B.; Shearmann, J.P.; Cooper, C.E. Exercise induced oxidative stress: Myths, realities and physiological relevance. *Sports Med.* **2005**, *35*, 1045–1062. [CrossRef] [PubMed]
51. Zuo, L.; Pannell, B.K. Redox characterization of functioning skeletal muscle. *Front. Physiol.* **2015**, *6*, 338. [CrossRef] [PubMed]
52. Merry, T.L.; Steinberg, G.R.; Lynch, G.S.; McConell, G.K. Skeletal muscle uptake during contraction is regulated by nitric oxide and ROS independently of AMPK. *Am. J. Physiol. Endocrinol. Metab.* **2009**, *298*, E577–E585. [CrossRef] [PubMed]
53. Powers, S.K.; Talbert, E.E.; Adhihetty, P.J. Reactive oxygen and nitrogen species as intracellular signals in skeletal muscle. *J. Physiol.* **2011**, *589*, 2129–2138. [CrossRef] [PubMed]
54. Bassel-Duby, R.; Olson, E.N. Signaling pathways in skeletal muscle remodeling. *Annu. Rev. Biochem.* **2006**, *75*, 19–37. [CrossRef] [PubMed]
55. Powers, S.K.; Duarte, J.; Kavazis, A.N.; Talbert, E.E. Reactive oxygen species are signalling molecules for skeletal muscle adaptation. *Exp. Physiol.* **2010**, *95*, 1–9. [CrossRef] [PubMed]
56. Malik, V.; Rodino-Klapac, L.R.; Mendell, J.R. Emerging drugs for Duchenne muscular dystrophy. *Expert Opin. Emerg. Drugs* **2012**, *17*, 261–277. [CrossRef]
57. Charles, A.-L.; Meyer, A.; Dal-Ros, S.; Auger, C.; Keller, N.; Ramamoorthy, T.G.; Zoll, J.; Metzger, D.; Schini-Kerth, V.; Geny, B. Polyphenols prevent ageing-related impairment in skeletal muscle mitochondrial function through decreased reactive oxygen species production. *Exp. Physiol.* **2013**, *98*, 536–545. [CrossRef] [PubMed]
58. Visser, S.B.; Kritchevsky, B.H.; Goodpaster, A.B.; Newman, M.; Nevitt, E. Leg muscle mass and composition in relation to lower extremity performance in men and women aged 70–79: The health, aging and body composition study. *J. Am. Geriatr. Soc.* **2002**, *50*, 897–904. [CrossRef] [PubMed]

59. Feng, J.; Navratil, M.; Thompson, L.V.; Arriaga, E.A. Estimating relative carbonyl levels in muscle microstructures by fluorescence imaging. *Anal. Bioanal. Chem.* **2008**, *391*, 2591–2598. [CrossRef] [PubMed]
60. Feng, J.; Xie, H.; Meany, D.L.; Thompson, L.V.; Arriaga, E.A.; Griffin, T.J. Quantitative proteomic profiling of muscle type-dependent and age-dependent protein carbonylation in rat skeletal muscle mitochondria. *J. Gerontol. A Biol. Sci. Med.Sci.* **2008**, *63*, 1137–1152. [CrossRef] [PubMed]
61. Braga, M.; Sinha Hikim, A.P.; Datta, S.; Ferrini, M.G.; Brown, D.; Kovacheva, E.L.; Gonzalez-Cadavid, N.F.; Sinha-Hikim, I. Involvement of oxidative stress and caspase 2-mediated intrinsic pathway signaling in age-related increase in muscle cell apoptosis in mice. *Apoptosis* **2008**, *13*, 822–832. [CrossRef] [PubMed]
62. Nakashima, Y.; Ohsawa, I.; Nishimaki, K.; Kumamoto, S.; Maruyama, I.; Suzuki, Y.; Ohta, S. Preventive effects of Chlorella on skeletal muscle atrophy in muscle-specific mitochondrial aldehyde dehydrogenase 2 activity-deficient mice. *BMC Complement. Altern. Med.* **2014**, *14*, 390. [CrossRef] [PubMed]
63. Beltran Valls, M.R.; Wilkinson, D.J.; Narici, M.V.; Smith, K.; Phillips, B.E.; Caporossi, D.; Atherton, P.J. Protein carbonylation and heat shock proteins in human skeletal muscle: Relationships to age and sarcopenia. *J. Gerontol. A Biol. Sci. Med. Sci.* **2014**, *70*, 174–181. [CrossRef] [PubMed]
64. Coto Montes, A.; Boga, J.A.; Bermejo Millo, C.; Rubio González, A.; Potes Ochoa, Y.; Vega Naredo, I.; Martínez Reig, M.; Romero Rizos, L.; Sánchez Jurado, P.M.; Solano, J.J.; et al. Potential early biomarkers of sarcopenia among independent older adults. *Maturitas* **2017**, *104*, 117–122. [CrossRef] [PubMed]
65. Bellanti, F.; Romano, A.D.; Lo Buglio, A.; Castriotta, V.; Guglielmi, G.; Greco, A.; Serviddio, G.; Vendemiale, G. Oxidative stress is increased in sarcopenia and associated with cardiovascular disease risk in sarcopenic obesity. *Maturitas* **2018**, *109*, 6–12. [CrossRef] [PubMed]
66. Gueugneau, M.; Coudy-Gandilhon, C.; Gourbeyre, O.; Chambon, C.; Combaret, L.; Polge, C.; Taillandier, D.; Attaix, D.; Friguet, B.; Maier, A.B.; et al. Proteomics of muscle chronological ageing in post-menopausal women. *BMC Genom.* **2014**, *15*, 1165. [CrossRef] [PubMed]
67. Franceschi, C.; Capri, M.; Monti, D.; Giunta, S.; Olivieri, F.; Sevini, F.; Panourgia, M.P.; Invidia, L.; Celani, L.; Scurti, M.; et al. Inflammaging and anti-inflammaging: A systemic perspective on aging and longevity emerged from studies in humans. *Mech. Ageing Dev.* **2007**, *128*, 92–105. [CrossRef] [PubMed]
68. Ventura, M.T.; Casciaro, M.; Gangemi, S.; Buquicchio, R. Immunosenescence in aging: Between immune cells depletion and cytokines. *Clin. Mol. Allergy* **2017**, *15*, 21. [CrossRef] [PubMed]
69. Goronzy, J.J.; Weyand, C.M. T cell development and receptor diversity during aging. *Curr. Opin. Immunol.* **2005**, *17*, 468–475. [CrossRef] [PubMed]
70. Taub, D.D.; Longo, D.L. Insight into thymic aging and regeneration. *Immunol. Rev.* **2005**, *205*, 72–93. [CrossRef] [PubMed]
71. Herndler-Brandstetter, D.; Cioca, D.P.; Grubeck-Loebensteiner, B. Immunizations in the elderly: Do they live up to their promise? *Wien. Med. Wochenschr.* **2006**, *156*, 130–141. [CrossRef] [PubMed]
72. Gruver, A.L.; Hudson, L.L.; Sempowski, G.D. Immunosenescence of ageing. *J. Pathol.* **2007**, *211*, 144–156. [CrossRef] [PubMed]
73. Wikby, A.; Ferguson, F.; Forsey, R.; Thompson, J.; Strindhall, J.; Lofgren, S.; Nilsson, B.O.; Ernerudh, J.; Pawelec, G.; Johansson, B. An immune risk phenotype, cognitive impairment, and survival in very late life: Impact of allostatic load in Swedish octogenarian and nonagenarian humans. *J. Gerontol. A Biol. Sci. Med. Sci.* **2005**, *60*, 556–565. [CrossRef] [PubMed]
74. De Mello-Coelho, V.; Cutler, R.G.; Bunbury, A.; Tammara, A.; Mattson, M.P.; Taub, D.D. Age-associated alterations in the levels of cytotoxic lipid molecular species and oxidative stress in the murine thymus are reduced by growth hormone treatment. *Mech. Ageing Dev.* **2017**, *167*, 46–55. [CrossRef] [PubMed]
75. Langhi, L.G.; Andrade, L.R.; Shimabukuro, M.K.; van Ewijk, W.; Taub, D.D.; Borojevic, R.; de Mello Coelho, V. Lipid-laden multilocular cells in the aging thymus are phenotypically heterogeneous. *PLoS ONE* **2015**, *10*, e0141516. [CrossRef] [PubMed]
76. Taub, D.D.; Murphy, W.J.; Longo, D.L. Rejuvenation of the aging thymus: Growth hormone- and ghrelin-mediated signaling pathways. *Curr. Opin. Pharmacol.* **2010**, *10*, 408–424. [CrossRef] [PubMed]
77. De Mello-Coelho, V.; Bunbury, A.; Rangel, L.B.; Giri, B.; Weeraratna, A.; Morin, P.J.; Bernier, M.; Taub, D.D. Fat-storing multilocular cells expressing CCR5 increase in the thymus with advancing age: Potential role for CCR5 ligands on the differentiation and migration of preadipocytes. *Int. J. Med. Sci.* **2010**, *7*, 1–14. [CrossRef]
78. Gautam, N.; Das, S.; Mahapatra, S.K.; Chakraborti, S.P.; Kundu, P.K.; Roy, S. Age associated oxidative damage in lymphocytes. *Oxid. Med. Cell. Longev.* **2010**, *3*, 275–282. [CrossRef] [PubMed]

79. Ma, X. Epidemiology of myelodysplastic syndromes. *Am. J. Med.* **2012**, *125*, S2–S5. [CrossRef] [PubMed]
80. Shumilov, E.; Flach, J.; Kohlmann, A.; Banz, Y.; Bonadies, N.; Fiedler, M.; Pabst, T.; Bacher, U. Current status and trends in the diagnostics of AML and MDS. *Blood Rev.* **2018**. [CrossRef] [PubMed]
81. Malcovati, L.; Della Porta, M.G.; Pascutto, C.; Invernizzi, R.; Boni, M.; Travaglino, E.; Passamonti, F.; Arcaini, L.; Maffioli, M.; Bernasconi, P.; et al. Prognostic factors and life expectancy in myelodysplastic syndromes classified according to WHO criteria: A basis for clinical decision-making. *J. Clin. Oncol.* **2005**, *23*, 7594–7603. [CrossRef] [PubMed]
82. Farquhar, M.J.; Bowen, D.T. Oxidative stress and the myelodysplastic syndromes. *Int. J. Hematol.* **2003**, *77*, 342–350. [CrossRef] [PubMed]
83. De Souza, G.F.; Barbosa, M.C.; Santos, T.E.; Carvalho, T.M.; de Freitas, R.M.; Martins, M.R.; Gonçalves, R.P.; Pinheiro, R.F.; Magalhães, S.M. Increased parameters of oxidative stress and its relation to transfusion iron overload in patients with myelodysplastic syndromes. *J. Clin. Pathol.* **2013**, *66*, 996–998. [CrossRef] [PubMed]
84. Gan, Z.S.; Wang, Q.Q.; Li, J.H.; Wang, X.L.; Wang, Y.Z.; Du, H.H. Iron Reduces M1 Macrophage Polarization in RAW264.7 Macrophages Associated with Inhibition of STAT1. *Mediat. Inflamm.* **2017**, *8570818*. [CrossRef] [PubMed]
85. Angelucci, E.; Cianciulli, P.; Finelli, C.; Mecucci, C.; Voso, M.T.; Tura, S. Unraveling the mechanisms behind iron overload and ineffective hematopoiesis in myelodysplastic syndromes. *Leuk. Res.* **2017**, *62*, 108–115. [CrossRef] [PubMed]
86. Ivars, D.; Orero, M.T.; Javier, K.; Díaz-Vico, L.; García-Giménez, J.L.; Mena, S.; Tormos, C.; Egea, M.; Pérez, P.L.; Arrizabalaga, B.; et al. Oxidative imbalance in low/intermediate-1-risk myelodysplastic syndrome patients: The influence of iron overload. *Clin. Biochem.* **2017**, *50*, 911–917. [CrossRef] [PubMed]
87. Ghoti, H.; Amer, J.; Winder, A.; Rachmilewitz, E.; Fibach, E. Oxidative stress in red blood cells, platelets and polymorphonuclear leukocytes from patients with myelodysplastic syndromes. *Eur. J. Haematol.* **2007**, *79*, 463–467. [CrossRef] [PubMed]
88. Rassool, F.V.; Gaymes, T.J.; Omidvar, N.; Brady, N.; Beurlet, S.; Pla, M.; Reboul, M.; Lea, N.; Chomienne, C.; Thomas, N.S.; et al. Reactive oxygen species, DNA damage, and error-prone repair: A model for genomic instability with progression in myeloid leukemia? *Cancer Res.* **2007**, *67*, 8762–8771. [CrossRef] [PubMed]
89. Smith, C.; Gasparetto, M.; Jordan, C.; Pollyea, D.A.; Vasiliou, V. The effects of alcohol and aldehyde dehydrogenases on disorders of hematopoiesis. *Adv. Exp. Med. Biol.* **2015**, *815*, 349–359. [CrossRef] [PubMed]
90. Gasparetto, M.; Smith, C.A. ALDHs in normal and malignant hematopoietic cells: Potential new avenues for treatment of AML and other blood cancers. *Chem. Biol. Interact.* **2017**, *276*, 46–51. [CrossRef] [PubMed]
91. Semlitsch, T.; Tillian, H.M.; Zarkovic, N.; Borovic, S.; Purtscher, M.; Hohenwarter, O.; Schaur, R.J. Differential influence of the lipid peroxidation product 4-hydroxynonenal on the growth of human lymphatic leukaemia cells and human peripheral blood lymphocytes. *Anticancer Res.* **2002**, *22*, 1689–1697. [PubMed]
92. Rinaldi, M.; Barrera, G.; Spinsanti, P.; Pizzimenti, S.; Ciafrè, S.A.; Parella, P.; Farace, M.G.; Signori, E.; Dianzani, M.U.; Fazio, V.M. Growth inhibition and differentiation induction in murine erythroleukemia cells by 4-hydroxynonenal. *Free Radic. Res.* **2001**, *34*, 629–637. [CrossRef] [PubMed]
93. Gasparetto, M.; Pei, S.; Minhajuddin, M.; Khan, N.; Pollyea, D.A.; Myers, J.R.; Ashton, J.M.; Becker, M.W.; Vasiliou, V.; Humphries, K.R.; et al. Targeted therapy for a subset of acute myeloid leukemias that lack expression of aldehyde dehydrogenase1A1. *Haematologica* **2017**, *102*, 1054–1065. [CrossRef] [PubMed]
94. Koelling, T.M.; Yeager, A.M.; Hilton, J.; Haynie, D.T.; Wiley, J.M. Development and characterization of a cyclophosphamide-resistant subline of acute myeloid leukemia in the Lewis × Brown Norway hybrid rat. *Blood* **1990**, *76*, 1209–1213. [PubMed]
95. Ran, D.; Schubert, M.; Pietsch, L.; Taubert, I.; Wuchter, P.; Eckstein, V.; Bruckner, T.; Zoeller, M.; Ho, A.D. Aldehyde dehydrogenase activity among primary leukemia cells is associated with stem cell features and correlates with adverse clinical outcomes. *Exp. Hematol.* **2009**, *37*, 1423–1434. [CrossRef] [PubMed]
96. Hassane, D.C.; Guzman, M.L.; Corbett, C.; Li, X.; Abboud, R.; Young, F.; Liesveld, J.L.; Carroll, M.; Jordan, C.T. Discovery of agents that eradicate leukemia stem cells using an in silico screen of public gene expression data. *Blood* **2008**, *111*, 5654–5662. [CrossRef] [PubMed]
97. Pimková, K.; Chrastinová, L.; Suttnar, J.; Štikarová, J.; Kotlín, R.; Hermák, J.E. Plasma Levels of Aminothiols, Nitrite, Nitrate, and Malondialdehyde in Myelodysplastic Syndromes in the Context of Clinical Outcomes and as a Consequence of Iron Overload. *Oxid. Med. Cell. Longev.* **2014**, *2014*, 416028. [CrossRef] [PubMed]

98. Gradinaru, D.; Margina, D.; Ilie, M.; Borsa, C.; Ionescu, C.; Prada, G.I. Correlation between erythropoietin serum levels and erythrocyte susceptibility to lipid peroxidation in elderly with type 2 diabetes. *Acta Physiol. Hung.* **2015**, *102*, 400–408. [CrossRef] [PubMed]
99. Esfahani, A.; Ghoreishi, Z.; Nikanfar, A.; Sanaat, Z.; Ghorbanihaghjo, A. Influence of chemotherapy on the lipid peroxidation and antioxidant status in patients with acute myeloid leukemia. *Acta Med. Iran.* **2012**, *50*, 454–458. [PubMed]
100. Brioche, T.; Lemoine-Morel, S. Oxidative Stress, Sarcopenia, Antioxidant Strategies and Exercise: Molecular Aspects. *Curr. Pharm. Des.* **2016**, *22*, 2664–2678. [CrossRef] [PubMed]
101. Espino, J.; Pariente, J.A.; Rodríguez, A.B. Oxidative stress and immunosenescence: Therapeutic effects of melatonin. *Oxid. Med. Cell. Longev.* **2012**, *2012*, 670294. [CrossRef] [PubMed]

2

Antioxidant Activities and Caffeic Acid Content in New Zealand Asparagus (*Asparagus officinalis*) Roots Extracts

Abbey Symes [1], Amin Shavandi [1], Hongxia Zhang [1], Isam A. Mohamed Ahmed [2], Fahad Y. Al-Juhaimi [2] and Alaa El-Din Ahmed Bekhit [1,*]

1 Department of Food Science, University of Otago, Dunedin 9054, New Zealand; abbeysymes77@gmail.com (A.S.); amin.shavandi@otago.ac.nz (A.S.); hongxia.zhang@postgrad.otago.ac.nz (H.Z.)

2 Department of Food Science and Nutrition, College of Food and Agricultural Sciences, King Saud University, Riyadh 11451, Saudi Arabia; isamnawa@yahoo.com (I.A.M.A.); faljuhaimi@ksu.edu.sa (F.Y.A.-J.)

* Correspondence: aladin.bekhit@otago.ac.nz

Abstract: *Asparagus officinalis* are perennial plants that require re-planting every 10–20 years. The roots are traditionally mulched in the soil or treated as waste. The *A. officinalis* roots (AR) contain valuable bioactive compounds that may have some health benefiting properties. The aim of this study was to investigate the total polyphenol and flavonoid contents (TPC and TFC, respectively) and antioxidant (2,2-diphenyl-1-picrylhydrazyl (DPPH), Oxygen Radical Absorbance Capacity (ORAC) and Ferric Reducing/Antioxidant Power (FRAP) assays) activities of New Zealand AR extract. The antioxidant activity decreased with a longer extraction time.

Keywords: asparagus roots; antioxidant activity; bioactive compounds

---

1. Introduction

Asparagus belongs to the *Asparagaceae* genus, which originated in the Eastern Mediterranean region and Asia. Asparagus is a versatile plant with a unique texture and flavour that has promoted its consumption worldwide. There are 22 different species of asparagus recorded in India [1]. Most of the research on the bioactive properties of asparagus extracts was carried out on extracts obtained from the shoots of *Asparagus officinalis* and the roots of *A. racemosus* [2,3]. Different parts of *A. racemosus* have been suggested to have health benefits such as improving the immune system and cancer prevention [4,5]. *A. officinalis* is mainly cultivated for the consumption of the shoot, but its roots have no value and very little research has been carried out on bioactives in the roots of this important plant.

A. officinalis can be harvested for up to 40 years or until their productivity and quality decline. The quality of asparagus declines over time due to diseases from microorganisms, such as *Fusarium*, *Phytophthora*, *Stemphylium*, *Phomopsis asparagi*, and *Cercospora asparagi* Sacc species, as well as the autotoxins that asparagus itself produces, which hinder the growth of new asparagus plants [6]. Therefore, the regeneration of the rootstock becomes necessary for productivity. Old asparagus roots are considered as a waste in many countries, including New Zealand, and are commonly left to rot in fields. However, asparagus waste, not including the roots, has been reported as a potential source of bioactive compounds such as saponins, polyphenols, and flavonoids [7]. These bioactive compounds could be extracted from the roots, hence utilising the roots in a manageable manner and offers the opportunity to add value to the production process. The roots also possess allopathic properties, which can prevent other asparagus plants from growing. Therefore, farmers could improve the re-growth of new asparagus by removing the allopathic potential of old roots, as well as increasing their income by selling the roots, allowing the recipients of the bioactive compounds to have access to a natural product with potential health benefits. Environmental factors such as temperature and exposure to UV and soil nutrients can affect the synthesis and the content of bioactives in plants. Therefore, the objective of this study was to determine the antioxidant activity of New Zealand *A. officinalis* root extracts obtained using methanol and ethanol as the most commonly used extraction solvents.

2. Materials and Methods

Methanol, ethanol, sodium carbonate, acetonitrile, trifluoroacetic acid, and sodium acetate were obtained from Fisher Scientific (Waltham, MA, USA). Gallic acid, sodium nitrite, rutin, 2,2-diphenyl-1-picrylhydrazyl (DPPH), fluorescein sodium salt, 6-hydroxy-2,5,7,8-tetramethylchroman-2-carboxylic acid (Trolox), 2,4,6-tris(2-pyridyl)-s-triazine (TPTZ), caffeic acid, saponin, and ferrous sulphate were obtained from Sigma-Aldrich (St. Louis, MO, USA). Folin-Ciocalteu reagent and di-sodium phosphate decahydrate were purchased from Merck Millipore Corporation (Billerica, MA, USA); aluminium chloride from Loba Chemie (Mumbai, India); sodium hydroxide and glacial acetic acid from VWR International, (Radnor, PA, USA), sodium dihydrogen orthophosphate 1-hydrate and ferric chloride from BDH Chemicals LTD (Poole, UK); 2,2′-azobis-2-methyl-propanimidamide dichloride (AAPH) from the Cayman Chemical Company (Ann Arbor, MI, USA). All chemicals used were of analytical grade.

2.1. *Preparation of Asparagus Roots*

New Zealand green and purple AR roots were obtained from a commercial farm in Palmerston (New Zealand) (40.3523° S, 175.6082° E) from plants that had been planted for 15 years. The *A. officinalis* roots (AR) were cleaned from soil and other contaminants were removed from the roots by thoroughly washing them with tap water and then rinsing them with deionized water [8]. Then the roots were dried using an oven (Contherm 2150, Contherm Scientific Limited, Upper Hut, New Zealand) at 60 °C for 72 h. The dried roots were then pulverized into a powder using a Jingangdikai JG100 grinder (Jingangdikai Co., Guandong, China) and sieved through a 40 mm mesh. The dried root powder samples were transferred into closed plastic containers and kept at −20 °C until further analysis.

2.2. *Extraction of Bioactive Compounds*

The effects of extraction solvent (water, methanol or ethanol), solvent concentration, number of extractions (reflect the number of extractions of the same sample) and extraction time on the yield and antioxidant activities of the extracts were investigated. A modified method of Fan et al. [9] was carried out for the extraction of bioactive compounds from the AR. The AR powder was extracted using deionized water, methanol or ethanol at different concentrations (50%, 70%, and 90%). The samples were extracted twice and all extractions were carried out with triplicate samples. For the first extraction, 10 g of the AR powder was combined with 200 mL of the extraction solvent in a flask. The samples were then wrapped in aluminium foil and placed into a shaking incubator (Ratek, Victoria, Australia) at 70 °C for 2 h shaking at a speed of 80 RPM. After 2 h, the samples were centrifuged (J2-21 M/E Beckman, Brea, CA, USA) at 10,000× g for 20 min and the supernatant was filtered using Whatman No 1 filter paper by vacuum. The methanol and ethanol in the extracted samples were removed using a Rotavapor® (Büchi, Chadderton, UK) at 40 °C, and then the samples were frozen at −80 °C before being freeze-dried (Labconco, Kansas City, MO, USA). The pellets from the centrifuge and filter steps were subjected to a second extraction as described above. The samples from both extractions were kept separate and referred to in the following sections as "extraction order". The samples were frozen at −80 °C and freeze-dried. This process was repeated using the same solvent: solid ratio, and extraction temperature using ethanol as the extraction solvent at a longer extraction time of 10 h. The yield was calculated using the following equation:

$$\text{Yield } (\%) = \frac{(\text{Weight of freeze} - \text{dried extract})}{\text{Weight of dried asparagus roots}} \times 100$$

2.3. Analysis of Asparagus Root Extracts

The samples were analysed for their TPC (Total phenolic content), TFC (Total phenolic content) and antioxidant activities using solutions prepared fresh on the day of analysis (1 mg/mL in 50% methanol), kept on ice and protected from light. All analyses were carried out in triplicate measurements.

2.4. Total Phenolic Content

To determine the TPC of the samples, the Folin-Ciocalteu colourimetric method was carried out using a plate reader (Biotek, Winooski, VT, USA) as described by Farasat et al. [10]. In a 96-well microplate, 20 μL of the extract was added, followed by 100 μL of Folin-Ciocalteu reagent (1:10) and 80 μL of sodium carbonate (7.5%). The plate was left in the dark at room temperature for 30 min, and the absorbance was read at 600 nm. Gallic acid was used to construct a standard curve (0–0.15 mg/mL), hence the polyphenol content of the samples was expressed as Gallic Acid Equivalents per gram of extract (mg GAE/g extract).

2.5. Total Flavonoid Content

The aluminium chloride colourimetric method of Herald et al. [11] was carried out using a plate reader to determine the TFC. In a 96-well microplate, 100 μL of distilled water, 10 μL of sodium nitrite (50 g/L), and 25 μL of the extract solution were added to each well. After 5 min of incubation in the dark at room temperature, 15 μL of aluminium chloride (100 g/L) was added and the mixture was left for a further 6 min in the dark at room temperature. Finally, 50 μL of sodium hydroxide (1 mol/L) and 50 μL of distilled water were added to the wells. The absorbance of the mixture was measured at 510 nm and rutin was used to construct a standard curve (1–0.05 mg/mL), hence the flavonoid content of the samples was expressed as rutin equivalent per gram of extract (mg RE/g extract).

2.6. Antioxidant Activity

2.6.1. Determination of DPPH Radical Scavenging Activity

The DPPH assay was conducted using the method described by De-Ancos et al. [12] using a plate reader. A 10 μL of the sample and 90 μL of deionized water were added to each well of a 96-well microplate. Then, in dimmed light, 100 μL of DPPH (78 mg/L) was added to each well. The plate was left in the dark at 25 °C for 30 min before the absorbance was measured at 517 nm. Gallic acid was used to construct a standard curve, and the DPPH scavenging activity was determined as DPPH inhibition (%) from the equation:

$$\text{DPPH Inhibition} = \frac{(1 - \text{test sample})}{\text{blank sample absorbance}} \times 100$$

2.6.2. Determination of Oxygen Radical Absorbance Capacity (ORAC)

The method of Huang et al. [13] was used to determine the ORAC. Phosphate buffer (75 mM, pH 7.4) was prepared and a stock solution of 1 mM of fluorescein sodium salt was made using the buffer, wrapped in aluminium foil and kept at 4 °C. This stock solution was diluted further to make a 10 nM solution, which was used on the day of the assay. The AAPH was made by dissolving 0.0646 g in 1 mL of the phosphate buffer. The 10 nM fluorescein and AAPH solutions were kept on ice in the dark until use and were made fresh daily. For the standard curve Trolox (0–150 mM) was prepared in phosphate buffer and used to construct the standard curve.

A 25 µL of the standard or sample and 150 µL of the 10 nM fluorescein were pipetted into a 96-well microplate in the dark. Then the plate was covered in parafilm and placed in the plate reader at 37 °C for 30 min. A 25 µL of APPH was added, the plate was shaken for 20 s, and the fluorescence was read at excitation at 485 nm and emission at 527 nm, at 1-min intervals over 1.5 h. The results were analysed by calculating the AUC, using the following equation:

$$AUC = 1 + \sum_{t_0=0\ \text{min}}^{t_i=90\ \text{min}} \frac{A_i}{A_0}$$

where A_0 is the initial fluorescence reading at t_0 and A_i is the reading at t_i hence, the final ORAC results were the difference between the area under the curve the blank and the samples. The results were expressed as mM Trolox equivalents per gram of extract (mM TE/g extract).

2.6.3. Ferric Reducing Ability Power (FRAP) Assay

The method of Benzie and Strain [14] was used with some modifications as reported by Teh et al. [15] so that it could be applied to a plate reader in a 96-well microplate. A FRAP solution was made in acetate buffer (300 mM, pH 3.6) that contained 10 mM TPTZ, 20 mM $FeCl_3$ and deionized water. The 10 mM TPTZ was made up in 10 mL of HCl (40 nM) and placed in a water bath at 50 °C until the compound was dissolved. The 20 mM $FeCl_3$ was made up in 10 mL of distilled water.

FRAP solution 100 mL of the acetate buffer (300 mM, pH 3.6), 10 mL of TPTZ (10 mM) and 10 mL of $FeCl_3$ were combined and kept at 37 °C until use. This solution was made fresh daily. For the standard curve, iron sulphate was used (0–1.5 mM). In a 96-well microplate, 10 µL of the standard (iron sulphate) or sample was added, followed by 200 µL of the FRAP solution. The plate was incubated at 37 °C for 4 min inside the plate reader. The results were expressed as mM iron sulphate equivalents per gram of extract (mM $FeSO_4$ E/g extract).

2.7. HPLC Analysis

Reverse phase HPLC [9] was used to separate and quantify the bioactive compounds extracted from the different extraction methods. All of the samples were filtered into 2 mL amber vials using a 0.45 µm nylon filter (Phenomenex, Torrance, CA, USA). The amber vials were then placed into the auto-sampler chamber, which was kept at 4 °C during the analysis. The HPLC used was an Agilent 1200 (Agilent Technologies, Santa Clara, CA, USA), with autosampler and Diode Array Detector (DAD). The column used was a Luna C18 (5 µm, 250 × 4.6 mm, Phenomenex, Torrance, CA, USA), with a 10 µm 4 × 3 mm C18 guard column (Phenomenex, Torrance, CA, USA). The column was maintained at 25 °C. The mobile phase consisted of Milli-Q water (A) and acetonitrile containing 0.02% v/v of trifluoroacetic acid (TFA) (B). Preliminary work using several standards (quercetin, rutin, gallic acid, ferulic acid, and caffeic acid) showed that the main compound in AR is caffeic acid. The caffeic acid content in the obtained extracts of the analytes was identified and quantified by comparing the retention time of the peak with a reference standard eluted under the same conditions.

2.8. Statistical Analysis

The statistical analysis was carried out using Minitab 16 Statistical Software (State College, PA, USA) using the general linear model (GLM) protocol. The investigated parameters were the TPC, TFC, caffeic acid and DPPH, ORAC and FRAP activities of AR extracts. For the solvent extraction method, a multivariate analysis of variance (ANOVA) was carried out to examine the effects of extraction solvent (methanol, ethanol, and water), solvent concentration (50%, 70%, and 90%), extraction order (1st and 2nd extraction) and their interactions on the measured parameters. The results for 2-h and 10-h extraction times using ethanol were analysed separately. Tukey's honestly significant difference

(HSD) post hoc test was used for multi comparison tests. A Pearson's correlation was also carried out to determine the correlations among the measured parameters.

3. Results and Discussion

In agreement with the literature, the conditions required for the optimal conventional extraction method of bioactive compounds from plant materials depended greatly on the extraction order and time, extraction solvent and concentration [16].

3.1. Extraction Time and Order on the Yield

There was a significant effect for the extraction order ($p < 0.05$) in both 2-h and 10-h extractions, where the 1st extraction had a significantly higher yield compared to the 2nd extraction (Table 1). A careful evaluation of the economics of the process needs to be considered as to whether it would be worthwhile for a 2nd extraction to be carried out (i.e., the yield and activity would have to provide enough incentive for the extra processing time and cost). The yield from 10-h 1st extraction was significantly higher than the 2-h comparable extraction ($p < 0.01$, data not shown). The obtained extracts reflected a mix of several cellular biomaterials, including carbohydrates. Therefore, it was important to evaluate the bioactivity of the extract rather than limiting the evaluation on crude extract, since the maximum amount of bioactive compounds extracted by the solvent may have varied due to differences in the compounds' affinity toward the various extraction solvents.

Table 1. The yield of extracts (Mean ± SEM) obtained using solvent extraction methods. [a,b] Within each extraction and [x–z] within each extraction time, values that do not share the same letter are significantly different ($p < 0.05$).

Extraction Time	Extraction Solvent	Extraction Order	Average Yield (%)
2-h	50% Methanol	1	42.4 ± 1.8 [a]
	70% Methanol	1	42.1 ± 1.8 [a]
	90% Methanol	1	41.8 ± 1.8 [a]
	50% Ethanol	1	44.0 ± 1.8 [a]
	70% Ethanol	1	44.3 ± 1.8 [a]
	90% Ethanol	1	36.4 ± 1.8 [a]
	Water	1	38.4 ± 1.8 [a]
	50% Methanol	2	3.2 ± 1.8 [b]
	70% Methanol	2	3.4 ± 1.8 [b]
	90% Methanol	2	3.0 ± 1.8 [b]
	50% Ethanol	2	3.6 ± 1.8 [b]
	70% Ethanol	2	5.1 ± 1.8 [b]
	90% Ethanol	2	7.0 ± 1.8 [b]
	Water	2	4.2 ± 1.8 [b]
10-h	50% Ethanol	1	53.6 ± 3.4 [x]
	70% Ethanol	1	60.1 ± 3.4 [x]
	90% Ethanol	1	29.8 ± 3.4 [y]
	50% Ethanol	2	12.8 ± 3.4 [z]
	70% Ethanol	2	6.4 ± 3.4 [z]
	90% Ethanol	2	7.2 ± 3.4 [z]

3.2. Effect of Extraction Solvent on TPC, TFC, and Antioxidant Activity

There were significant effects for the extraction solvents during 2-h extraction time on the TPC, TFC and FRAP activity ($p < 0.001$) but not the DPPH scavenging (DPPH) and ORAC activities (Tables 2 and 3). There were no differences between ethanol and methanol for TFC and FRAP activity. Given that methanol led to a small increase (about 5–7%) in TPC and with the known toxicity of methanol, it was decided that ethanol was the best extraction solvent as it would be more acceptable as an extraction solvent for health reasons [17–19]. The best extraction solvent to extract the maximum amount of bioactive compounds is dependent on the type of plant matrix in question [16]. Different amounts of antioxidant compounds were extracted by methanol, ethanol and water from plants materials, which was depended on the polarity, density and pH [16]. Hence, different antioxidant compounds have varying optimal extraction conditions. Although polyphenols and flavonoids are polar compounds, they express maximum extraction potential when are extracted from a solvent containing a combination of polar and non-polar substances [20]. Therefore, it was possible that different compounds were extracted in the different extraction solvents. The best extraction solvent determined in this research is in agreement with the literature on the extraction of bioactives from asparagus, as ethanol was found to be the most popular extraction solvent [2,3,9,21,22]. Methanol was found to be the optimum extraction solvent when it was used as pure methanol in a Soxhlet system [23,24]. During preliminary trials, a Soxhlet extraction method was carried out; however, it was found to be time-consuming and required a high amount of solvent, which resulted in high cost and a lot of organic waste to manage. Ideally, the best method needed for this type of research should be simple and easy to carry out, so that the commercialization pathway is affordable and commercially viable. Therefore, the ethanol extraction process was chosen for further investigations.

The extraction was carried out using two extractions times; 2-h and 10-h. The 2-h and 10-h extraction times resulted in different ($p < 0.05$) antioxidant activities (Figure 1). For the TPC, ORAC, and FRAP, a 2-h extraction had higher activities compared to 10-h extraction. For the TFC and DPPH activity, the opposite was true. Fan et al. [9] investigated a range of extraction times up to 2.5 h and concluded that an extraction time of 2-h was sufficient to extract the maximum amount of antioxidant compounds from asparagus residue. From time 0 to 2.5 h, it was found that the amount of antioxidants extracted increased until it reached a constant value at 2 h and then decreased slightly with the increase in extraction time. This was not found in this research, as the amount of antioxidants extracted from the 10-h extraction was not less than the 2-h extraction. Solana, Boschiero, Dall'Acqua, and Bertucco [24] determined that in whole *A. officinalis* and found a longer extraction time (4 h) allowed more phenolic acids to be extracted.

In the present study, a long extraction time resulted in a lower amount of total polyphenols (Figure 1a). This was in agreement with Shi et al. [25] findings in grape seeds. Oxidation of the polyphenols during the long processing time may have resulted in polymerised insoluble compounds and reduced total polyphenols [25].

There was a significant effect for the extraction order ($p < 0.05$) in both 2-h and 10-h extractions, where the 1st extraction had a significantly higher yield compared to the 2nd extraction. The yield from the 10-h 1st extraction was significantly higher ($p < 0.05$) than the 2-h comparable extraction. The use of a 2nd extraction step appears to be important as it led to up to 20% recovery of yield, such as with 90% ethanol (Table 1). Other materials in the literature determined that a two-step extraction process resulted in the maximum amount of antioxidant compounds [25–27].

In the 2-h extraction, TPC per gram extract from the 1st and 2nd extractions were not different and a similar trend was found with TFC. However, ORAC and FRAP activities were affected ($p < 0.05$) by the extraction order (Figure 1). For the 10-h extraction, higher TPC and TFC ($p < 0.05$) were found in extracts from the 2nd extraction compared to the 1st extraction (Figure 1). Nawaz, Shi, Mittal, and Kakuda [27] investigated the optimal number of extractions to recover the maximum amount of polyphenols from grape seeds. The authors found that two extractions were ideal for that purpose. They found that the diffusion rate of the solute from the grape seeds decreased with increasing number of extractions. The extraction of bioactive is regulated by the diffusion of the extraction solvent into the matrix particles, where the driving force is the difference in pressure; and also by the diffusion of the antioxidant compounds from the matrix into the extraction solvent, where the driving force is the concentration difference [27]. As more antioxidant compounds were removed in the 1st extraction step, the concentration difference would have decreased, resulting in less compounds being extracted. Additional antioxidant compounds were extracted in the 2nd extraction due to disruption of the matrix during the 1st extraction, allowing the solvent in the 2nd extraction to diffuse more easily and extract more bioactives [28]. Hence, several researchers found a 3rd extraction is not justified (Nawaz, Shi, Mittal and Kakuda [27]; Cacace and Mazza [29]. In terms of yield, a 2nd extraction step would require economical evaluation in terms of benefit-cost relationship.

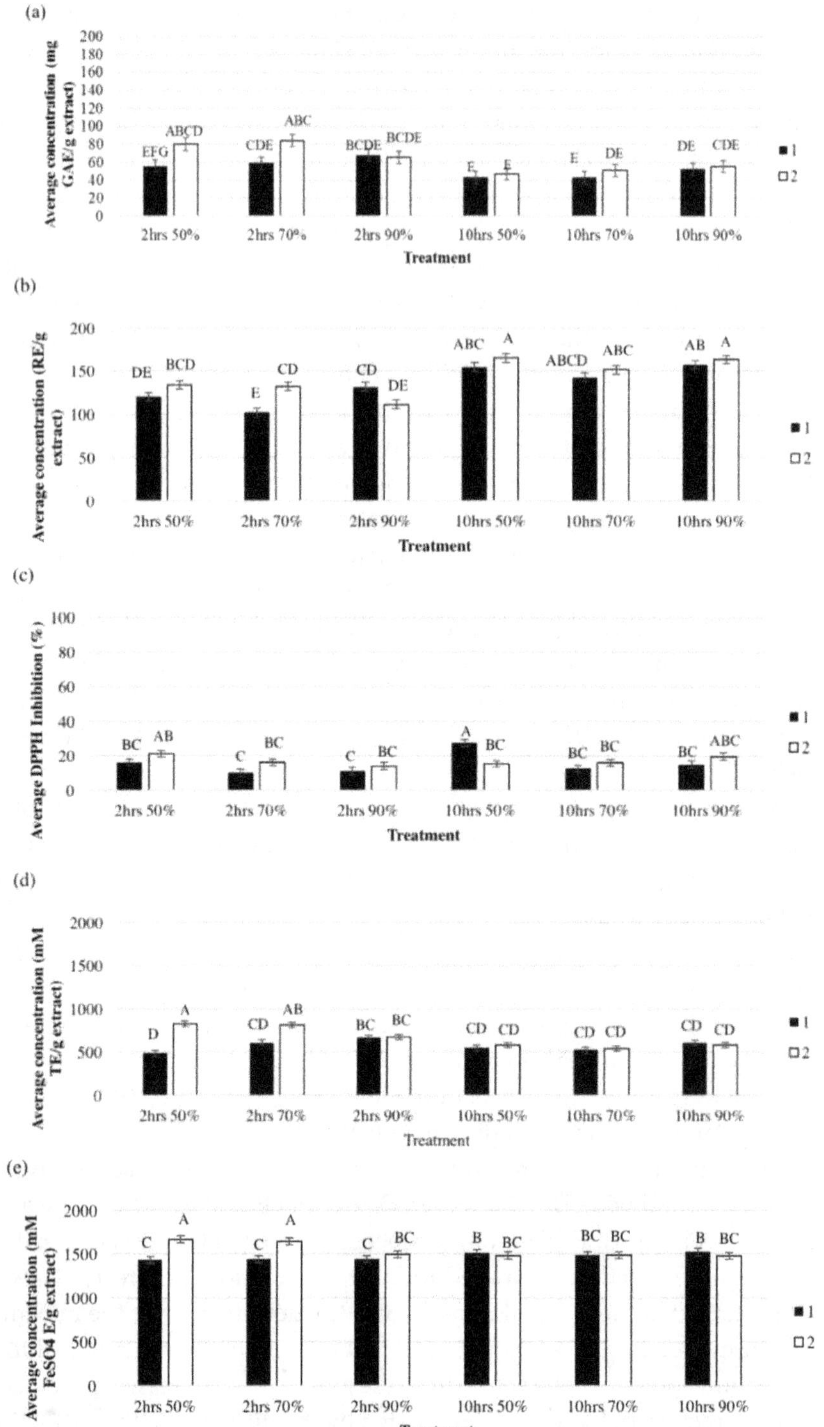

Figure 1. The effect of ethanol concentration, extraction order and extraction time on total phenolic content (**a**); total flavonoid content (**b**); 2,2-diphenyl-1-picrylhydrazyl (DPPH) scavenging activity (**c**); Oxygen Radical Absorbance Capacity (ORAC) activity (**d**); and Ferric Reducing/Antioxidant Power (FRAP) activity (**e**) of the extract obtained from asparagus root powder after 2 and 10-h extraction time. Bars that do not share the same letter are significantly different ($p < 0.05$).

Table 2. Summary of antioxidant activities of asparagus root extract obtained from 2-h extraction. $^{a–h}$ Values that do not share the same letter are significantly different ($p < 0.05$).

Solvent	Total Polyphenols (mg GAE/g Extract)		Total Flavonoids (mg RE/g Extract)		DPPH Inhibition %		ORAC Antioxidant Activity (mM TE/g Extract)		FRAP Antioxidant Activity (mM $FeSO_4$ E/g Extract)		Caffeic Acid (mg/g Extract)	
	Order		Order		Order		Order		Order		Order	
	1	2	1	2	1	2	1	2	1	2	1	2
Methanol 50%	61.5 ^{efg}	78.8 ^{efg}	128.6 ^{d}	126.6 ^{d}	23.6 ^{d}	40.8 ^{abcd}	557.6 ^{de}	596.9 ^{ade}	1445.0 ^{d}	1572.5 ^{bc}	2.5 ^{ab}	2.7 ^{ab}
Methanol 70%	67.9 ^{efg}	84.7 ^{defg}	122.5 ^{de}	127.7 ^{d}	47.0 ^{a}	42.3 ^{abcd}	776.1 ^{abc}	676.5 ^{abcd}	1439.8 ^{d}	1632.1 ^{ab}	2.2 ^{ab}	2.7 ^{ab}
Methanol 90%	64.9 ^{efg}	91.4 ^{def}	118.0 ^{de}	123.3 ^{de}	39.9 ^{abcd}	29.1 ^{abcd}	591.1 ^{de}	699.3 ^{abcd}	1451.0 ^{d}	1638.4 ^{ab}	2.6 ^{ab}	2.5 ^{ab}
Ethanol 50%	56.1 ^{h}	80.2 ^{efg}	120.4 ^{de}	134.0 ^{d}	41.8 ^{abcd}	38.3 ^{abcd}	481.1 ^{e}	829.5 ^{a}	1435.1 ^{d}	1668.6 ^{a}	1.7 ^{b}	2.8 ^{a}
Ethanol 70%	59.1 ^{efg}	84.2 ^{defg}	102.1 ^{e}	132.3 ^{d}	27.1 ^{cd}	41.2 ^{abcd}	604.3 ^{de}	811.8 ^{ab}	1438.3 ^{d}	1646.3 ^{a}	1.7 ^{b}	3.0 ^{a}
Ethanol 90%	68.4 ^{efg}	65.7 ^{efg}	131.9 ^{de}	119.4 ^{d}	26.1 ^{abcd}	32.1 ^{abcd}	661.2 ^{abcd}	670.7 ^{abcd}	1439.8 ^{d}	1494.0 ^{d}	3.0 ^{a}	2.3 ^{ab}
Water	52.0 ^{g}	63.7 ^{defg}	109.3 ^{de}	110.9 ^{de}	41.5 ^{abcd}	23.8 ^{d}	593.2 ^{de}	655.6 ^{abcd}	1422.4 ^{d}	1487.6 ^{d}	2.1 ^{ab}	2.1 ^{ab}

Gallic Acid Equivalents (GAE); Rutin Equivalent (RE); 2,2-diphenyl-1-picrylhydrazyl (DPPH); Trolox Equivalents (TE); Oxygen Radical Absorbance Capacity (ORAC); Ferric Reducing/Antioxidant Power (FRAP).

Table 3. *p*-Values found for the effects of conventional extraction parameters on the total polyphenol content, total flavonoid content, and antioxidant activity (DPPH, ORAC and FRAP) of extracts obtained from AR ($p < 0.05$ indicates significance).

Time	Factor	Total Polyphenols	Total Flavonoids	DPPH Inhibition %	ORAC	FRAP
2 h	Extraction Solvent	0.000	0.000	0.270	0.127	0.000
	Concentration	0.161	0.200	0.012	0.131	0.218
	Extraction Order	0.000	0.000	0.100	0.000	0.000
	Extraction Solvent Concentration	0.600	0.011	0.002	0.005	0.000
	Extraction Solvent × Extraction Order	0.641	0.095	0.001	0.000	0.000
	Concentration × Extraction Order	0.154	0.053	0.339	0.021	0.099
	Extraction Solvent × Concentration × Extraction Order	0.071	0.039	0.002	0.000	0.000
10 h	Concentration	0.000	0.000	0.000	0.040	0.662
	Extraction Order	0.000	0.000	0.298	0.613	0.101
	Concentration × Extraction Order	0.001	0.163	0.000	0.526	0.413
Comparing 2 h and 10 h	Extraction Time	0.000	0.000	0.015	0.000	0.002
	Concentration	0.279	0.000	0.000	0.610	0.000
	Extraction Order	0.000	0.000	0.160	0.000	0.000
	Extraction Time × Concentration	0.060	0.499	0.451	0.059	0.000
	Extraction Time × Extraction Order	0.005	0.000	0.014	0.000	0.000
	Concentration × Extraction Order	0.336	0.004	0.010	0.000	0.000
	Extraction Time × Concentration × Extraction Order	0.489	0.073	0.004	0.013	0.000

3.3. *Effect of Extraction Time and Order on the Antioxidant Compounds*

The optimal condition to extract TPC involved a 2-h extraction and the use of 70% ethanol. In all cases, the 2nd extraction had slightly more, but insignificant TPC compared to the 1st extraction, except for 2-h 50% ethanol (Figure 1a). For TFC, the 10-h extraction had more TFC compared with the 2-h extraction. The optimal conditions for TFC extraction were 10-h extraction using 50% ethanol. Similar to the TPC, the 2nd extraction had slightly more, but insignificant TFC compared to the 1st extraction, with the exception of 2-h 70% ethanol treatment.

The optimal conditions for the extraction of DPPH inhibition activity were using a 10-h extraction with 50% ethanol. Under these conditions, the extract from the 1st extraction significantly ($p < 0.05$) had more antioxidant activity compared to the 2nd extraction. The optimal conditions for the extraction of ORAC antioxidant activity were 2-h extraction using 70% ethanol, which had significantly ($p < 0.05$) higher ORAC activity compared to the 10-h extraction. Even though the 2-h and 50% ethanol had the highest ($p < 0.05$) ORAC antioxidant activity in the 2nd extraction, the 2-h and 70% ethanol treatment resulted in a combined higher ORAC activity.

The 2-h 50% and 70% ethanol treatments had significantly ($p < 0.05$) higher FRAP antioxidant activity compared to the other treatments. The optimal conditions for extracts for that activity were 2-h at 50% ethanol. The 2nd extraction had more FRAP antioxidant activity compared to the 1st extraction in most cases (Figure 1e). This could be due to the matrix of the AR, as the 1st extraction would have disrupted the matrix, allowing the 2nd extraction to easily remove more antioxidants [27]. Furthermore, the removal of carbohydrates and other soluble compounds during the first extraction can help more specific extraction of antioxidants. To determine the optimal conditions to extract antioxidant compounds from AR, the extraction yields were calculated and are shown in Table 1. There were no effects ($p > 0.05$) for the solvent or the solvent concentration on the yield of AR extracts (Table 1).

3.4. *Effect of Extraction Order and Solvent Type on Antioxidant Activity*

The interaction between extraction order and extraction solvent investigated for the 2-h extraction, as the 10-h extraction only examined the use of one solvent "ethanol". The extraction order and extraction solvent and their interaction had significant ($p < 0.05$) effects on the antioxidant activities of the extracts, which was dependent on the antioxidant assay used (Tables 2 and 3). The 1st extraction did not have a significant effect ($p > 0.05$) on DPPH inhibition activity compared to the 2nd extraction for all the solvents used. For the ORAC activity, only the 50% and 70% 2nd extraction of ethanol were significantly higher ($p < 0.05$) than the other extractions. Ethanol 90% and water 1st extracts had significantly ($p < 0.05$) lower FRAP activity than their 2nd counterpart extracts. The 2nd methanol (50%, 70%, and 90%) and ethanol (50% and 70%) extracts had significantly ($p < 0.05$) higher FRAP activity found compared to water and ethanol 90% extracts. In general, methanol and ethanol extracts were similar in their antioxidant activity, while water extracts were significantly ($p < 0.05$) lower in most cases.

3.5. *Effect of Solvent Concentration*

Methanol and ethanol at different concentrations extracted the same amounts of TFC that were not different from water (Table 2). It is worth mentioning that the differences between ethanol and methanol in terms of TFC were less than 5–6%, which economically may not be attractive to justify the use of a toxic chemical such as methanol. Methanol 70% extract had the highest DPPH radical scavenging and ORAC activity (Figure 1 and Table 2). The FRAP activity of water and 90% ethanol extracts were lower than the other treatment with the exception of 50% methanol extract (Figure 1). Generally, 70% methanol and 50% ethanol were good extraction solvents for antioxidants of AR, and water was the least effective extraction solvent. In the 10-h extraction method, only ethanol was used since generally little differences were observed between ethanol and methanol in 2-h extraction. The optimal solvent concentration for the extraction of antioxidant compounds from plants depends on the matrix of the plant and the properties of the antioxidant compounds [16]. Optimal ethanol concentration used for the extraction of bioactives from different asparagus types and parts ranged from 50% to 80% [2,3,9,21,22], which is in agreement with the findings in this study. This wide range of concentrations could be due to the polarity of the antioxidant compounds, and the affinity they have towards the extraction solvent [16]. Different solvent concentrations may be able to diffuse in the AR structure and extract different types and amounts of antioxidant compounds. Shi, Yu, Pohorly, Young, Bryan, and Wu [25] and Fan, Yuan, Wang, Gao, and Huang [9] reported that a concentration of 50% ethanol was optimal as it allowed the maximum amount of the water-soluble polyphenols to be extracted. Furthermore, 50% ethanol has been known to be effective at extracting flavonoids [30], which is in accordance with the findings of this study.

3.6. Effect of Extraction Order and Solvent Concentration on the Antioxidant Activity

Only FRAP activity in 2-h extracts was significantly ($p < 0.05$) affected by the extraction order and the 2nd extraction had higher FRAP activity compared to the 1st extraction in all the solvents. In the 10-h extraction, TPC and DPPH activity were affected by the extraction order and solvent concentration ($p < 0.05$). Extracts obtained from the 90% solvent concentration significantly had higher TPC compared to 50% and 70% (Figure 1). There was an effect for the extraction order on TPC which was observed in 70% solvent concentration only. For the DPPH, 50% ethanol the first extraction had the highest DPPH scavenging activity (Figure 1). This could have been due to the antioxidants responsible for the inhibition of DPPH being more favourable to be extracted by 50% ethanol due to the polarity [16]. The concentration did not greatly influence the extraction of antioxidant compounds, apart from DPPH. This is in agreement with the findings of Diankov et al. [31] who found a negligible concentration effect when extracting antioxidant compounds in lemon peels.

3.7. Pearson Correlations for the Measured Activities in AR Extract

Pearson correlations analysis was carried out on the 2-h extraction and the 10-h extraction to examine the influence of extraction time on these relationships (Table 4). In the 2-h extraction, there were many positive correlations ($p < 0.05$). The DPPH assay and flavonoids had a positive correlation. This meant that the TFC were affecting DPPH inhibition activity. The FRAP and ORAC assays both had positive correlations to polyphenols and flavonoids, therefore the polyphenols and flavonoids contributed towards the FRAP and ORAC antioxidant activities. The FRAP and ORAC assays also had a positive correlation with each other. This meant that these two methods may have targeted the same type of antioxidant. The positive correlation between antioxidants was in agreement with previous findings for basil leaves [16] and spinach [32].

Table 4. Pearson's Overall Correlation between the Antioxidant Assays in the 2-h Extraction ($p < 0.05$ indicates significance).

Extraction Time	Antioxidant Assay		Polyphenols	Flavonoids	DPPH	ORAC
2-h	Flavonoids	Pearson's coefficient	0.322			
		p-value	0.000			
	DPPH Inhibition %	Pearson's coefficient	0.110	0.269		
		p-value	0.228	0.003		
	ORAC	Pearson's coefficient	0.201	0.199	0.162	
		p-value	0.025	0.028	0.076	
	FRAP	Pearson's coefficient	0.455	0.338	0.084	0.450
		p-value	0.000	0.000	0.353	0.000
10-h	Flavonoids	Pearson's coefficient	0.433			
		p-value	0.001			
	DPPH Inhibition %	Pearson's coefficient	−0.165	−0.110		
		p-value	0.232	0.428		
	ORAC	Pearson's coefficient	0.171	0.280	−0.161	
		p-value	0.217	0.041	0.244	
	FRAP	Pearson's coefficient	0.003	0.109	−0.007	−0.075
		p-value	0.982	0.432	0.962	0.587

3.8. Analysis of AR Extract Using HPLC

Caffeic acid is a hydrocinnamic acid, and it contributes towards the autotoxicity in *A. officinalis* roots [33]. The major phenolic peak detected in *A. officinalis* roots is controversial with rutin [34] or caffeic acid [33,35] being alternatively reported as the highest phenolic compound in the roots of *A. officinalis* L. Although literature reported the presence of rutin in *A. officinalis* this was not reflected in the results of this study, as rutin was not found. This could have been due to the preparation conditions of *A. officinalis* AR samples, as Makris and Rossiter [36] found rutin degraded when *A. officinalis* spears were chopped. As shown in Table 2, after 2-h extraction the amount of caffeic acid was not affected by the solvent type ($p > 0.05$). Ethanol concentration and extraction order affected the caffeic acid content (Table 2), where 90% ethanol extract had higher caffeic acid content than the 50% and 70% ethanol extracts in the 1st extraction. Similarly, using 90% ethanol, 2.4 (mg/g extract) of caffeic acid was obtained after 10 h that was significantly higher than the 1.5 and 1.3 mg/g extract obtained with 50% and 70% ethanol, respectively. Studies have shown that caffeic acid and its derivatives exhibit significant biological activities such as antioxidants to control lipid peroxidation [37] and have a potential therapeutic effect in treating neurodegenerative diseases [38].

4. Conclusions

The antioxidant activities of green asparagus root were determined using conventional hydro-alcohol extraction methods. It was concluded that one extraction was sufficient to extract the majority of antioxidant compounds as a 2nd extraction had a significantly lower yield and so would not have been worthwhile, in respect to the time and extraction solvent required. The optimal conditions were found to be using 50% ethanol for 2-h, with a yield of 44%. The 2-h extraction time allowed more TPC, ORAC, and FRAP activities to be obtained. Although more flavonoids were found in the 10-h extraction, they did not appear to contribute more towards these antioxidant activities. Rutin was not found in New Zealand *A. officinalis* roots and caffeic acid was found to be the dominant phenolic in AR extracts. The extraction method developed in this study was simple and easy to carry out. Therefore, this method would enable the use of asparagus roots as a valuable-by product and hence prevent them from being a waste.

Acknowledgments: The authors would like to thank Rod Philip (Palmerston asparagus Co.) for the kind donation of the samples. Also, the authors extend their appreciation to the International Scientific Partnership Program ISPP at King Saud University for funding this research work through ISPP# 0073).

Author Contributions: Abbey Symes and Alaa El-Din Ahmed Bekhit conceived and designed the experiments; Abbey Symes and Hongxia Zhang performed the experiments; Alaa El-Din Ahmed Bekhit and Isam A. Mohamed Ahmed analysed the data; Amin Shavandi contributed reagents and materials; Alaa El-Din Ahmed Bekhit, Amin Shavandi and Fahad Y. Al-Juhaimi wrote the paper.

Conflicts of Interest: The authors declare no conflict of interest.

References

1. Kamat, J.P.; Boloor, K.K.; Devasagayam, T.P.; Venkatachalam, S. Antioxidant properties of *Asparagus racemosus* against damage induced by γ-radiation in rat liver mitochondria. *J. Ethnopharmacol.* **2000**, *71*, 425–435. [CrossRef]
2. Fuentes-Alventosa, J.M.; Jaramillo-Carmona, S.; Rodríguez-Gutiérrez, G.; Rodríguez-Arcos, R.; Fernández-Bolaños, J.; Guillén-Bejarano, R.; Espejo-Calvo, J.; Jiménez-Araujo, A. Effect of the extraction method on phytochemical composition and antioxidant activity of high dietary fibre powders obtained from asparagus by-products. *Food Chem.* **2009**, *116*, 484–490. [CrossRef]
3. Hossain, M.I.; Sharmin, F.A.; Akhter, S.; Bhuiyan, M.A.; Shahriar, M. Investigation of cytotoxicity and in-vitro antioxidant activity of *Asparagus racemosus* root extract. *ICPJ* **2012**, *1*, 250–257. [CrossRef]
4. Agrawal, A.; Sharma, M.; Rai, S.K.; Singh, B.; Tiwari, M.; Chandra, R. The effect of the aqueous extract of the roots of *Asparagus racemosus* on hepatocarcinogenesis initiated by diethylnitrosamine. *Phytother. Res.* **2008**, *22*, 1175–1182. [CrossRef] [PubMed]

5. Dahanukar, S.; Thatte, U.; Pai, N.; Mose, P.; Karandikar, S. Protective effect of *Asparagus racemosus* against induced abdominal sepsis. *Research* **1986**, *24*, 125–128.
6. Elena, K. First report of *Phomopsis asparagi* causing stem blight of asparagus in Greece. *Plant Pathol.* **2006**, *55*, 300. [CrossRef]
7. Fuentes-Alventosa, J.; Jaramillo-Carmona, S.; Rodríguez-Gutiérrez, G.; Guillén-Bejarano, R.; Jiménez-Araujo, A.; Fernández-Bolaños, J.; Rodríguez-Arcos, R. Preparation of bioactive extracts from asparagus by-product. *FBP* **2013**, *91*, 74–82. [CrossRef]
8. Sahu, R.; Saxen, J. Screening of total phenolic and flavonoid content in conventional and non-conventional species of Curcuma. *J. Pharmacogn. Phytochem.* **2013**, *2*, 176–179.
9. Fan, R.; Yuan, F.; Wang, N.; Gao, Y.; Huang, Y. Extraction and analysis of antioxidant compounds from the residues of *Asparagus officinalis* L. *J. Food Sci. Technol.* **2015**, *52*, 2690–2700. [CrossRef] [PubMed]
10. Farasat, M.; Khavari-Nejad, R.-A.; Nabavi, S.M.B.; Namjooyan, F. Antioxidant activity, total phenolics and flavonoid contents of some edible green seaweeds from northern coasts of the Persian Gulf. *Iran. J. Pharm. Res.* **2014**, *13*, 163–170. [PubMed]
11. Herald, T.J.; Gadgil, P.; Tilley, M. High-throughput microplate assays for screening flavonoid content and DPPH-scavenging activity in sorghum bran and flour. *J. Sci. Food Agric.* **2012**, *92*, 2326–2331. [CrossRef] [PubMed]
12. De-Ancos, B.; Sgroppo, S.; Plaza, L.; Cano, M.P. Possible nutritional and health-related value promotion in orange juice preserved by high-pressure treatment. *J. Sci. Food Agric.* **2002**, *82*, 790–796. [CrossRef]
13. Huang, D.; Ou, B.; Hampsch-Woodill, M.; Flanagan, J.A.; Prior, R.L. High-throughput assay of oxygen radical absorbance capacity (ORAC) using a multichannel liquid handling system coupled with a microplate fluorescence reader in 96-well format. *J. Agric. Food Chem.* **2002**, *50*, 4437–4444. [CrossRef] [PubMed]
14. Benzie, I.F.; Strain, J. The ferric reducing ability of plasma (frap) as a measure of "antioxidant power": The frap assay. *Anal. Biochem.* **1996**, *239*, 70–76. [CrossRef] [PubMed]
15. Teh, S.S.; Niven, B.E.; Bekhit, A.E.D.A.; Carne, A.; Birch, E.J. The use of microwave and pulsed electric field as a pretreatment step in ultrasonic extraction of polyphenols from defatted hemp seed cake (*Cannabis sativa*) using response surface methodology. *Food Bioprocess Technol.* **2014**, *7*, 3064–3076. [CrossRef]
16. Złotek, U.; Mikulska, S.; Nagajek, M.; Świeca, M. The effect of different solvents and number of extraction steps on the polyphenol content and antioxidant capacity of basil leaves (*Ocimum basilicum* L.) extracts. *Saudi J. Biol. Sci.* **2016**, *23*, 628–633.
17. Carter, W.P.; Pierce, J.A.; Luo, D.; Malkina, I.L. Environmental chamber study of maximum incremental reactivities of volatile organic compounds. *Atmos. Environ.* **1995**, *29*, 2499–2511. [CrossRef]
18. McMartin, K.E.; Ambre, J.J.; Tephly, T.R. Methanol poisoning in human subjects: Role for formic acid accumulation in the metabolic acidosis. *Am. J. Med.* **1980**, *68*, 414–418. [CrossRef]
19. Perini, M.; Camin, F. Δ18o of ethanol in wine and spirits for authentication purposes. *J. Food Sci.* **2013**, *78*, C839–C844. [CrossRef] [PubMed]
20. Boussetta, N.; Lesaint, O.; Vorobiev, E. A study of mechanisms involved during the extraction of polyphenols from grape seeds by pulsed electrical discharges. *Innov. Food Sci. Emerg. Technol.* **2013**, *19*, 124–132. [CrossRef]
21. Guillén, R.; Rodríguez, R.; Jaramillo, S.; Rodríguez, G.; Espejo, J.A.; Fernández-Bolaños, J.; Heredia, A.; Jiménez, A. Antioxidants from asparagus spears: Phenolics. *Acta Hortic.* **2008**, *776*, 247–253. [CrossRef]
22. Lee, E.J.; Yoo, K.S.; Patil, B.S. Development of a rapid HPLC-UV method for simultaneous quantification of protodioscin and rutin in white and green asparagus spears. *J. Food Sci.* **2010**, *75*, C703–C709. [CrossRef] [PubMed]
23. Lee, J.H.; Lim, H.J.; Lee, C.W.; Son, K.H.; Son, J.K.; Lee, S.K.; Kim, H.P. Methyl protodioscin from the roots of *Asparagus cochinchinensis* attenuates airway inflammation by inhibiting cytokine production. *Evid.-Based Complement. Altern. Med.* **2015**, *2015*, 640846. [CrossRef] [PubMed]
24. Solana, M.; Boschiero, I.; Dall'Acqua, S.; Bertucco, A. A comparison between supercritical fluid and pressurized liquid extraction methods for obtaining phenolic compounds from *Asparagus officinalis* L. *J. Supercrit. Fluids* **2015**, *100*, 201–208. [CrossRef]
25. Shi, J.; Yu, J.; Pohorly, J.; Young, J.C.; Bryan, M.; Wu, Y. Optimization of the extraction of polyphenols from grape seed meal by aqueous ethanol solution. *J. Food Agric. Environ.* **2003**, *1*, 42.

26. Bekhit, A.E.-D.A.; Cheng, V.J.; Harrison, R.; Ye, Z.; Bekhit, A.A.; Ng, T.; Kong, L. Technological aspects of by-product utilization. In *Valorization of Wine Making By-Products*; Chapter 4; CRC Press: Boca Raton, FL, USA, 2016; p. 117.
27. Nawaz, H.; Shi, J.; Mittal, G.S.; Kakuda, Y. Extraction of polyphenols from grape seeds and concentration by ultrafiltration. *Sep. Purif. Technol.* **2006**, *48*, 176–181. [CrossRef]
28. Renard, C.M.; Baron, A.; Guyot, S.; Drilleau, J.-F. Interactions between apple cell walls and native apple polyphenols: Quantification and some consequences. *Int. J. Biol. Macromol.* **2001**, *29*, 115–125. [CrossRef]
29. Cacace, J.; Mazza, G. Mass transfer process during extraction of phenolic compounds from milled berries. *J. Food Eng.* **2003**, *59*, 379–389. [CrossRef]
30. Bazykina, N.; Nikolaevskii, A.; Filippenko, T.; Kaloerova, V. Optimization of conditions for the extraction of natural antioxidants from raw plant materials. *Pharm. Chem. J.* **2002**, *36*, 46–49. [CrossRef]
31. Diankov, S.; Karsheva, M.; Hinkov, I. Extraction of natural antioxidants from lemon peels. Kinetics and antioxidant capacity. *J. Chem. Technol. Met.* **2011**, *46*, 315–319.
32. Payne, A.C.; Mazzer, A.; Clarkson, G.J.J.; Taylor, G. Antioxidant assays—Consistent findings from FRAP and ORAC reveal a negative impact of organic cultivation on antioxidant potential in spinach but not watercress or rocket leaves. *Food Sci. Nutr.* **2013**, *1*, 439–444. [CrossRef] [PubMed]
33. Miller, H.G.; Ikawa, M.; Peirce, L.C. Caffeic acid identified as an inhibitory compound in asparagus root filtrate. *HortScience* **1991**, *26*, 1525–1527.
34. Huang, X.F.; Luo, J.; Zhang, Y.; Kong, L.Y. Chemical constituents of *Asparagus officinalis*. *Chin. J. Nat. Med.* **2006**, *4*, 181–184.
35. Lake, R.; Falloon, P.; Cook, D. Replant problem and chemical components of asparagus roots. *N. Z. J. Crop Hortic. Sci.* **1993**, *21*, 53–58. [CrossRef]
36. Makris, D.P.; Rossiter, J.T. Domestic processing of onion bulbs (*Allium cepa*) and asparagus spears (*Asparagus officinalis*): Effect on flavonol content and antioxidant status. *J. Agric. Food Chem.* **2001**, *49*, 3216–3222. [CrossRef] [PubMed]
37. Son, S.; Lewis, B.A. Free radical scavenging and antioxidative activity of caffeic acid amide and ester analogues: Structure-Activity relationship. *J. Agric. Food Chem.* **2002**, *50*, 468–472. [CrossRef] [PubMed]
38. Fu, W.; Wang, H.; Ren, X.; Yu, H.; Lei, Y.; Chen, Q. Neuroprotective effect of three caffeic acid derivatives via ameliorate oxidative stress and enhance pka/creb signaling pathway. *Behav. Brain Res.* **2017**, *328*, 81–86. [CrossRef] [PubMed]

3

The Addition of Manganese Porphyrins during Radiation Inhibits Prostate Cancer Growth and Simultaneously Protects Normal Prostate Tissue from Radiation Damage

Arpita Chatterjee [1], Yuxiang Zhu [1], Qiang Tong [1,2], Elizabeth A. Kosmacek [1], Eliezer Z. Lichter [1] and Rebecca E. Oberley-Deegan [1,*]

1 Department of Biochemistry and Molecular Biology, University of Nebraska Medical Center, Omaha, NE 68198, USA; arpita.chatterjee@unmc.edu (A.C.); yuxiang.zhu@unmc.edu (Y.Z.); qiangtong@hust.edu.cn (Q.T.); elizabeth.kosmacek@unmc.edu (E.A.K.); Eliezer.lichter@unmc.edu (E.Z.L.)

2 Department of Gastrointestinal Surgery, Union Hospital, Tongji Medical College, Huazhong University of Science and Technology, Wuhan 430022, China

* Correspondence: becky.deegan@unmc.edu

Abstract: Radiation therapy is commonly used for prostate cancer treatment; however, normal tissues can be damaged from the reactive oxygen species (ROS) produced by radiation. In separate reports, we and others have shown that manganese porphyrins (MnPs), ROS scavengers, protect normal cells from radiation-induced damage but inhibit prostate cancer cell growth. However, there have been no studies demonstrating that MnPs protect normal tissues, while inhibiting tumor growth in the same model. LNCaP or PC3 cells were orthotopically implanted into athymic mice and treated with radiation (2 Gy, for 5 consecutive days) in the presence or absence of MnPs. With radiation, MnPs enhanced overall life expectancy and significantly decreased the average tumor volume, as compared to the radiated alone group. MnPs enhanced lipid oxidation in tumor cells but reduced oxidative damage to normal prostate tissue adjacent to the prostate tumor in combination with radiation. Mechanistically, MnPs behave as pro-oxidants or antioxidants depending on the level of oxidative stress inside the treated cell. We found that MnPs act as pro-oxidants in prostate cancer cells, while in normal cells and tissues the MnPs act as antioxidants. For the first time, in the same in vivo model, this study reveals that MnPs enhance the tumoricidal effect of radiation and reduce oxidative damage to normal prostate tissue adjacent to the prostate tumor in the presence of radiation. This study suggests that MnPs are effective radio-protectors for radiation-mediated prostate cancer treatment.

Keywords: prostate cancer; manganese porphyrin; radiation; ROS; lipid oxidation

---

1. Introduction

One of the most common treatments for prostate cancer is radiation therapy. Increased production of reactive oxygen species (ROS) is reported during and after radiation therapy [1]. Radiation-mediated ROS, specifically hydroxyl radicals, cause cytotoxic effects in tumor cells, which inhibits tumor growth [2]. However, some tumor cells escape this initial ROS-mediated cell death and become adapted to the elevated ROS levels, which can cause radio-resistance [3,4]. During radiation, normal tissue adjacent to the tumor, can be damaged directly by radiation or indirectly through bystander effects, which can result in fibrosis and loss of tissue function over time. These events collectively lead to side effects that reduce the quality of life of prostate cancer patients [5,6].

Radiation-mediated side effects are caused by the ongoing production of free radicals in non-targeted normal tissues [7,8]. The majority of free radicals initially arise from the lysis of water molecules. However, free radicals and ROS are released hours to days after radiation. These sources are likely from NADPH oxidases and damaged mitochondria. The acute and chronic elevation of ROS results in damage of DNA, protein and lipids. One such reaction is the non-enzymatic peroxidation of polyunsaturated fatty acids catalyzed by free radicals. Lipid peroxidation is a self propagating chain reaction and the initial oxidation of only a few lipids can result in damage to lipid bilayers, ultimately destabilizing functional and protective membranes, which can cause severe tissue damage. The chemical by-product of this lipid peroxidation is 4-hydroxynonenal (4-HNE), which forms adducts to the histidine, cysteine and lysine residues of proteins, amino group containing lipids and to guanosine moieties of DNA [9]. Therefore, under oxidative stress, such as radiation, the excess load of free radicals leads to lipid peroxidation as measured by the production of 4-HNE.

Given the pivotal role of ROS in inducing and propagating normal tissue damage following radiotherapy, a ROS scavenger could be an effective radioprotector. The use of a radioprotector, which can prevent tumor adjacent normal tissue damage during radiation therapy without hindering the radiation-mediated inhibition of tumor growth, would be beneficial for prostate cancer patients undergoing radiation therapy. We have previously described that manganese porphyrins (MnPs: MnTE-2-PyP or MnTnBuOE-2-PyP, Figure 1A,B), which are ROS scavengers, can inhibit the growth of either prostate or colon cancer cells in combination with radiation or chemotherapeutic agents in vitro [10,11]. We have also reported that MnPs protect prostate and colon fibroblasts from radiation-induced damage in vitro [10,12]. We have previously shown that, MnTE-2-PyP protects from radiation damage to normal urogenital tissues in rats [13]. Others have shown that MnTE-2-PyP does not protect prostate cancer cells from radiation killing in hind flank tumor models [14]. However, no one has examined the ability of MnPs in combination with radiation to inhibit tumor growth, while simultaneously protecting normal tissues from radiation damage in a prostate cancer model.

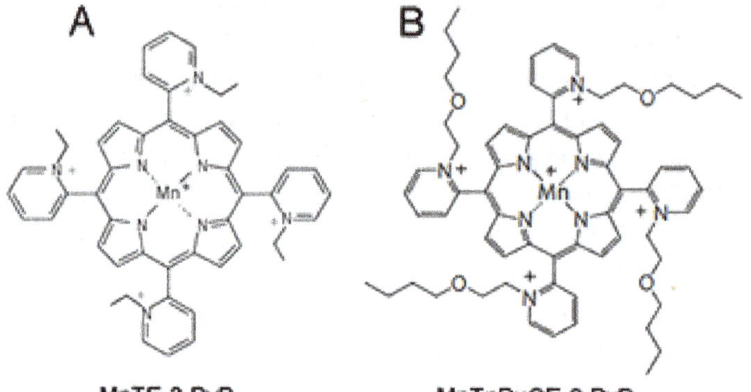

A

MnTE-2-PyP

B

MnTnBuOE-2-PyP

Figure 1. Structure of the two manganese porphyrins, (**A**) MnTE-2-PyP and (**B**) MnTnBuOE-2-PyP. These two porphyrins mimic the active site of native SOD enzymes.

An intriguing question in the field has been, "How do MnPs have different effects on cancer vs. normal cells?" Batinic-Haberle et al. have proposed that MnPs act differently in a normal cell as compared to a tumor cell due to different redox environments of the cells [15]. If the affected cell has inadequate antioxidant defenses, the manganese metal at the active site of the porphyrin may become oxidized and, in turn, act as an oxidizing agent rather than a reducing agent in this environment. Thus, a more oxidizing environment will likely cause the MnPs to act as pro-oxidants and a more balanced redox environment, will cause the MnPs to behave as mild antioxidants. We have previously shown that in normal prostate fibroblasts, MnTE-2-PyP scavenges superoxide and reduces overall ROS in these irradiated cells [12]. Others have shown that when cancer cells are treated with MnPs in combination with ascorbate or other chemotherapeutic drugs, the cancer cells become more oxidatively stressed and results in cell death [16–19]. However, no one has characterized the effects of these MnPs alone in cells with different basal redox environments.

In the initial disease stage, prostate cancer is dependent on androgens for tumor growth and the tumor growth can be reduced by the removal of androgens [20,21]. As the disease progresses, the tumors become androgen independent and more oxidatively stressed [22]. Therefore, the survival strategies in initial vs. late stage tumor cells are different. We have reported that MnTE-2-PyP can inhibit the growth of both androgen dependent (LNCaP) and independent (PC3) cell lines in the presence of radiation in vitro [11]. Therefore, MnPs could potentially be used in combination with radiation in both androgen dependent and androgen independent tumor models.

To test this hypothesis, we have orthotopically implanted human prostate cancer cell lines (LNCaP or PC3) into the prostates of athymic nude mice. After tumor development, mice were irradiated with X-rays in the presence or absence of MnPs. MnP treatment continued until animals were sacrificed or died. We found that MnP treatment, when combined with radiation, significantly enhanced the antitumor effect of radiation and promoted overall life span of mice in both prostate tumor models. We also measured the ability of MnPs to mitigate radiation-generated 4-HNE levels in the tumor and normal tissue regions that are adjacent to the tumor in both orthotopic cancer models. In both tumor types, we observed increased 4-HNE levels when MnPs were combined with radiation. In contrast, in normal prostate glandular regions neighboring the tumor tissues, we found that both MnPs reduced 4-HNE formation as compared to the irradiated alone animals. These results indicate that the addition of MnPs can maintain normal redox homeostasis in the normal tissue adjacent to the tumor and protect it from radiation damage, while enhancing oxidative stress in the tumors when combined with radiation.

In this study, we also investigated the role of MnPs on superoxide levels and overall redox environment in the prostate cancer cells in vitro. We found that the MnPs behave quite differently in the two prostate cancer cells. In the less aggressive LNCaP cells, we found that both MnPs do not increase hydrogen peroxide levels. In contrast, in PC3 cells, which are highly aggressive, the addition of the MnP resulted in a significant increase in hydrogen peroxide levels, which resulted in the oxidation of protein thiols. We found that LNCaP cells have twice as much catalase activity as PC3 cells, and we postulate that peroxide removal may be a key factor in regulating the activity of the MnPs.

2. Materials and Methods

2.1. Cell Lines

PC3 and LNCaP cells were purchased from American Type Culture Collection (ATCC, Manassas, VA, USA). Constitutive luciferase expressing PC3 cells (PC3-Luc) were purchased from Applied Biological Materials Inc. (ABM, Richmond, BC, Canada).

To generate constitutive luciferase expressing LNCaP cells (LNCaP-Luc), 50 μL of pre-made lentiviral expression plasmid for firefly luciferase (LVP020-PBS, Amsbio, Cambridge, MA, USA) was transfected into LNCaP cells at 50% confluency. After 72 h of transfection, transfected cells were selectively cultured for two weeks in puromycin (0.4 μg/mL) containing media. Constitutive expression of luciferase was monitored every week using the Tropix LucScreen Assay (Applied Biosystem, Foster City, CA, USA, cat. T2300) and GFP production was observed using a fluorescence microscope (Leica, DM4000 B LED, Buffalo Grove, IL, USA).

Both cell types were cultured in RPMI-1640 media containing, 10% (for PC3) or 5% (for LNCaP) fetal bovine serum (FBS) and 1% penicillin/streptomycin. Cultures were maintained at 37 °C and 5% CO_2.

2.2. Primary Prostate Fibroblast Isolation and Culture Conditions

Prostates were collected from six to eight-week-old C57BL/6 mice [12]. After mincing the prostates, they were digested by 5 mg/mL of collagenase I (Thermo Fisher Scientific, Waltham, MA, USA, cat. 17100017) for 30 min at 37 °C [23]. Tissue fragments were then cultured for 2–3 weeks in Dulbecco's Minimal Essential Media (DMEM, Hyclone, Logan, UT, USA) supplemented with 10% fetal bovine serum (FBS), 1% penicillin/streptomycin and 1% non-essential amino acids. After 5 days of culture, all the cells were fibroblasts. The purity of the cells were determined by ERTR7 (Santa Cruz, cat. sc-73355), a fibroblast marker and Keratin17 (Cell Signaling cat. 4543) an epithelial cell marker. All experiments were repeated in triplicate using primary fibroblasts cells collected from prostates of different mice.

2.3. *Animal Husbandry*

Six to eight week old, male, athymic mice or C57Bl/6 mice (Charles River Laboratories, Wilmington, MA, USA) were used for experiments. Animals were housed five animals per cage in standard mouse cages in the animal facility at the University of Nebraska Medical Center (UNMC, Omaha, NE, USA) and were exposed to a 12 h light/12 h dark cycle and fed and watered ad libitum. All experimental protocols were reviewed and approved by the UNMC Institutional Animal Care (Omaha, NE, USA) and Use Committee (14-054-08-FC).

2.4. *Orthotopic Implantation of Tumor Cells*

Athymic mice were anesthetized by continuous flow of 2.5% isoflurane with oxygen using a mouse anesthesia machine. A one cm midline incision was made in the lower abdomen after cleaning the skin with an iodine solution. To expose the prostate gland, seminal vesicles and bladder were gently retracted. PC3-Luc or LNCaP-Luc cells (50 μL containing 2.0×10^6 cells in 50% Matrigel) were injected into the dorsal prostatic lobe using a 30-gauge needle. The peritoneal tissues were closed in two layers with absorbable catgut sutures (cat. 563B, Surgical Specialties, Tijuana, Mexico) and the skin was closed with wound clips (cat. 1111C15, Thomas Scientific, Swedesboro, NJ, USA). Buprenorphine (0.1 mg/kg, Reckitt Benckiser Healthcare (UK) Ltd., Hull, UK) was administrated by intraperitoneal route just after the surgery followed by three doses at six, twenty-four and forty-eight h after surgery. Sterile surgical procedures were maintained for the entire process. Wound clips were removed after ten days and animals were monitored for infection or distress.

2.5. *Bio-Luminescence Imaging*

D-Luciferin potassium salt (100 mg/kg, PerkinElmer, cat. 122799, Waltham, MA, USA) was dissolved in sterile PBS and injected intraperitoneally into the tumor bearing mice 15 min prior to imaging. For imaging the luciferase expressing tumors, mice were anesthetized using 2.5% isoflurane with oxygen and placed in the Xenogen IVIS Spectrum bioluminescence imaging system (PerkinElmer, MA, USA). Images were acquired and analyzed by Living Image 4.5.1 software (Caliper Life Sciences, Hopkinton, MA, USA) with an exposure time of one second. Regions of interest (ROI) were determined to encompass the area with the most intense light, and signal intensity was calculated based on a measurement of photons/s/cm^2/sr.

2.6. *Radiation and MnP Administration Protocol*

Scheme/timeline used for LNCaP or PC3 tumor models:

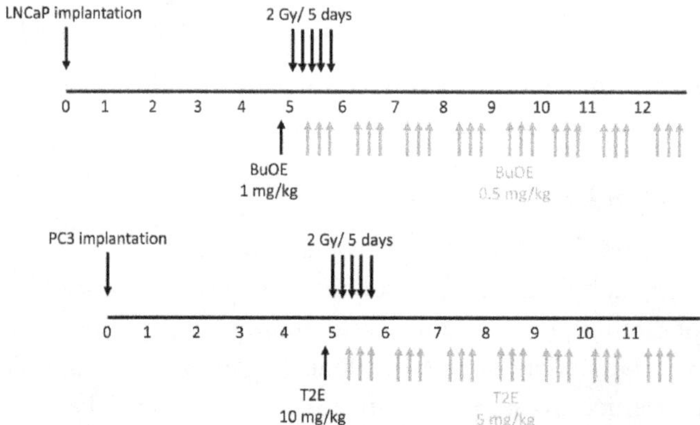

Five weeks after surgery, tumors were imaged as described in the bioluminescence imaging section. Animals bearing very large tumors, no tumors, or very small tumors were excluded from the rest of the study. The average tumor size was 200 mm^3. Forty mice (10 mice per group) from the PC3-Luc cell implanted group and 32 mice (8 mice per group) from the LNCaP-Luc implanted group were used for further experiments. This ensured that all the tumors were similar size before starting the treatment protocol. The mice were divided into four treatment groups for PC3 and LNCaP models: 1. PBS only 2. MnPs only 3. Radiation only and 4. Radiation + MnPs. Both PC3 and LNCaP tumors were irradiated with X-rays (2 Gy per day, for five sequential days) to their lower abdomen using lead shielding (Rad Source RS-2000 Biological System). A single dose of PBS (for controls) or 1 mg/kg MnTnBuOE-2-PyP (BuOE) for LNCaP bearing mice, or 10 mg/kg MnTE-2-PyP (T2E) for PC3 bearing mice was administrated 24 h prior to the first radiation dose. MnTE-2-PyP and MnTnBuOE-2-PyP were kind gifts from Dr. James Crapo (National Jewish Health, Denver, CO, USA). During and after irradiation for both tumor types, half of the mice from each of irradiated and non-irradiated groups were treated with MnPs intraperitoneally, three times a week. The maintenance dosing was half the pre-radiation loading doses reported above. The control mice from each of radiated and non-radiated groups were treated with an equal volume of PBS, three times a week.

2.7. *Tumor Harvesting, Tumor Size Measurement and Enumerating Metastatic Lesions*

From LNCaP-Luc implanted mice, three mice from each of the four groups were sacrificed and the tumors were harvested three weeks post-irradiation. In the case of PC3-Luc implantation, five mice from each of the four groups were sacrificed and the tumors were harvested two weeks post-radiation. PC3 cells grow more quickly than LNCaP cells, which is why LNCaP cells were allowed to grow an additional week after implantation. The width and length of the excised tumor was measured with calipers and the volume was estimated according to the formula: $[(\text{width})^2 \times \text{length}/2]$. After measurement of the primary tumor, half of the tumor was flash frozen and stored at −80 °C. The other half was fixed in 4% formalin followed by 70% ethanol. These tissues were paraffin embedded and 7 μm sections were cut and placed on slides for immunostaining by the Tissue Science Facility at the University of Nebraska Medical Center (Omaha, NE, USA).

The number of metastatic nodules at the distal sites were enumerated for every animal by visual inspection and verified as true metastases using the LucScreen assay. The animals were placed in one of four groups: no observable metastases, 1 metastatic nodule, 2 metastatic nodules, and 3 or more metastatic nodules.

2.8. *Tumor Growth and Overall Animal Survival*

The remaining animals were continuously administered MnTnBuOE-2-PyP or MnTE-2-PyP or PBS, three times a week until sacrifice. Animals were imaged every week to monitor tumor size using the Xenogen IVIS Spectrum bioluminescence imaging system after injection of D-Luciferin potassium salt, as described above. The average signal intensity per tumor was calculated for every animal group and plotted over time.

Animals were euthanized when the tumor volume began to influence health status and/or mobility. For survival curve analysis, total life span in days after irradiation was calculated and plotted against percent survival in all groups. Kaplan Meier survival analysis was performed using GraphPad prism 6.0.5 software (La Jolla, CA, USA).

2.9. *Tumor Lysate Preparations and Western Blot*

Frozen tumor samples were minced and homogenized (Pro scientific, Oxford, CT, USA) in lysis buffer [120 mM NaCl, 50 mM Tris-HCl, 5 mM EDTA, 1% NP-40 and complete protease inhibitor cocktail tablets (1 tablet/50 mL, cat. 11697498001; Roche Diagnostics, Indianapolis, IN, USA)]. After incubation on ice for 30 min, the tissue homogenates were sonicated for 8–10 pulses at 80% amplitude. Lysates were then centrifuged for 15 min at 12,000× *g* and protein concentrations of the supernatants were determined by using the Bradford Assay (Amresco, cat. E530). Tumor tissue lysate (40 µg) was electrophoresed on a 4–12% gel, transferred to a nitrocellulose membrane, and blocked in 5% milk for two hours. To examine PCNA expression, membranes were incubated overnight at 4 °C with a PCNA antibody (BD Transduction laboratories, cat. 610665, 1:1000 dilution). Mouse secondary antibodies (1:10,000 dilution, cat. A24524; Invitrogen, Carlsbad, CA, USA) were incubated for one hour and the blots were developed using ECL (cat. 80196, Pierce ECL2 western blotting substrate) and exposed to film. Densitometry was performed on the blots using ImageJ analysis software 1.50i (National Institutes of Health, Bethesda, MD, USA).

2.10. *Immunohistochemistry*

Fixed tumor tissue that also contained normal prostate tissue, was paraffin embedded and sectioned by the Tissue Science Facility at the University of Nebraska Medical Center. Sections were then immunostained for a marker of oxidative stress, 4-hydroxynonenal (4-HNE). Tissues were de-paraffinized in xylenes and rehydrated through graded alcohols. For antigen retrieval, slides were heated to 95 °C in 0.01 M sodium citrate buffer (pH 6.0) with 0.05% Tween 20. Slides were then allowed to cool in phosphate buffer (pH 7.0) for 30 min. For blocking, 4-HNE staining required the use of a M.O.M. ™ kit (Vector Labs, Burlingame, CA, USA, cat. BMK-2202) and was used according to the manufacturer's directions. Following blocking, tissue sections were incubated with a primary antibody (4-HNE, 1:50, R&D Systems, Minneapolis, MN, USA, cat. MAB3249) overnight at 4 °C in a humidified chamber. The following day, slides were washed in Super Sensitive Wash Buffer (BioGenex Laboratories, Fremont, CA, USA, cat. HK583-5K) and stained with a secondary antibody conjugated to AlexaFluor555 (1:100, goat anti-mouse, Invitrogen, cat. A21422). Slides were mounted under coverslips with ProLong™ Gold Antifade with DAPI (Invitrogen, cat. P36931). Areas of normal prostate glandular tissue were imaged using a Leica DM 4000B LED fluorescent microscope, followed by analysis with ImageJ. The normal prostate glandular region and the tumor tissue were selected for further analysis. The epithelial cell layer, omitting the glandular lumen area, was manually traced and the intensity of 4-HNE staining was measured. Tumor tissues were manually traced and the intensity of 4-HNE staining was measured. Average raw integrated intensity per unit area was calculated. Statistical significance was determined using 1-way ANOVA followed by post hoc Tukey's multiple correction test.

2.11. *Measurement of Superoxide*

To measure the superoxide production, PC3 or LNCaP cells were seeded at a concentration of 0.5×10^6 cells/flask in the presence or absence of MnTE-2-PyP (30 µM) or MnTnBuOE-2-PyP (0.5 µM) or an equal volume of PBS overnight. In some cases, cells were irradiated with 2 Gy of X-rays, then harvested by trypsinization 48 h post-radiation. After washing, cells were stained with dihydroethidium (DHE, 5 µM) for 20 min at 37 °C in the dark and then subjected to flow cytometric analysis using a LSRII Green 532 Flow Cytometer (BD Biosciences, San Jose, CA, USA). In order to measure superoxide specifically, 405/570 nm excitation/emission was used. Data was analyzed using FACSDiVa analysis software v8.0.2 (BD Biosciences, San Jose, CA, USA).

2.12. *Detection of Intracellular Hydrogen Peroxide Levels*

PC3 or LNCaP cells were seeded in chamber slides (ThermoFisher Scientific, cat. 05031780) and treated with PBS, MnTnBuOE-2-PyP (0.5 µM), or MnTE-2-PyP (30 µM) overnight. In some cases, cells were irradiated with 2 Gy of X-rays 24 h before hydrogen peroxide staining began. Cells were then treated with DMSO or Peroxy Orange 1 (15 µM, Fisher Scientific, cat. 4944) for one hour in the dark at 37 °C. The fluorescence was detected by a Leica DM 4000B LED fluorescent microscope with the Ex/Em at 555 nm/565 nm. An average of five images were taken for each condition. The average intensity per cell was calculated based on a minimum number of 100 cells for each condition, and analysis was performed using ImageJ.

2.13. Detection of Thiol Oxidation

The method of detecting thiol oxidation levels has been described previously [24]. Briefly, cells were treated with PBS, MnTnBuOE-2-PyP (0.5 μM), or MnTE-2-PyP (30 μM) for three days. In some cases, 24 h before harvest, the cells were exposed to 2 Gy of irradiation with or without MnP treatment. Cells were homogenized in lysis buffer (120 mM NaCl, 50 mM Tris-HCl, 5 mM EDTA, 1% NP-40 and complete protease inhibitor cocktail) and incubated for 10 min on ice. Lysates were centrifuged at 4 °C for 7 min at 12,000× *g*, and the supernatants were collected. Protein concentrations were measured by the Bradford assay. The final concentration of each sample was adjusted to 1 mg/mL. Lysates were then treated with distilled water, or 1 mM DTT, or 1 mM diamide at room temperature for 30 min. To isolate proteins with reduced thiols, protein lysate (20 μg) was mixed with 970 μL of binding buffer (0.1% SDS in PBS) and 5 μL of 30 μM *N*-(Biotinoyl)-*N*′-(Iodoacetyl)Ethylenediamine (BIAM) (Invitrogen, Carlsbad, CA, USA, cat. B1591). The whole reaction system was incubated for 30 min at room temperature in the dark. The reaction was terminated by the addition of 50 μL of 500 mM β-mercaptoethanol. Streptavidin-agarose beads (100 μL) (ThermoFisher Scientific, cat. SE243295) were then mixed with samples for one hour at room temperature. The streptavidin-agarose-bound complex was washed four times by adding 1 mL of binding buffer and centrifuged at 850× *g*. Samples were boiled at 75 °C for 10 min with 4 μL of 10× reducing agent, 10 μL 4× loading dye, and 26 μL distilled water. Samples were run on the Bolt^{TM} 4–12% Bis-Tris Plus gels (Invitrogen, cat. NW04120BOX) and transferred to the nitrocellulose membrane (Invitrogen, cat. IB23001). The western blots were probed with an streptavidin-HRP antibody (1:10,000) (ThermoFisher Scientific, cat. QG223359) and bands were detected with ECL reagent.

2.14. Catalase Activity Staining Assay

Catalase activity staining assay was performed as described before [24]. Briefly, cells were treated with PBS or MnTE-2-PyP (30 μM) or MnTnBuOE-2-PyP (0.5 μM) overnight. In some cases, cells were irradiated with 2 Gy and harvested 24 h later. Cells were homogenized in lysis buffer (120 mM NaCl, 50 mM Tris-HCl, 5 mM EDTA, 1% NP-40 and complete protease inhibitor cocktail) and incubated for 10 min on ice. Lysates were centrifuged at 4 °C for 7 min at 12,000× *g*, and the supernatants were collected. Protein concentrations were measured by the Bradford assay. To measure catalase activity, proteins (30 μg) were loaded onto the 10% Mini-PROTEAN TGX precast gel (Bio-Rad, Hercules, CA, USA, cat. 4561033) and run at 100 V for 2 h at 4 °C. The gel was extensively rinsed with distilled water three times, for 10 min each and then soaked in 0.003% H_2O_2 for 10 min. The staining solution (2% ferric chloride and 2% potassium ferricyanide in distilled water) was poured onto the gel. The achromatic bands are indicative of catalase activity. Gel images were inverted and densitometry of the bands were performed using Image J.

2.15. Statistical Analysis

GraphPad Prism 6.0.5 was used for all the statistical analyses. Mean and standard deviation values from three independent experiments were used for statistical analysis for all the experiments performed. Unless otherwise described, significant differences between the groups was determined by a 1-way ANOVA test followed by a post hoc Tukey's test for multiple comparisons or a student's *t*-test. For the non-invasive tumor size measurement, linear regression modeling was used to determine differences between slopes. For survival analysis, a Kaplan Meier curve was plotted. The percent survival and median survival in days were documented and compared between groups by using the Mantel-Cox test.

3. Results

3.1. MnTnBuOE-2-PyP Inhibits Growth of PC3 and LNCaP Cells In Vitro

Our laboratory has previously shown that MnTE-2-PyP (30 μM) inhibits colony formation of both PC3 and LNCaP cells by ~50% in vitro [11]. We wanted to determine whether MnTnBuOE-2-PyP had similar effects on prostate cancer growth. We found that MnTnBuOE-2-PyP (0.5 μM) significantly inhibited PC3 colony growth by 30% and LNCaP growth by 50% (Figure 2). Thus, MnTE-2-PyP and MnTnBuOE-2-PyP have similar inhibitory effects on prostate cancer growth in vitro.

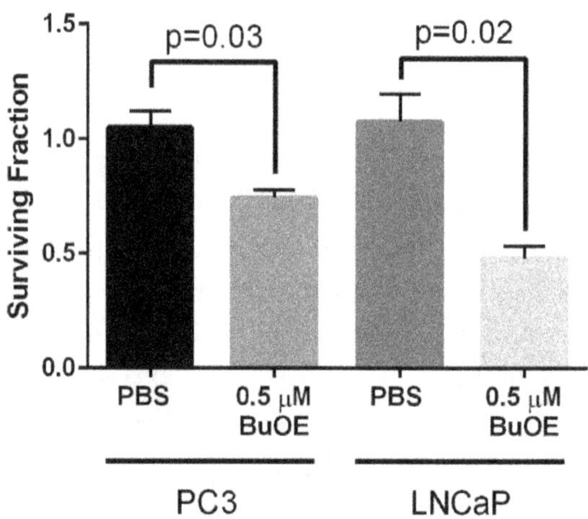

Figure 2. MnTnBuOE-2-PyP inhibits colony formation of prostate cancer cells. Clonogenic assays were performed on PC3 or LNCaP cells with or without MnTnBuOE-2-PyP (0.5 μM). The addition of MnTnBuOE-2-PyP significantly inhibited growth of both prostate cancer cell lines. Data represent mean ± SD from three independent experiments.

3.2. MnPs Decrease Primary Tumor Volume

We next wanted to determine the effects of these drugs on prostate cancer in vivo and in combination with radiation. MnTnBuOE-2-PyP is in phase I clinical trials for glioblastoma and head and neck cancer patients as a radioprotector. The most common prostate cancer diagnosed in human patients are androgen sensitive tumors [25]. These tumor types are routinely treated with radiation, so we investigated the effects of MnTnBuOE-2-PyP in an orthotopic model of androgen sensitive prostate cancer, the LNCaP cancer model. Since most of the published work on MnPs and prostate cancer has been done with MnTE-2-PyP, we also investigated the effect of MnTE-2-PyP in a more aggressive PC3 prostate cancer model. MnTnBuOE-2-PyP is much more lipophilic than MnTE-2-PyP but they have essentially the same rate constant for dismuting superoxide to hydrogen peroxide [26]. Thus, MnTnBuOE-2-PyP is needed at about 1/10 the dose of MnTE-2-PyP to observe similar changes in cells and animals [26]. Therefore, the dosing of both cells and animals with MnTE-2-PyP is about 10 times more than what is used for MnTnBuOE-2-PyP for the experiments performed in this current study.

Five weeks following orthotopic implantation of LNCaP or PC3 cells into the mouse prostates, the lower abdominal area of the mice in the RAD groups, were irradiated with X-rays (2 Gy/day, for 5 consecutive days). After irradiation, either PBS or MnP (MnTnBuOE-2-PyP or MnTE-2-PyP) was injected three times a week. After two weeks post-radiation (for PC3) or three weeks post-radiation (for LNCaP), mice ($n = 3$ for LNCaP and $n = 5$ for PC3) were sacrificed and tumors excised. Combined treatment of MnPs with radiation decreased the average tumor volume by 92.3% in LNCaP tumors and 80.0% in PC3 tumors as compared to the PBS treated group (Figure 3A,B). Whereas, radiation alone decreased the average tumor volume by 64.0% and 50.0% in the respective tumor models. Therefore, the addition of MnPs significantly enhanced the anti-tumor activity of radiation, by 28.25% (in the

LNCaP model) and 29.96% (in the PC3 model) (Figure 3A,B). MnPs significantly decreased tumor volumes in the presence of radiation in both of the prostate cancer models at this early time point.

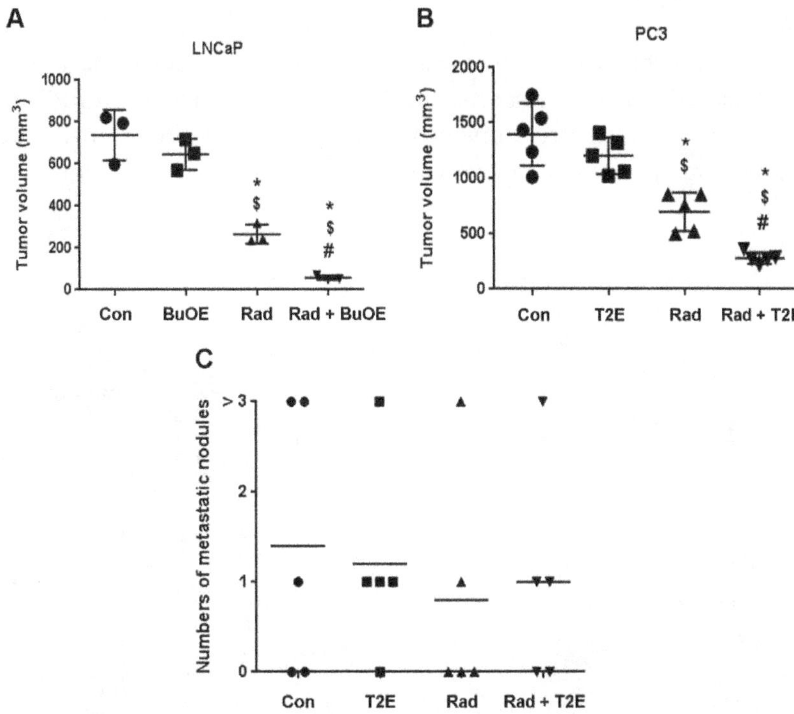

Figure 3. MnPs decrease primary tumor volume. (**A**) LNCaP (**B**) or PC3 cells were orthotopically implanted into mouse prostates. Five weeks post-implantation, the lower abdominal area of mice in the RAD groups, were irradiated with X-rays (2 Gy/day for 5 days). After irradiation, PBS or MnTnBuOE-2-PyP (BuOE, 0.5 mg/kg) (**A**) or MnTE-2-PyP (T2E, 5 mg/kg) (**B**) was injected three times a week. After three (**A**) or two (**B**) weeks of treatment, tumors were harvested and the volumes were calculated. (**C**) After sacrificing the mice, the number of metastatic nodules in the peritoneal cavity were measured and documented visually in PC3 tumor bearing mice. Significance among tumor sizes were determined using a 1-way ANOVA followed by the post hoc Tukey's for multiple comparisons test. The symbol (*) denotes a significant difference as compared to control group; the symbol ($) denotes a significant difference as compared to the BuOE or T2E group; and the symbol (#) denotes a significant difference when compared to the RAD group, (n = 3 for all four groups in the LNCaP model and n = 5 for all the groups in the PC3 model).

3.3. MnPs Do Not Increase Metastasis

Metastatic prostate cancer is the major cause of prostate cancer related deaths. The American Cancer Society reported in 2017, the five-year survival rate of prostate cancer patients with distant metastasis is only 28%. Therefore, it was necessary to examine the effect of MnPs on metastasis. During the tumor harvest two weeks (for PC3) or three weeks (for LNCaP) after irradiation, the number of metastatic nodules was documented. In the LNCaP tumor model, no metastatic nodules were observed in any of the groups (data not shown). In contrast, for the PC3 model, metastatic nodules were observed in the inguinal lymph nodes, liver, peritoneal cavity and upper digestive tract. We found no significant differences in the numbers of metastatic nodules among any of the groups (Figure 3C). This study suggests that MnPs do not affect metastatic progression of the PC3 tumors.

3.4. MnPs Decrease Primary Tumor Growth Over Time

Luciferase expressing tumor cells were tracked by injecting the tumor bearing animals with luciferin followed by bio-imaging once a week after irradiation throughout the life span of the mouse.

The luminescence signal reflects the number of luciferase expressing cancer cells, which corresponds to tumor size. The average luminescence signal intensity for each group was plotted against time. Using linear regression modeling, the curves were fit to the data and the slopes of the curves were analyzed (Figure 4A,B). Not surprisingly, we found that in both models, radiation decreased tumor growth when compared to the PBS control group. Tumor growth was further significantly inhibited in the groups treated with radiation in the presence of MnPs, (p value = 0.008 in LNCaP and p value = 0.013 in PC3) as compared to the irradiated alone groups (Figure 4A,B). This study revealed that MnPs treatment further inhibited prostate tumor growth in combination with radiation.

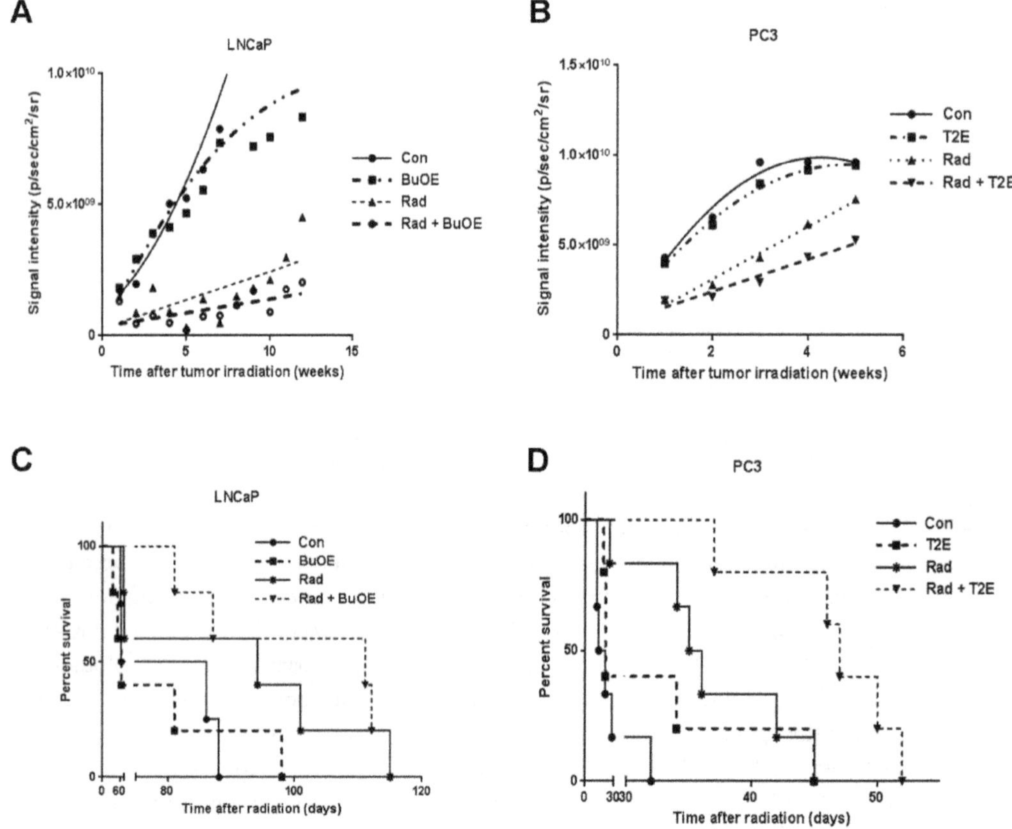

Figure 4. MnPs decrease the tumor growth rate and increases survival of tumor bearing mice. LNCaP or PC3 cells were orthotopically implanted into mouse prostates. Five weeks after implantation, the lower abdominal area of mice in the RAD groups, were irradiated with X-rays (2 Gy/day for 5 days). After irradiation, PBS or MnTnBuOE-2-PyP (BuOE, 0.5 mg/kg) or MnTE-2-PyP (T2E, 5 mg/kg) was injected three times a week during the life span of the mouse. Tumor sizes were measured once a week by non-invasive imaging. (**A**) LNCaP tumor growth; (**B**) PC3 tumor growth. All the data points were statistically analyzed by linear regression modeling. Tumor growth rate in the LNCaP model was significantly reduced in RAD + BuOE group as compared to the RAD only group (p value = 0.008). In the PC3 model, tumor growth rate was significantly reduced in the RAD + T2E group as compared to the RAD only group (p value = 0.013). Radiation significantly reduced the tumor growth rate in both models; (**C**) Survival curve for mice bearing LNCaP tumors; (**D**) Survival curve for mice bearing PC3 tumors. Kaplan-Meier survival curves were plotted and median life span in days after therapy was calculated in all groups. Differences between median survival was determined by the Log-rank (Mantel-Cox) test. In both tumor models, radiation increased the median survival as compared to controls and RAD + MnP treatment further increased the median survival as compared to the RAD only group. In the LNCaP model, these increases were not statistically significant but in the PC3 model, these increases were significant. LNCaP model: n = 4 for PBS only group, n = 5 for all other groups. PC3 model: n = 6 for PBS and RAD only groups, n = 5 for T2E and RAD + T2E groups.

3.5. MnPs in Combination with Radiation Increases Median Survival

To determine the effect of MnPs on the survival of prostate cancer tumor bearing mice, we have generated Kaplan-Meier survival curves for each treatment group (Figure 4C,D). In the LNCaP model, median survival was 64, 75, 94, and 111 days in control, MnTnBuOE-2-PyP, radiation, and MnTnBuOE-2-PyP combined with radiation groups, respectively (Figure 4C). In the PC3 model, control, MnTE-2-PyP, radiation, and MnTE-2-PyP combined with radiation groups have median survivals of 17.5, 21, 35.5 and 47 days respectively (Figure 4D). In both tumor models, MnPs increased the survival of the mice in the presence of radiation. Median survival of LNCaP bearing mice was further increased by seventeen days when animals were treated with radiation in combination with MnTnBuOE-2-PyP as compared to irradiated alone mice. However, this increase in median survival was not significantly different between these groups. In the PC3 tumor model, the median survival of irradiated mice was increased significantly by eighteen days as compared to control (p value = 0.0030). Median survival of the mice in the irradiated and MnTE-2-PyP treated group was significantly increased by twelve days as compared to the irradiated only group (p value = 0.0080). (Figure 4C,D). Thus, our study revealed that MnPs do not interfere with the anti-tumor action of radiation but rather enhance post-radiation median survival in both models of prostate cancer.

3.6. MnPs, in Combination with Radiation, Decrease Prostate Cancer Cell Proliferation

As MnPs decrease tumor progression and tumor volume, we tested whether MnPs can affect proliferation of tumor cells by performing western blots for the expression of the proliferation cell nuclear antigen (PCNA) in the tumor lysates obtained 2–3 weeks post-radiation. In LNCaP tumors, expression of PCNA was markedly reduced by radiation, or when radiation was combined with MnTnBuOE-2-PyP as compared to controls, but this decrease was not statistically significant (p value = 0.0504 and 0.0566 in the case of RAD only and RAD + BuOE group respectively). This may be partly due to the small sample size (n = 3) for each group. In the PC3 tumor model, MnTE-2-PyP, in combination with radiation, significantly decreased PCNA expression (p value = 0.0311, Figure 5).

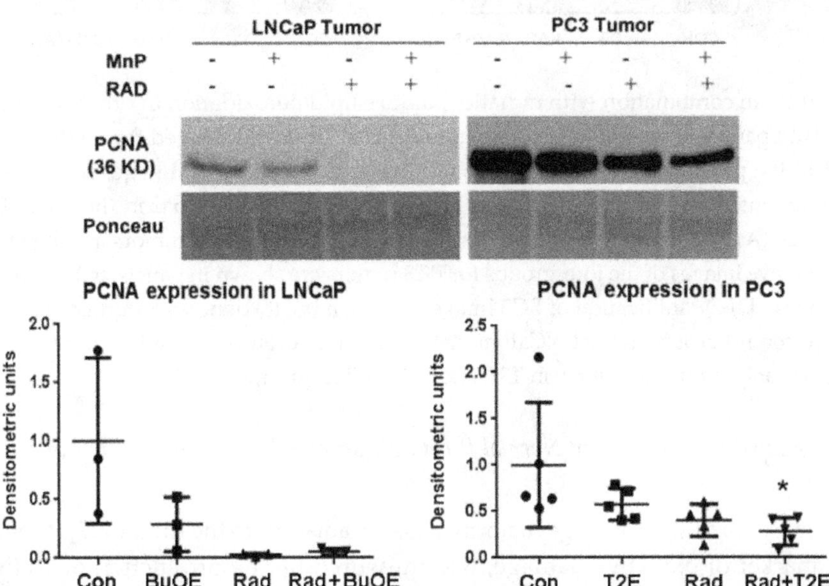

Figure 5. In combination with radiation, MnPs decrease PCNA expression. After harvesting the tumor, 40 μg of tumor lysates (n = 3 for LNCaP and n = 5 for PC3) were used to measure the expression levels of PCNA by western blot. Ponceau staining was used to confirm equal protein loading. Densitometry was quantified using ImageJ. Significant change in PCNA expression level was calculated by a 1-way ANOVA followed by post hoc Tukey's multiple correction test. The symbol (*) denotes a significant difference as compared to controls.

3.7. MnPs Enhance Lipid Oxidation in Prostate Cancer Tissues in Combination with Radiation Therapy

Lipid oxidation, as indicated by 4-HNE staining, was significantly enhanced three weeks after radiation therapy for LNCaP tumors or two weeks after radiation exposure for PC3 tumors from irradiated mice treated with MnPs (Figure 6). Radiation alone resulted in significant lipid peroxidation in PC3 tumors but not in LNCaP tumors, although there was a trend of increased 4-HNE staining in these animals (Figure 6). The addition of either MnTE-2-PyP or MnTnBuOE-2-PyP alone did not significantly affect lipid peroxidation in the tumor tissues, although there was a trend of increased 4-HNE levels (Figure 6). PC3 tumors had higher levels of 4-HNE overall as compared to LNCaP cells, indicating that PC3 cells are more oxidatively stressed than LNCaP cells, even at baseline.

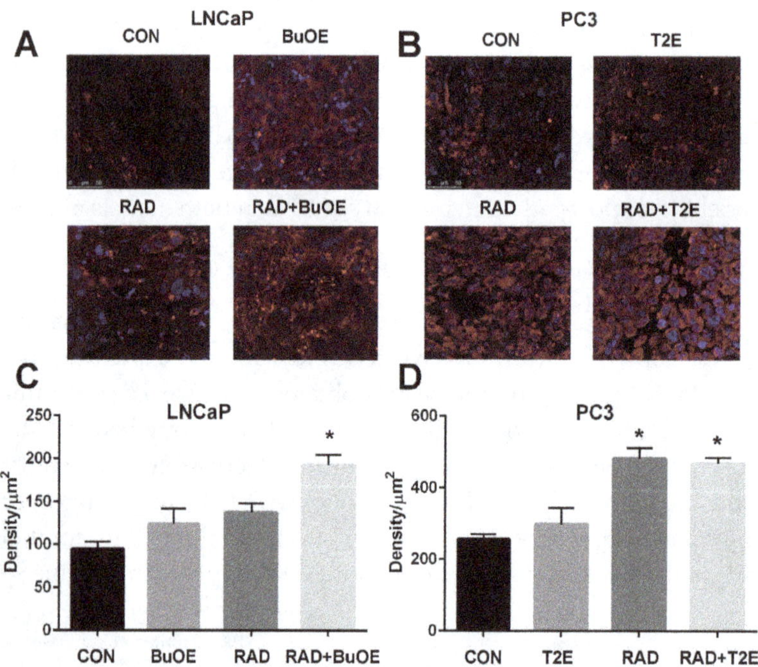

Figure 6. MnPs, in combination with radiation, induce lipid peroxidation in prostate cancer tissues. Formalin fixed paraffin embedded prostate tissue was stained and imaged for 4-HNE. 4-HNE was quantified in the prostate tumor tissues. Images were analyzed using ImageJ software. Average raw integrated intensity per unit area was plotted. The magnification bar in the lower left panels denotes 50 μm. (**A**) Representative images of the four groups for LNCaP tumors are shown in panels; (**B**) Representative images of the four groups for PC3 tumors are shown in panels; (**C**) Quantification of LNCaP images; (**D**) Quantification of PC3 images. The symbol (*) denotes a significant difference as compared to control group. In the LNCaP model, $n = 3$ for all groups. In the PC3 model, $n = 4$ in PBS only and RAD only groups and $n = 5$ in T2E and RAD + T2E groups.

3.8. MnPs Reduce Lipid Peroxidation in Normal Prostate Tissues Adjacent to Prostate Cancer after Radiotherapy

Radiation causes oxidative damage to normal tissues adjacent to the tumor [27]. Lipid peroxidation, a well-known marker of oxidative damage, was measured by the production of 4-HNE. To further demonstrate that MnPs are radioprotectors, we quantified the levels of 4-HNE in the normal prostate glandular tissues adjacent to the tumor from both prostate cancer models. Radiation caused a significant increase in 4-HNE levels in the prostate glands of both LNCaP and PC3 tumor models as compared to controls (Figure 7). In the LNCaP tumor model, radiation significantly increased 4-HNE levels in normal tissues as compared to controls (p value < 0.0001). MnTnBuOE-2-PyP treatment significantly decreased 4-HNE levels in normal tissues in irradiated mice as compared to the RAD only group (p value = 0.0009, Figure 7). In the PC3 tumor model, radiation significantly increased 4-HNE levels in normal tissues as compared to controls (p value = 0.0318). MnTE-2-PyP reduced 4-HNE levels, but the differences were not statistically significant as compared to irradiated alone animals.

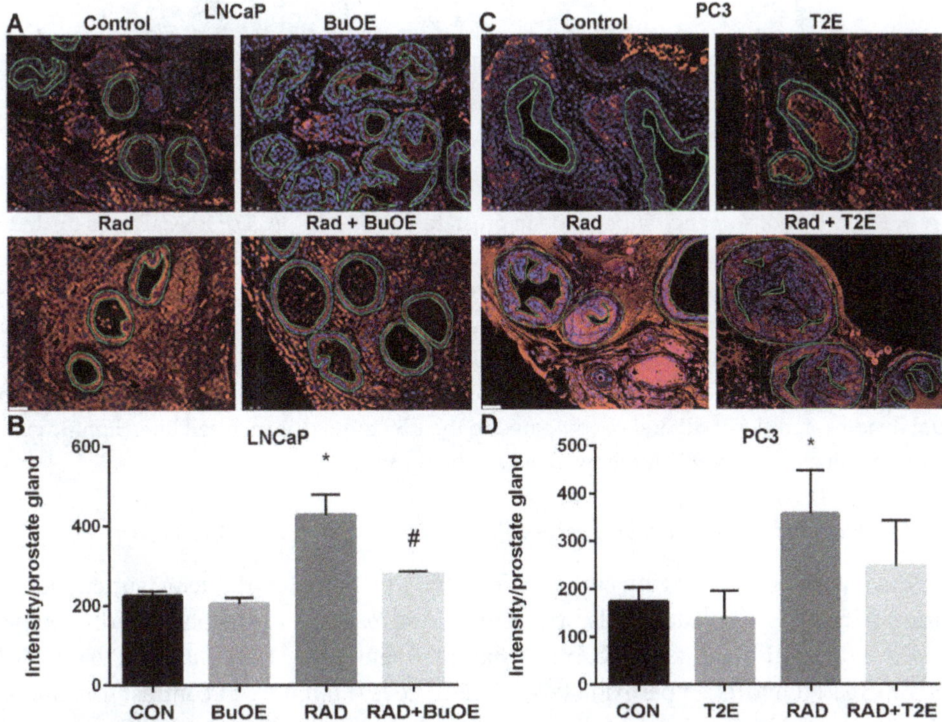

Figure 7. MnPs decrease radiation-induced lipid peroxidation in normal prostate tissues adjacent to the tumor. Formalin fixed paraffin embedded prostate tissue was stained and imaged for 4-HNE. 4-HNE was quantified in the epithelial cells of the normal prostate glands (outlined in images). (**A**) Representative images of the four groups for LNCaP tumors; (**B**) Quantification of LNCaP images; (**C**) Representative images of the four groups for PC3 tumors; (**D**) Quantification of PC3 images. Images were analyzed using ImageJ software. Average raw integrated intensity per unit area was plotted. The magnification bar in the lower left panels denotes 50 μm. The symbol (*) denotes a significant difference as compared to control group and the symbol (#) denotes a significant difference when compared to the RAD group. In the LNCaP model, n = 3 for all groups. In the PC3 model, n = 4 in PBS only and RAD only groups and n = 5 in T2E and RAD + T2E groups.

3.9. MnPs Affect Superoxide Levels Differently in PC3 Cells as Compared to LNCaP Cells

MnPs are superoxide scavengers, but in certain cell types they can also act as pro-oxidants [26]. In our animal model, the MnP are acting as antioxidants by reducing 4-HNE levels in normal tissues (Figure 7), but enhancing 4-HNE in tumor tissues (Figure 6). To determine what role MnPs were playing in the prostate cancer redox state, we measured DHE activation. Excitation at 405 nm can specifically measure the by-product of DHE and superoxide [12]. We have previously published that MnTE-2-PyP significantly inhibits superoxide in normal primary prostate fibroblast by 2-fold [12]. In contrast to normal cells, MnP treatment did not result in superoxide scavenging (Figure 8). In fact, there was a trend of both MnP treatment causing a small increase in superoxide levels in the cancer cells, but this was not significant (Figure 8). Radiation (2 Gy) resulted in a significant elevation of superoxide levels in both LNCaP and PC3 cells; however, this overall increase was more pronounced in the LNCaP cells. The addition of the MnP with radiation had no effect on these increased levels of superoxide (Figure 8). PC3 cells had a significant higher percentage of cells producing superoxide at baseline as compared to LNCaP cells, again indicating that PC3 cells are more oxidatively stressed than LNCaP cells.

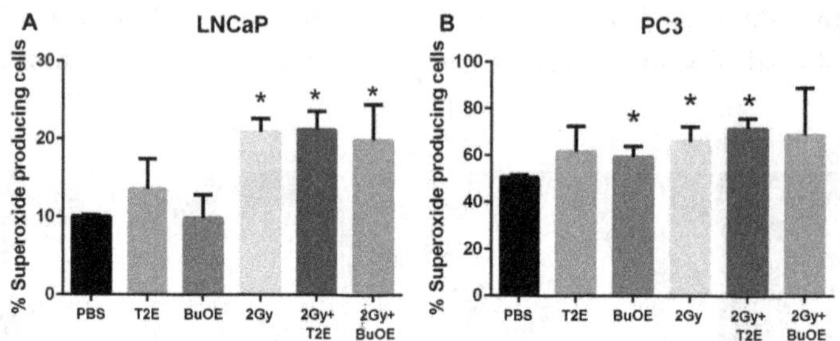

Figure 8. MnPs do not scavenge superoxide in prostate cancer cells. PC3 or LNCaP cells treated with MnTE-2-PyP (30 μM), or MnTnBuOE-2-PyP (0.5 μM) or an equal volume of PBS. In some cases, cells were irradiated (2 Gy) in the presence or absence of the respective MnPs. Cells were stained with DHE and subjected to flow cytometric analysis. (**A**) Percent superoxide producing cells (405 nm) in LNCaP cells; (**B**) Percent superoxide producing cells (405 nm) in PC3 cells. The data are representative of three independent experiments and are presented as the mean ± the standard deviation. The (*) symbol denotes significant difference compared to the PBS group for each cell line. Significance was determined using 1-way ANOVA followed by a student *t*-test.

3.10. MnPs Enhance Hydrogen Peroxide Levels in PC3 Cells But Not LNCaP Cells

Since MnPs were not scavenging superoxide or the MnPs are not reducing superoxide as quickly as it is being produced in the cancer cells, we wanted to investigate the levels of hydrogen peroxide in the cancer cells with MnP treatment. We found that treatment with MnTnBuOE-2-PyP or MnTE-2-PyP significantly increased hydrogen peroxide levels in PC3 cells (Figure 9). In contrast, treatment with the MnPs did not enhance intracellular hydrogen peroxide levels in LNCaP cells (Figure 9). Radiation alone or in combination with MnP had little effect on hydrogen peroxide levels in both cell lines. However, in PC3 cells, radiation in combination with MnTnBuOE-2-PyP or MnTE-2-PyP resulted in a significant enhancement of hydrogen peroxide levels as compared to untreated PC3 cells (Figure 9). In normal prostate fibroblasts, MnP treatment did not result in increased hydrogen peroxide levels either (data not shown).

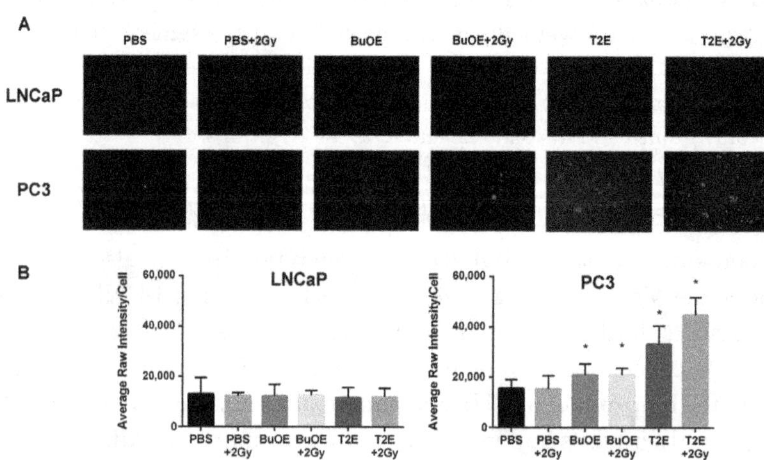

Figure 9. MnTE-2-PyP and MnTnBuOE-2-PyP significantly enhance intracellular hydrogen peroxide in PC3 cells but not in LNCaP cells. (**A**) Representative images of LNCaP (top panel) and PC3 (bottom panel) cells treated with either MnTE-2-PyP (30 μM), MnTnBuOE-2-PyP (0.5 μM) or PBS ± radiation (2 Gy) and stained with peroxy orange 1 (PO1), a probe that fluoresces in the presence of hydrogen peroxide; (**B**) Quantification of the PO1 staining in LNCaP and PC3 cells treated with either MnTE-2-PyP, MnTnBuOE-2-PyP or PBS ± radiation (2 Gy). The symbol (*) denotes a significant difference as compared to control group (PBS for each respective cell line). Data represent mean ± SD from three independent experiments.

3.11. MnPs Enhance Thiol Oxidation in PC3 Cells But Not LNCaP Cells

Hydrogen peroxide can directly oxidize thiol containing amino acids. Therefore, we wanted to determine if these increased hydrogen peroxide levels had an effect on thiol oxidation of intracellular proteins in PC3 cells. Using a *N*-(Biotinoyl)-*N′*-(Iodoacetyl)Ethylenediamine (BIAM) assay, where the BIAM binds only to reduced thiols, we found that MnTE-2-PyP or MnTnBuOE-2-PyP treated PC3 cells had significantly fewer reduced thiols present in the cell lysate as compared to untreated cells (Figure 10A). This indicates that MnP treatment results in oxidation of thiols in PC3 cells. Radiation (2 Gy) had little effect on thiol oxidation. In accordance with the hydrogen peroxide data, MnPs did not cause oxidation of thiols in LNCaP cells (Figure 10B). The addition of MnPs to normal primary prostate fibroblast cells also did not result in the oxidation of thiols (Figure 10C).

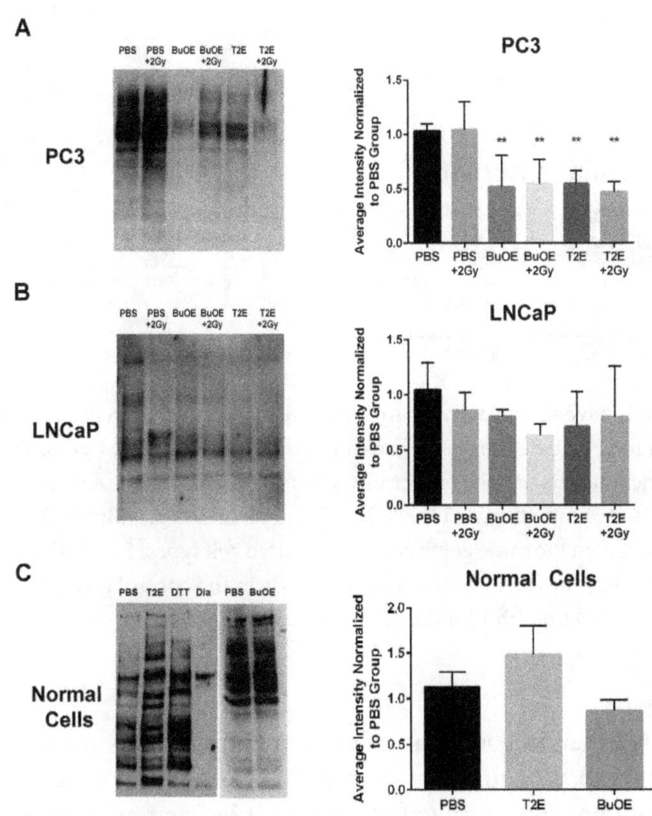

Figure 10. MnTE-2-PyP and MnTnBuOE-2-PyP enhance thiol oxidation in PC3 cells but not in LNCaP cells or normal cells. (Left Panels) Representative images of total reduced thiols by binding to BIAM beads from whole cell lysates treated with MnTE-2-PyP, MnTnBuOE-2-PyP or PBS ± radiation. (Right Panels) (**A**) LNCaP cells. (**B**) PC3 cells. (**C**) Normal cells. Densitometric analysis was performed on three separate blots as shown to the right of each blot. As a control, the lysates were treated with the reducing agent dithiothreiotol (DTT) or the oxidizing agent diamide (Dia). MnTE-2-PyP and MnTnBuOE-2-PyP enhance thiol oxidation in PC3 cells ± radiation but not in LNCaP cells or normal prostate fibroblasts. The symbol (*) denotes a significant difference as compared to control group (PBS for each respective cell line). Data represent mean ± SD from three independent experiments.

3.12. LNCaP Cells Have Twice as Much Catalase Activity as PC3 Cells and MnP Treatment Does Not Affect Catalase Activity

Because there was such a difference observed in hydrogen peroxide levels in PC3 cells as compared to LNCaP cells treated with MnPs, we investigated the baseline catalase activity in these two cell lines. LNCaP cells had significantly higher levels (2-fold greater) of catalase activity as compared to PC3 cells

(Figure 11). Radiation alone or MnP treatment alone had no effect on catalase activity. The combination of radiation with MnPs also had no effect on catalase activity in either cell line (Figure 11).

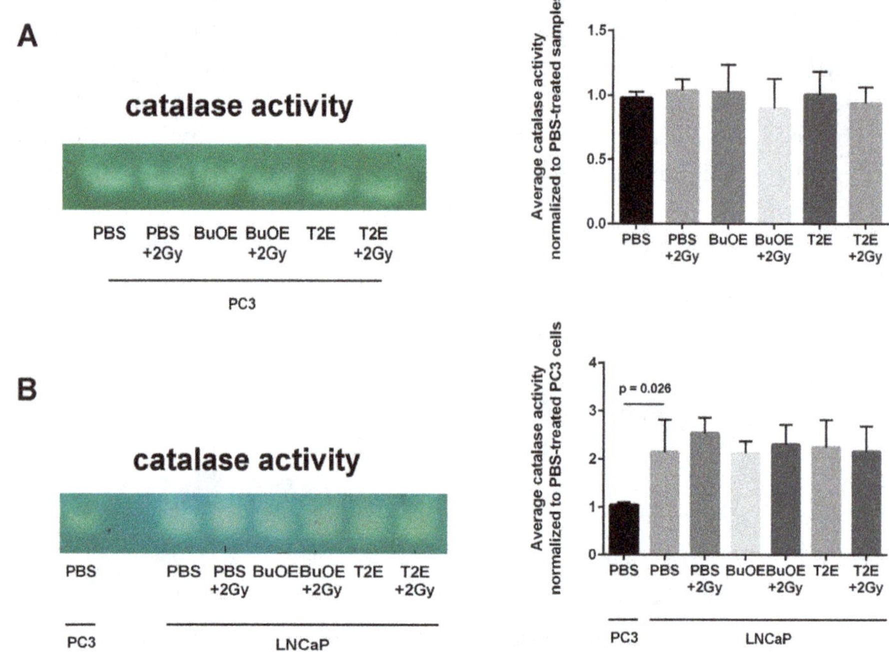

Figure 11. LNCaP cells have significantly more catalase activity than PC3 cells. (**A**) Left: A representative catalase activity gel for PC3 cells treated ± radiation and/or ± MnTE-2-PyP or ± MnTnBuOE-2-PyP. Right: Densitometric analysis of catalase activity gels; (**B**) Left: A representative catalase activity gel for LNCaP cells treated ± radiation and/or ± MnTE-2-PyP or ± MnTnBuOE-2-PyP. PC3 cells treated with PBS are also loaded on the same gel to compare the two cell types. Right: Densitometric analysis of catalase activity gels. The mean OD of the reactive bands in the control group was normalized to 1.0. Data represent mean ± SD from three independent experiments.

4. Discussion

This study revealed that, in combination with radiation, MnPs decrease primary tumor size by inhibiting the proliferation of tumor cells in both LNCaP and PC3 orthotopic prostate tumor models. Thus, the overall median survival of the tumor bearing mice, treated with radiation and MnPs, was significantly increased. MnPs had no effect on metastatic progression, which is one of the major causes of prostate cancer related deaths. This study also demonstrated that MnPs protect tumor adjacent normal prostate tissue from radiation-induced lipid peroxidation. We also observed that the tumor redox environment affects the activity of the MnPs. In the oxidizing tumor environment, the MnPs do not scavenge superoxide, if anything there is a trend to increased amounts of superoxide levels in the prostate cancer cells. In contrast, in normal prostate cells we have previously shown that MnPs reduce superoxide levels in normal cells alone and in combination with radiation [12]. We speculate that the superoxide molecules autodismute into hydrogen peroxide. In LNCaP cells, there are two-fold higher levels of catalase activity as compared to PC3 cells. Thus, the hydrogen peroxide made in LNCaP cells when treated with MnPs is adequately scavenged and thiol oxidation is not observed in these cells. In contrast, PC3 cells cannot compensate for the increased levels of hydrogen peroxide with MnP treatment and the result is increased thiol oxidation. We only measured catalase activity; there could be differences in other peroxide removing enzymes as well between LNCaP and PC3 cells. This will be a future direction of these studies.

In combination with radiation therapy, or other chemotherapeutic agents, MnPs have been reported as anti-tumor agents. In a head and neck cancer model, MnTnBuOE-2-PyP sensitized tumor tissue to radiation [28]. In combination with other chemotherapeutic agents, MnTnBuOE-2-PyP acted as a pro-apoptotic molecule in glioblastoma multiforme [29]. Clonogenic survival of human pancreatic cancer cells was significantly decreased by MnP treatment in combination with ascorbate and gemcitabine [30]. We have reported previously that MnPs inhibit growth of prostate and colon cancer cells in combination with radiation or chemotherapies [10,11]. There have also been many studies that show MnTE-2-PyP or MnTnBuOE-2-PyP protect normal tissues from radiation damage in a variety of models [10,12]. However, no one has shown that the administration of MnPs protects normal tissues but not cancer tissues in the presence of radiation simultaneously.

We have observed that both MnPs do not scavenge superoxide, or are unable to scavenge superoxide at a rate equivalent to its production in cancer cells. In fact, there is a trend for a slight increase in superoxide levels in cancer cells treated with MnPs. Both MnPs have been reported to enhance oxidative stress in cancer cells [16–18,29,31]. It has been theorized that the SOD mimics act as pro-oxidants in oxidizing environments, such as cancer cells, because the Mn metal itself becomes oxidized. In the native SOD protein, the metal active site is surrounded by a large protein, which protects the metal from reacting with anything but superoxide. Thus, SOD enzymes generally do not act as pro-oxidants under any conditions. However, the SOD mimics are very small molecules and the manganese metal is able react with a variety of small oxidizing molecules. Therefore, instead of donating electrons to reduce free radicals (as is observed in normal cells and is normally thought as to how SOD mimics function), the SOD mimic instead steals electrons and in the process oxidizes these molecules. Thus, the SOD mimic acts a pro-oxidant when the surrounding environment oxidizes the metal. We postulate that the SOD mimics are behaving as such in the cancer cells.

Superoxide and hydrogen peroxide levels are key factors in determining how cancer cells will respond to therapeutic agents [32]. Superoxide can promote cell cycle progression and tumor vessel formation. Low levels of hydrogen peroxide leads to caspase dependent cell death, while, high levels of hydrogen peroxide can activate caspase independent apoptosis as well as necrotic cell death [33]. MnPs were proposed as therapeutic molecules against cancer cells because they can lower superoxide levels and potentially increase the hydrogen peroxide levels in cancer cells [32,34]. We found that in combination with radiation, MnTE-2-PyP or MnTnBuOE-2-PyP increases hydrogen peroxide levels in the PC3 cells [24]. In contrast, the MnPs do not increase hydrogen peroxide levels in LNCaP cells because LNCaP cells contain more of the hydrogen peroxide scavenging enzyme, catalase. Therefore, it is possible that in PC3 but not in LNCaP cells, MnPs can activate the hydrogen peroxide mediated mechanism of cell growth arrest.

It has previously been demonstrated that MnPs inhibit tumor growth in combination with ascorbate because MnPs oxidize ascorbate to peroxides, which increases steady state levels of hydrogen peroxide and hydroxyl anions [35] and leads to a caspase independent cancer cell death [16,36]. MnTE-2-PyP has also been reported to cause metabolic quiescence, which could account for the reduction in tumor cell growth observed in MnTE-2-PyP treated cancer cells [37]. We showed that MnTE-2-PyP and MnTnBuOE-2-PyP regulates thiol oxidation of redox sensitive proteins in PC3 cells. Presumably, some of these oxidized proteins could alter signaling molecules and potentially affect cell fate determination. Activity of cell cycle regulatory kinases and phosphatases are regulated by modulation of their oxidation state [38]. Thus, these proteins are potential targets of MnP-mediated cell growth arrest. One or any combination of these mechanisms could be considered as probable causes of MnP-mediated tumor growth arrest in PC3 models. Identification of the oxidized proteins in PC3 cells are planned for future experiments.

In our study, MnPs enhanced the anti-tumor effect of radiation. This data is also supported by another study showing that MnTE-2-PyP significantly controls tumor growth by decreasing the vascular density of the tumor [39]. Previously, C57BL/6 mice bearing RM-9 prostate tumors that were treated with MnTE-2-PyP showed reduced tumor growth due to activation of the immune system, specifically elevation of T helper, cytotoxic T cells and Natural Killer T cells [14]. Since we were using athymic mice to grow the human prostate cancer cells orthotopically, we did not observe these changes to the immune system. Therefore, we speculate that if we used a syngeneic mouse cancer model or a humanized mouse model, we may observe an increase in anti-tumor T cells and this may further inhibit the prostate cancer growth. These important studies need to be done to investigate the role of the immune system in MnP treatment of cancer in combination with radiation.

It has previously been reported that MnTE-2-PyP reduces the PCNA levels in a skin cancer model [40]. In our study, we also observed a reduction of PCNA by MnPs when combined with radiation in both tumor models. In replicating cells, PCNA acts as a harbor for the DNA replication-initiation protein machinery on the replication fork [41]. Depletion in PCNA causes a stall in DNA replication, which ultimately leads to an accumulation of cells in the S phase of the cell cycle [42]. Therefore, reduction of PCNA in both of the tumor types by MnP treatment and radiation, suggests probable growth arrest of tumor cells. This is likely another mechanism by which MnPs cause reduction of tumor size in combination with radiation.

There are vast differences in cell signaling and survival strategies in prostate cancer cells from early and late stages of prostate cancer. In the early stage, prostate tumor cells are confined to the prostate and the cancer cells are dependent on androgens for survival [43]. As the disease progresses, the tumor cells lose their dependency on external androgen for their survival [44–46]. Either, the cancer cells produce intracellular androgen for their survival or they utilize a ligand independent activation of the androgen receptor, which leads to activation of downstream survival mechanisms [47]. The androgen deprivation therapy fails at this point of disease progression. Therefore, the treatment protocols for early and late stages of prostate cancer vary differently. LNCaP cells are responsive to androgens and are not invasive. PC3 cells on the other hand are androgen independent and are highly metastatic. Therefore, LNCaP and PC3 cells can be considered representatives of early and late stages of prostate cancer, respectively. In our study, in combination with radiation, MnTE-2-PyP and MnTnBuOE-2-PyP inhibited tumor growth and protected the normal tissues in both prostate orthotopic models. Therefore, it can be concluded that in combination with radiation therapy, MnPs can inhibit both early non-metastatic and late-castration resistant prostate cancer growth.

In prostate cancer, the majority of patients receive radiation therapy. One of the major disadvantages of radiation is that it causes oxidative damage in the normal tissue adjacent to the tumor. Radiation enhances superoxide-mediated myofibroblast and senescent phenotypes in fibroblasts [48,49]. Radiotherapy for prostate cancer causes fibrosis and the dysfunction of the normal tissues in the radiation field and nearby tissues such as prostate, bladder, seminal vesicles, and bowel. Our study revealed that, MnP treatment during and after radiation, caused a significant reduction in radiation-mediated production of 4-HNE, a marker of lipid oxidation, in the tumor adjacent normal prostate glandular region. The MnTnBuOE-2-PyP treated animals were more protected from radiation damage than MnTE-2-PyP treated animals. This is probably due to the location of the MnPs inside the cells. MnTnBuOE-2-PyP is more lipophilic as compared to MnTE-2-PyP, so MnTnBuOE-2-PyP is likely in higher concentrations in the lipids than MnTE-2-PyP and, thus, is better able to protect from lipid oxidation [50].

There is a scarcity of effective radioprotectors for prostate cancer patients. Using antioxidants as radioprotectors has been controversial because it is feared that tumor tissue will be protected from radiation killing. In previous clinical trials, cancer patients receiving supplementation of β-carotene; or vitamins A, B, C, E, D3, or K3; or selenium; or cysteine and glutathione did not protect tumors with routine radiation or chemotherapy treatment [51]. However, there has been a lack of efficacy showing that vitamin supplementation protects normal tissues from radiation damage. This is likely due to these vitamins being poor ROS scavengers, not localizing to the area where free radicals are produced and were not given at high enough concentrations to be efficacious as free radical scavengers. Our study further illustrates that the redox active molecules, MnTE-2-PyP and MnTnBuOE-2-PyP, are not only effective radioprotectors, but also inhibit cancer growth in combination with radiation therapy. Thus, this study suggests that use of MnPs during and post-radiation in prostate cancer can significantly enhance the protection of normal tissues against side effects associated with prostate cancer therapy, while simultaneously inhibiting prostate cancer tumor growth. We believe that the addition of MnPs will result in better treatment of prostate cancer and improve the overall quality of life of patients undergoing radiation therapy for prostate cancer.

Acknowledgments: National Institutes of Health Grants (1R01CA178888), NIH SP20 GM103480 COBRE, Fred and Pamela Buffet Cancer Center Support Grant (P30CA036727) and National Natural Science Foundation of China (81172186) supported this study.

Author Contributions: Arpita Chatterjee wrote the majority of this manuscript and conducted experiments in Figures 2–8 of the manuscript. Yuxiang Zhu conducted experiments presented in Figures 5–11. Qiang Tong helped to conduct experiments presented in Figures 2–4 of the manuscript. Elizabeth A. Kosmacek helped to conduct and analyze experiments presented in Figures 2–8 of the manuscript and helped edit the manuscript. Eliezer Z. Lichter helped to analyze Figures 6 and 7 of the manuscript. Rebecca E. Oberley-Deegan developed and oversaw the project, helped conduct experiments 2–7 in the manuscript and helped to edit the manuscript.

Conflicts of Interest: There are no conflicts of interest for the authors except Rebecca Oberley-Deegan. Oberley-Deegan is a consultant with BioMimetix Pharmaceutical, Inc. and holds equities in BioMimetix Pharmaceutical, Inc.

References

1. Mikkelsen, R.B.; Wardman, P. Biological chemistry of reactive oxygen and nitrogen and radiation-induced signal transduction mechanisms. *Oncogene* **2003**, *22*, 5734–5754. [CrossRef] [PubMed]
2. Riley, P.A. Free radicals in biology: Oxidative stress and the effects of ionizing radiation. *Int. J. Radiat. Biol.* **1994**, *65*, 27–33. [CrossRef] [PubMed]
3. Kim, Y.S.; Kang, M.J.; Cho, Y.M. Low production of reactive oxygen species and high DNA repair: Mechanism of radioresistance of prostate cancer stem cells. *Anticancer Res.* **2013**, *33*, 4469–4474. [PubMed]
4. Sun, C.; Wang, Z.H.; Liu, X.X.; Yang, L.N.; Wang, Y.; Liu, Y.; Mao, A.H.; Liu, Y.Y.; Zhou, X.; Di, C.X.; et al. Disturbance of redox status enhances radiosensitivity of hepatocellular carcinoma. *Am. J. Cancer Res.* **2015**, *5*, 1368–1381. [CrossRef]
5. Elliott, S.P.; Malaeb, B.S. Long-term urinary adverse effects of pelvic radiotherapy. *World J. Urol.* **2011**, *29*, 35–41. [CrossRef] [PubMed]
6. Sullivan, L.; Williams, S.G.; Tai, K.H.; Foroudi, F.; Cleeve, L.; Duchesne, G.M. Urethral stricture following high dose rate brachytherapy for prostate cancer. *Radiother. Oncol.* **2009**, *91*, 232–236. [CrossRef] [PubMed]
7. Herskind, C.; Westergaard, O. Variable protection by OH scavengers against radiation-induced inactivation of isolated transcriptionally active chromatin: The influence of secondary radicals. *Radiat. Res.* **1988**, *114*, 28–41. [CrossRef] [PubMed]
8. Maier, P.; Wenz, F.; Herskind, C. Radioprotection of normal tissue cells. *Strahlenther. Onkol.* **2014**, *190*, 745–752. [CrossRef] [PubMed]
9. Schaur, R.J. Basic aspects of the biochemical reactivity of 4-hydroxynonenal. *Mol. Asp. Med.* **2003**, *24*, 149–159. [CrossRef]
10. Kosmacek, E.A.; Chatterjee, A.; Tong, Q.; Lin, C.; Oberley-Deegan, R.E. MnTnBuOE-2-PyP protects normal colorectal fibroblasts from radiation damage and simultaneously enhances radio/chemotherapeutic killing of colorectal cancer cells. *Oncotarget* **2016**, *7*, 34532–34545. [CrossRef] [PubMed]
11. Tong, Q.; Weaver, M.R.; Kosmacek, E.A.; O'Connor, B.P.; Harmacek, L.; Venkataraman, S.; Oberley-Deegan, R.E. MnTE-2-PyP reduces prostate cancer growth and metastasis by suppressing p300 activity and p300/HIF-1/CREB binding to the promoter region of the PAI-1 gene. *Free Radic. Biol. Med.* **2016**, *94*, 185–194. [CrossRef] [PubMed]
12. Chatterjee, A.; Kosmacek, E.A.; Oberley-Deegan, R.E. MnTE-2-PyP Treatment, or NOX4 Inhibition, Protects against Radiation-Induced Damage in Mouse Primary Prostate Fibroblasts by Inhibiting the TGF-Beta 1 Signaling Pathway. *Radiat. Res.* **2017**, *187*, 367–381. [CrossRef] [PubMed]
13. Oberley-Deegan, R.E.; Steffan, J.J.; Rove, K.O.; Pate, K.M.; Weaver, M.W.; Spasojevic, I.; Frederick, B.; Raben, D.; Meacham, R.B.; Crapo, J.D.; et al. The antioxidant, MnTE-2-PyP, prevents side-effects incurred by prostate cancer irradiation. *PLoS ONE* **2012**, *7*, e44178. [CrossRef] [PubMed]
14. Makinde, A.Y.; Luo-Owen, X.; Rizvi, A.; Crapo, J.D.; Pearlstein, R.D.; Slater, J.M.; Gridley, D.S. Effect of a metalloporphyrin antioxidant (MnTE-2-PyP) on the response of a mouse prostate cancer model to radiation. *Anticancer Res.* **2009**, *29*, 107–118. [PubMed]

15. Batinic-Haberle, I.; Spasojevic, I. Complex chemistry and biology of redox-active compounds, commonly known as SOD mimics, affect their therapeutic effects. *Antioxid. Redox Signal.* **2014**, *20*, 2323–2325. [CrossRef] [PubMed]
16. Evans, M.K.; Tovmasyan, A.; Batinic-Haberle, I.; Devi, G.R. Mn porphyrin in combination with ascorbate acts as a pro-oxidant and mediates caspase-independent cancer cell death. *Free Radic. Biol. Med.* **2014**, *68*, 302–314. [CrossRef] [PubMed]
17. Jaramillo, M.C.; Briehl, M.M.; Batinic-Haberle, I.; Tome, M.E. Manganese (III) meso-tetrakis N-ethylpyridinium-2-yl porphyrin acts as a pro-oxidant to inhibit electron transport chain proteins, modulate bioenergetics, and enhance the response to chemotherapy in lymphoma cells. *Free Radic. Biol. Med.* **2015**, *83*, 89–100. [CrossRef] [PubMed]
18. Jaramillo, M.C.; Briehl, M.M.; Crapo, J.D.; Batinic-Haberle, I.; Tome, M.E. Manganese porphyrin, MnTE-2-PyP^{5+}, Acts as a pro-oxidant to potentiate glucocorticoid-induced apoptosis in lymphoma cells. *Free Radic. Biol. Med.* **2012**, *52*, 1272–1284. [CrossRef] [PubMed]
19. Tovmasyan, A.; Sampaio, R.S.; Boss, M.K.; Bueno-Janice, J.C.; Bader, B.H.; Thomas, M.; Reboucas, J.S.; Orr, M.; Chandler, J.D.; Go, Y.M.; et al. Anticancer therapeutic potential of Mn porphyrin/ascorbate system. *Free Radic. Biol. Med.* **2015**, *89*, 1231–1247. [CrossRef] [PubMed]
20. Huggins, C. Endocrine-induced regression of cancers. *Science* **1967**, *156*, 1050–1054. [CrossRef] [PubMed]
21. Huggins, C. Endocrine-induced regression of cancers. *Cancer Res.* **1967**, *27*, 1925–1930. [CrossRef] [PubMed]
22. Recouvreux, M.V.; Wu, B.; Gao, A.C.; Zonis, S.; Chesnokova, V.; Bhowmick, N.; Chung, L.W.; Melmed, S. Androgen receptor regulation of local growth hormone in prostate cancer cells. *Endocrinology* **2017**, *158*, 2255–2268. [CrossRef] [PubMed]
23. Seluanov, A.; Vaidya, A.; Gorbunova, V. Establishing primary adult fibroblast cultures from rodents. *J. Vis. Exp.* **2010**. [CrossRef] [PubMed]
24. Tong, Q.; Zhu, Y.; Galaske, J.W.; Kosmacek, E.A.; Chatterjee, A.; Dickinson, B.C.; Oberley-Deegan, R.E. MnTE-2-PyP modulates thiol oxidation in a hydrogen peroxide-mediated manner in a human prostate cancer cell. *Free Radic. Biol. Med.* **2016**, *101*, 32–43. [CrossRef] [PubMed]
25. Scher, H.I.; Sawyers, C.L. Biology of progressive, castration-resistant prostate cancer: Directed therapies targeting the androgen-receptor signaling axis. *J. Clin. Oncol.* **2005**, *23*, 8253–8261. [CrossRef] [PubMed]
26. Batinic-Haberle, I.; Tovmasyan, A.; Spasojevic, I. An educational overview of the chemistry, biochemistry and therapeutic aspects of Mn porphyrins—From superoxide dismutation to HO-driven pathways. *Redox Biol.* **2015**, *5*, 43–65. [CrossRef] [PubMed]
27. Maier, P.; Hartmann, L.; Wenz, F.; Herskind, C. Cellular Pathways in Response to Ionizing Radiation and Their Targetability for Tumor Radiosensitization. *Int. J. Mol. Sci.* **2016**, *17*, 102. [CrossRef] [PubMed]
28. Ashcraft, K.A.; Boss, M.K.; Tovmasyan, A.; Roy Choudhury, K.; Fontanella, A.N.; Young, K.H.; Palmer, G.M.; Birer, S.R.; Landon, C.D.; Park, W.; et al. Novel Manganese-Porphyrin Superoxide Dismutase-Mimetic Widens the Therapeutic Margin in a Preclinical Head and Neck Cancer Model. *Int. J. Radiat. Oncol. Biol. Phys.* **2015**, *93*, 892–900. [CrossRef] [PubMed]
29. Yulyana, Y.; Tovmasyan, A.; Ho, I.A.; Sia, K.C.; Newman, J.P.; Ng, W.H.; Guo, C.M.; Hui, K.M.; Batinic-Haberle, I.; Lam, P.Y. Redox-Active Mn Porphyrin-based Potent SOD Mimic, MnTnBuOE-2-PyP(5+), Enhances Carbenoxolone-Mediated TRAIL-Induced Apoptosis in Glioblastoma Multiforme. *Stem Cell Rev.* **2016**, *12*, 140–155. [CrossRef] [PubMed]
30. Cieslak, J.A.; Strother, R.K.; Rawal, M.; Du, J.; Doskey, C.M.; Schroeder, S.R.; Button, A.; Wagner, B.A.; Buettner, G.R.; Cullen, J.J. Manganoporphyrins and ascorbate enhance gemcitabine cytotoxicity in pancreatic cancer. *Free Radic. Biol. Med.* **2015**, *83*, 227–237. [CrossRef] [PubMed]
31. Batinic-Haberle, I.; Keir, S.T.; Rajic, Z.; Tovmasyan, A.; Bigner, D.D. Lipophilic Mn porphyrins in the treatment of brain tumors. *Free Radic. Biol. Med.* **2011**, *51*, S119–S120. [CrossRef]
32. Azzolin, V.F.; Cadoná, F.C.; Machado, A.K.; Berto, M.D.; Barbisan, F.; Dornelles, E.B.; Glanzner, W.G.; Gonçalves, P.B.; Bica, C.G.; da Cruz, I.B. Superoxide-hydrogen peroxide imbalance interferes with colorectal cancer cells viability, proliferation and oxaliplatin response. *Toxicol. In Vitro* **2016**, *32*, 8–15. [CrossRef] [PubMed]
33. Tochigi, M.; Inoue, T.; Suzuki-Karasaki, M.; Ochiai, T.; Ra, C.; Suzuki-Karasaki, Y. Hydrogen peroxide induces cell death in human TRAIL-resistant melanoma through intracellular superoxide generation. *Int. J. Oncol.* **2013**, *42*, 863–872. [CrossRef] [PubMed]

34. Berto, M.D.; Bica, C.G.; de Sá, G.P.; Barbisan, F.; Azzolin, V.F.; Rogalski, F.; Duarte, M.M.; da Cruz, I.B. The effect of superoxide anion and hydrogen peroxide imbalance on prostate cancer: An integrative in vivo and in vitro analysis. *Med. Oncol.* **2015**, *32*, 251. [CrossRef] [PubMed]
35. Tian, J.; Peehl, D.M.; Knox, S.J. Metalloporphyrin synergizes with ascorbic acid to inhibit cancer cell growth through fenton chemistry. *Cancer Biother. Radiopharm.* **2010**, *25*, 439–448. [CrossRef] [PubMed]
36. Rawal, M.; Schroeder, S.R.; Wagner, B.A.; Cushing, C.M.; Welsh, J.L.; Button, A.M.; Du, J.; Sibenaller, Z.A.; Buettner, G.R.; Cullen, J.J. Manganoporphyrins increase ascorbate-induced cytotoxicity by enhancing H_2O_2 generation. *Cancer Res.* **2013**, *73*, 5232–5341. [CrossRef] [PubMed]
37. Delmastro-Greenwood, M.M.; Votyakova, T.; Goetzman, E.; Marre, M.L.; Previte, D.M.; Tovmasyan, A.; Batinic-Haberle, I.; Trucco, M.M.; Piganelli, J.D. Mn porphyrin regulation of aerobic glycolysis: Implications on the activation of diabetogenic immune cells. *Antioxid. Redox Signal.* **2013**, *19*, 1902–1915. [CrossRef] [PubMed]
38. Menon, S.G.; Goswami, P.C. A redox cycle within the cell cycle: Ring in the old with the new. *Oncogene* **2007**, *26*, 1101–1109. [CrossRef] [PubMed]
39. Moeller, B.J.; Batinic-Haberle, I.; Spasojevic, I.; Rabbani, Z.N.; Anscher, M.S.; Vujaskovic, Z.; Dewhirst, M.W. A manganese porphyrin superoxide dismutase mimetic enhances tumor radioresponsiveness. *Int. J. Radiat. Oncol. Biol. Phys.* **2005**, *63*, 545–552. [CrossRef] [PubMed]
40. Zhao, Y.; Chaiswing, L.; Oberley, T.D.; Batinic-Haberle, I.; St Clair, W.; Epstein, C.J.; St Clair, D. A mechanism-based antioxidant approach for the reduction of skin carcinogenesis. *Cancer Res.* **2005**, *65*, 1401–1405. [CrossRef] [PubMed]
41. Choe, K.N.; Moldovan, G.L. Forging Ahead through Darkness: PCNA, Still the Principal Conductor at the Replication Fork. *Mol. Cell* **2017**, *65*, 380–392. [CrossRef] [PubMed]
42. Zhao, H.; Lo, Y.H.; Ma, L.; Waltz, S.E.; Gray, J.K.; Hung, M.C.; Wang, S.C. Targeting tyrosine phosphorylation of PCNA inhibits prostate cancer growth. *Mol. Cancer Ther.* **2011**, *10*, 29–36. [CrossRef] [PubMed]
43. Denmeade, S.R.; Lin, X.S.; Isaacs, J.T. Role of programmed (apoptotic) cell death during the progression and therapy for prostate cancer. *Prostate* **1996**, *28*, 251–265. [CrossRef]
44. Harris, W.P.; Mostaghel, E.A.; Nelson, P.S.; Montgomery, B. Androgen deprivation therapy: Progress in understanding mechanisms of resistance and optimizing androgen depletion. *Nat. Clin. Pract. Urol.* **2009**, *6*, 76–85. [CrossRef] [PubMed]
45. Karantanos, T.; Corn, P.G.; Thompson, T.C. Prostate cancer progression after androgen deprivation therapy: Mechanisms of castrate resistance and novel therapeutic approaches. *Oncogene* **2013**, *32*, 5501–5511. [CrossRef] [PubMed]
46. Marques, R.B.; Dits, N.F.; Erkens-Schulze, S.; van Weerden, W.M.; Jenster, G. Bypass mechanisms of the androgen receptor pathway in therapy-resistant prostate cancer cell models. *PLoS ONE* **2010**, *5*, e13500. [CrossRef] [PubMed]
47. Feldman, B.J.; Feldman, D. The development of androgen-independent prostate cancer. *Nat. Rev. Cancer* **2001**, *1*, 34–45. [CrossRef] [PubMed]
48. Sabin, R.J.; Anderson, R.M. Cellular Senescence—Its role in cancer and the response to ionizing radiation. *Genome Integr.* **2011**, *2*, 7. [CrossRef] [PubMed]
49. Yarnold, J.; Brotons, M.C. Pathogenetic mechanisms in radiation fibrosis. *Radiother. Oncol.* **2010**, *97*, 149–161. [CrossRef] [PubMed]
50. Tovmasyan, A.; Sheng, H.; Weitner, T.; Arulpragasam, A.; Lu, M.; Warner, D.S.; Vujaskovic, Z.; Spasojevic, I.; Batinic-Haberle, I. Design, mechanism of action, bioavailability and therapeutic effects of mn porphyrin-based redox modulators. *Med. Princ. Pract.* **2013**, *22*, 103–130. [CrossRef] [PubMed]
51. Simone, C.B., 2nd; Simone, N.L.; Simone, V.; Simone, C.B. Antioxidants and other nutrients do not interfere with chemotherapy or radiation therapy and can increase kill and increase survival, Part 2. *Altern. Ther. Health Med.* **2007**, *13*, 40–47. [PubMed]

4

Quantification of Phenolic Compounds and In Vitro Radical Scavenging Abilities with Leaf Extracts from Two Varieties of *Psidium guajava* L.

Julio César Camarena-Tello [1], Héctor Eduardo Martínez-Flores [2,*], Ma. Guadalupe Garnica-Romo [3], José Saúl Padilla-Ramírez [4], Alfredo Saavedra-Molina [5], Osvaldo Alvarez-Cortes [6], María Carmen Bartolomé-Camacho [2] and José Octavio Rodiles-López [2]

1. Programa Institucional de Doctorado en Ciencias Biológicas, Universidad Michoacana de San Nicolás de Hidalgo, Morelia 58240, Mich., Mexico; cama.de.arena@hotmail.com
2. Facultad de Químico Farmacobiología, Universidad Michoacana de San Nicolás de Hidalgo, Morelia 58240, Mich., Mexico; carbarcam@hotmail.com (M.C.B.-C.); tavarodiles@hotmail.com (J.O.R.-L.)
3. Facultad de Ingeniería Civil, Universidad Michoacana de San Nicolás de Hidalgo, Morelia 58240, Mich., Mexico; ggarnica@umich.mx
4. Instituto Nacional de Investigaciones Forestales, Agrícolas y Pecuarias, Centro de Investigación Regional Norte-Centro, Campo Experimental Pabellón, Pabellón de Arteaga 20660, Aguascalientes, Mexico; padilla.saul@inifap.gob.mx
5. Instituto de Investigaciones Químico Biológicas, Universidad Michoacana de San Nicolás de Hidalgo, Morelia 58030, Mich., Mexico; saavedra@umich.mx
6. Departamento de Bioquímica, Instituto Tecnológico de Morelia, Morelia 58120, Mich., Mexico; oalvarezc@tecmor.mx

* Correspondence: hmartinez@umich.mx

Abstract: Guava leaf (*Psidium guajava* L.) extracts are used in both traditional medicine and the pharmaceutical industry. The antioxidant compounds in *P. guajava* leaves can have positive effects including anti-inflammatory, anti-hyperglycemic, hepatoprotective, analgesic, anti-cancer effects, as well as protecting against cardiovascular diseases. In the present study, phenolic compounds and in vitro antioxidant capacity were measured in extracts obtained with polar and non-polar solvents from leaves of two varieties of guava, Calvillo Siglo XXI and Hidrozac. The quantity of total phenolics and total flavonoids were expressed as equivalents of gallic acid and quercetin, respectively. Hydroxyl radical, **2,2′-azino-bis(3-ethylbenzothiazoline-6-sulphonic acid)** (ABTS), 2,2-diphenyl-1-picrylhydrazyl (DPPH), and Oxygen Radical Absorbance Capacity using fluorescein (ORAC-FL) in vitro tests were used to assess the radical scavenging abilities of the extracts. The total phenolics were higher in the aqueous fraction of the variety Calvillo Siglo XXI, while in the Hidrozac variety total phenolics were higher in the acetone and chloroform fractions. Total flavonoids were higher in all fractions in the variety Calvillo Siglo XXI. Total phenolics showed a highly positive correlation for ORAC-FL, and a moderately positive correlation with hydroxyl radicals. Finally, total flavonoids showed a slightly positive correlation for ORAC-FL and hydroxyl radicals. Both varieties of guava leaf extract showed excellent antioxidant properties.

Keywords: *Psidium guajava*; ORAC; DPPH; ABTS; total polyphenols; total flavonoids; nano spray-dryer

---

1. Introduction

Psidium guajava L. is a small tree that belongs to the Myrtaceae family. Guava is the common name used for species of *P. guajava*. The guava tree is distributed in tropical and subtropical regions of

America, the Caribbean, Asia, Africa, and the Pacific islands [1]. The primary producers of guava fruit are India, China, Thailand, Pakistan, and Mexico [2,3].

Currently, most of the commercialized orchards of guava fruits in Mexico present a great phenotypic, genetic, and morphological diversity due to propagation methods. This variability affects the productive potential of the guava crop, as well as the uniformity and quality of the harvested fruit. To improve the productivity of the guava crop in Mexico, the germplasms of different varieties has been selected and evaluated, which will be registered and commercially released as clonal varieties [4–7].

Different parts of guava trees are widely used as food and in folk medicine around the world [8]. Díaz-De-Cerio [9] reported that several studies have shown that guava leaves present anti-hyperglycemic and anti-hyperlipidemic activities. In Mexico, a phytodrug QG-5® is being produced from leaves of *Psidium guajava folia,* variety [10]. The activities present in extracts of guava leaves are mainly due to phenolic compounds.

Water and organic solvents such as chloroform, hexane, ethyl acetate, acetone, methanol, and ethanol are the most commonly used solvents for extracting phenolic compounds from leaves of different species of trees or plants. The nature of the sample as well as the polarity of the solvents are two of the main factors that influence the solubility of phenolic compounds [11–14].

Seo et al. [15] described that water, followed by ethanol and finally methanol, are the best solvents used to obtain extracts with high antioxidant capacity, in leaves of *Psidium guajava*. A study conducted by Nantitanon et al. [16] found that the extraction of phenolic compounds with greater antioxidant activity were obtained using the ultrasound process, followed by maceration with agitation, maceration without agitation, and finally soxhlet extraction. In other studies, the antioxidant properties related to phenolic compounds also were documented in extracts of branches, leaves, fruits, and seeds of guava trees [17,18].

According to reports, in the aforementioned studies, different solvents can be used for the extraction of phenolic compounds from guava leaves, but there is a possibility that these extracts present a risk to consumers. With respect to the toxicity of guava leaf extracts, Chen et al. [19] documented that ethanol and acetone extracts at concentrations greater than 100 μg/mL and 50 μg/mL, respectively, may present cytotoxicity, while aqueous extracts at concentrations lower than 500 μg/mL do not represent cytotoxicity.

The main phenolic compounds reported in guava leaves extracts are gallic acid, catechin, chlorogenic acid, caffeic acid, epicatechin, rutin, quercetin, kaempferol, and luteolin [20]. The phenolic compounds in guava leave extracts may vary depending on the variety, the way to dry the leaves, extraction technique, and the maturity of the leaves [16,21,22].

Consumption of antioxidants significantly decreases the adverse effects of some reactive oxygen and nitrogen species in the human body. The antioxidant capacity of the extracts can be measured by in vitro assays, which can be classified as either assays based on hydrogen atom transfer (HAT) or assays based on electron transfer (ET). The oxygen radical absorbance capacity (ORAC) is classified as HAT type assay, while 2,2-diphenyl-1-picrylhydrazyl (DPPH), total phenols, **2,2′-azino-bis(3-ethylbenzothiazoline-6-sulphonic acid)** (ABTS), and hydroxyl radicals are classified as electron transfer (ET)-type assays [23,24].

Total phenols, DPPH, hydroxyl radicals, and ABTS are the main assays that are carried out with the extracts of leaves form different varieties of *Psidium guajava*. Siwarungson et al. [22] used three varieties of *Psidium guajava* grown in Thailand, measuring total phenols, DPPH, and hydroxyl radicals. Jeong et al. [21] measured total phenolic compounds, ABTS, and DPPH in three varieties of *Psidium guajava* cultivated in Korea. These assays are used due to the versatility of the samples that can be analyzed from cell lines to nutrition lines, since it shows a premise of the structure and its relationship in the antioxidant activity of the compounds contained in the samples [25,26].

The objective of the present work was to quantify total polyphenols, total flavonoids, and the in vitro radical scavenging abilities of extracts obtained from Calvillo Siglo XXI and Hidrozac variety guava leaves. Currently, in Mexico these varieties do not have information regarding their content of total polyphenols, total flavonoids, and their antioxidant activity of their leaves. The only study that counts in Mexico of the variety Hidrozac and Calvillo is with its antioxidant activity of its fruit [27].

These varieties were registered in Mexico by the INIFAP (National Institute of Forestry, Agricultural and Livestock Research, Pabellón de Arteaga, Aguascalientes, México) in 2009 [4]. A difference between these two varieties is that Hidrozac produces pink pulp fruit while Calvillo Siglo XXI produces yellow pulp fruit. In the present work, it was found that there were significant differences in the amount of phenolic compounds and the radical scavenging abilities of Calvillo Siglo XXI and Hidrozac varieties. The correlation between total polyphenols and the radical scavenging abilities of the hydroxyl radicals and the ORAC test was positive.

2. Materials and Methods

2.1. Materials

Samples

The guava leaves were collected at the experimental site "Los cañones" of the INIFAP (National Institute of Forestry, Agricultural and Livestock Research), which is located in the municipality of Huanusco, Zacatecas, Mexico. Samples were collected 4 September 2015 and 24 August 2016. The coordinates of the collection site are longitude 21° 44.7′ N and 102° 58.0′ W to 1508 masl. Two varieties were selected, which are registered in the catalogue of vegetal varieties from 2009. Calvillo Siglo XXI no. GUA-005-160709 which produces yellow pulp fruits and Hidrozac no. GUA-002-160709 which produces pink pulp fruit. The collected leaves were dried in the shade and milled with a knife mill (PULVEX model 200, PULVEX SA. CV., Mexico City, Mexico) using a 0.8 mm diameter mesh. The ground material was stored in plastic bags in the dark at 22 °C prior to extraction.

2.2. Methods

2.2.1. Extractions

In all cases, regardless of the solvent used, the guava leaves were macerated under discontinuous stirring, with double extraction period (24 h × 2) at a solvent: sample ratio 10:1 (*v*/*w*). The samples collected in 2015 were subjected to extractions with solvents of different polarities: chloroform, acetone and water. For the extracts of the leaves collected in 2016, the samples were macerated only with water. The use of chloroform and acetone, and water, was to know the performance of the extracts before different solvents, and to know their composition in terms of total phenolic compounds and total flavonoids, as well as their antioxidant capacity. However, for the study of the leaves collected in 2016, it was decided to work only with water as a solvent, since it is the extract that would not present a possible toxicological effect, having the prospect of testing it on living organisms. In this way, we can have comparisons between the extracts obtained from the leaf collected both in 2015 and in 2016 using water as a solvent. Chloroform and acetone were recovered in a rotary evaporator (BM200, Yamato Scientific America Inc., Santa Clara, CA, USA) at 35 °C in a water bath, and the residual material was dried at 40 °C. The aqueous extract was dried using a nano spray dryer (B-90, BÜCHI Labortechnik AG, Flawil, Switzerland) using the following conditions: inlet temperature 105 °C, outlet temperature 38 °C, 90% sprinkler, and a 7 μm spray cap. Briefly, the liquid sample was fed to the spray head and droplets were generated by a piezoelectric driven actuator in a stainless steel membrane with holes of 7.0 μm inside the spray cap. The droplets were dried and the particles collected by electrostatic charging to deflect them to the collecting electrode. Nanometric particles were then collected. The dried extracts obtained for each solvent were stored in glass jars in the dark until use.

2.2.2. Total Phenolics

The total phenolic compounds were quantified using the methodology of Singleton et al. [28] and Taga et al. [29] with some modifications. 100 μg/mL of extracts was dissolved in 80% MeOH. Then, 100 μL of the solution was added to 100 μL of Folin–Ciocalteu reagent (1 N). This mix was stirred. After 3 min at rest, 2 mL of 2% *m/v* Na_2CO_3 was added and stirred and incubated in the dark for 30 min. Absorbance was then measured at 750 nm in a spectrophotometer UV–vis (LAMBDA 365, PerkinElmer, Inc., Waltham, MA, USA). The results were expressed as milligrams equivalent of gallic acid per gram of extract (mg GAE/g). Determinations were carried out in triplicate. A calibration curve was constructed using gallic acid at 0–4 μg.

2.2.3. Total Flavonoids

Quantification of flavonoids was carried out using the methodology of Dewanto et al. [30] with some modifications. 100 μg per mL of extracts were dissolved in 80% MeOH. After, 250 μL of the solution were added to 1.250 μL of H_2O, and 75 μL of $NaNO_2$ at 5% m/v. After 6 min 150 μL of 10% m/v $AlCl_3$ was added. After another 5 min 500 μL of 1 M NaOH and 275 μL of H_2O were added. Subsequently, absorbance was measured at 510 nm in a UV–vis spectrophotometer (LAMBDA 365, PerkinElmer, Inc., Waltham, MA, USA). Results were expressed as milligrams equivalent of quercetin per gram of extract (mg QE/g) and determinations were made in triplicate. A calibration curve was constructed using quercetin at 0–30 μg.

2.2.4. Hydroxyl Radicals

The ability to scavenge hydroxyl radicals was determined using the methodology of Smirnoff and Cumbes [31] and Zhang et al. [32], with some modifications. 8 mM $FeSO_4$, 3 Mm $C_7H_6O_3$, and 2% H_2O_2 were prepared with distilled water. The extracts were dissolved in **dimethyl sulfoxide** (DMSO) at a concentration of 500–3000 μg/mL. The reaction mixture consisted of 667 μL of extract, 200 μL of $FeSO_4$, 167 μL of H_2O_2, and 667 μL of $C_7H_6O_3$. The mixture was placed in a water bath for 30 min at 37 °C, before 299 μL of distilled water was added and the absorbance was measured (A1) at a wavelength of 510 nm on a UV–vis spectrophotometer (LAMBDA 365, PerkinElmer, Inc., Waltham, MA, USA). The ability to scavenge hydroxyl radicals was calculated using the following formula (1) used by Fu et al. [33]

$$\text{HO}\,\% = \frac{\text{A0} - (\text{A1} - \text{A2})}{\text{A0}} \times 100\% \quad (1)$$

where A0 is the absorbance of the control group (the sample solution was replaced with dilution solvent) and A2 the absorbance of the blank (H_2O and sample solution). The half maximal inhibitory concentration (IC_{50}) was calculated.

2.2.5. ABTS

The ABTS was measured according to the methodology of Re et al. [34] and Tachakittirungrod et al. [35] with some modifications. A calibration curve was generated with Trolox and results were expressed as TEAC (trolox equivalent antioxidant capacity). ABTS was dissolved in distilled water at a concentration of 7 mM and mixed with a 2.45 mM solution of potassium persulfate in water. The mixture was left to stand for 15 h in the dark to generate the radical solution ($ABTS\bullet^+$). For the tests, a fraction of the radical solution ($ABTS\bullet^+$) was prepared by adding MeOH until an absorbance of 0.7 ± 0.2 at a wavelength of 750 nm was reached. 180 μL of the radical solution ($ABTS\bullet^+$) was then mixed with 20 μL of extracts. After 5 min, absorbance was measured at a wavelength of 750 nm in a UV–vis spectrophotometer (LAMBDA 365, PerkinElmer, Inc., Waltham, MA, USA). The extracts were dissolved in MeOH at a concentration of 1 mg/mL.

2.2.6. DPPH

The assay was based on the method described by Brand-Williams [36], with some modifications. The reagents used as well as all the extracts were diluted with MeOH. The concentration of DPPH was 6×10^{-5} M and ascorbic acid was prepared at concentrations of 50–200 μg/mL. The extracts were prepared at concentrations of 50–1000 μg/mL. For the test, 100 μL of extract or ascorbic acid were mixed with 1900 μL of DPPH solution and held in the dark for 15 min. Absorbance was measured at a wavelength of 515 nm in a UV–vis spectrophotometer (LAMBDA 365, PerkinElmer, Inc., Waltham, MA, USA). Ascorbic acid was used as a control and was quantified at the half maximal inhibitory concentration (IC_{50}).

2.2.7. Oxygen Radical Absorbance Capacity Using Fluorescein (ORAC-FL)

The ORAC-FL test was conducted using the method described by Dávalos et al. [37] and Ou et al. [38] with some modifications. A 75 mM phosphate buffer solution (PH 7.4) was prepared. This buffer was used to prepare 70 nM fluorescein, 12 nM 2,2′-Azobis(2-amidinopropane) dihydrochloride (AAPH), and 2–8 μM Trolox. The extracts were diluted with 80% MeOH at a concentration of 10 μg/mL. The test was performed in a 96 well microplate. 120 μL of fluorescein was mixed with 20 μL of sample or trolox and incubated for 30 min at 37 °C. Subsequently, 60 μL of AAPH was added immediately. The fluorescence was measured every minute for 120 min, stirring automatically before each reading. A blank was prepared by replacing the antioxidant with phosphate buffer solution.

The area under the curve of fluorescence was calculated with Equation (2),

$$\mathrm{AUC} = 1 + \sum_{i=1}^{i=120} f_i/f_0 \tag{2}$$

where f_0 is the initial fluorescence read at time 0 and f_i is the fluorescence read at the time i. The net area under the curve (AUC) of samples was calculated by subtracting the AUC from the blank. Regression equations between net AUC and antioxidant concentration were calculated for all samples. A calibration curve was prepared with Trolox. The results were expressed as micromolar equivalents of Trolox for each microgram of extract (μM TE/μg). The measurements of fluorescence were performed at a temperature of 37 °C with an excitation wave of 485 nm and an emission wave of 520 nm in a spectral scanning multimode reader (Thermo Fisher Scientific, Waltham, MA, USA).

2.2.8. Statistical Analysis

All experiments were done in triplicate. The values were presented as the average ± SD (n = 3). Significant differences in the groups were determined by the analysis of variance using the Tukey Test HSD (honest significant difference) by homogeneous groups, calculated with Statistica software (version 7 Statistica Ink., Palo Alto, CA 94304, USA). $p < 0.05$ was considered statistically significant. Excel 2016 software (Microsoft Office 365, One Microsoft Way, Redmond, WA, USA) and JMP8 software (SAS, Cary, NC, USA) were used for correlation analysis.

3. Results

3.1. Total Phenolic and Total Flavonoid Compounds

Total polyphenols and total flavonoids were quantified in the aqueous, acetone, and chloroform extracts of both varieties of guava leaves.

3.1.1. Total Phenolic Compounds

Table 1 shows results of total phenolic compounds. Acetone had the greatest quantity of phenolic compounds for both varieties, followed by the aqueous fraction, and finally the chloroform fraction.

Between the two varieties, the chloroform extracts were statistically equivalent. In the acetone fraction, the extracts of Hidrozac had more phenolic compounds (374.63 mg GAE/g extract), whereas in the aqueous fraction Calvillo Siglo XXI had a greater quantity (242.10 mg GAE/g extract). The total phenolic compounds in the extract of the acetone fraction for both varieties was more than double the 141 mg EAG/g measured by You et al. [18] who also extracted with acetone for one night following maceration. The phenolic compounds obtained in our aqueous extracts were greater than those quantified by Seo et al. [15] from extracts boiled for 4 h in guava leaves (140 mg gallic acid equivalent (GAE)/g).

Table 1. Total polyphenols in the aqueous, acetone, and chloroform extracts of Calvillo Siglo XXI and Hidrozac leaves. The average values (±SD) are expressed as milligrams equivalent of gallic acid per gram of extract (mg GAE/g).

Extracts		Phenolic Compounds mg GAE/g Extract
Water 2016	Calvillo Siglo XXI	285.21 ± 35.54 [c,d]
	Hidrozac	256.76 ± 9.62 [c]
Water 2015	Calvillo Siglo XXI	242.10 ± 13.33 [c]
	Hidrozac	187.01 ± 9.24 [b]
Acetone 2015	Calvillo Siglo XXI	314.03 ± 8.05 [d]
	Hidrozac	374.63 ± 29.92 [e]
Chloroform 2015	Calvillo Siglo XXI	71.69 ± 3.69 [a]
	Hidrozac	100.03 ± 2.37 [a]

Different letters indicate significant differences ($p < 0.05$).

3.1.2. Total Flavonoids

Table 2 shows total extracted flavonoids. The extract with the greatest quantity of flavonoids, in general, was the acetone fraction, followed by the aqueous fraction, and finally the chloroform fraction. Between the two varieties, total flavonoid content in the chloroform fraction was statistically equivalent, while in the aqueous fraction and in the acetone fraction, Calvillo Siglo XXI had a greater quantity of total flavonoids. Total flavonoids in the aqueous fraction measured in our study was greater than the 50 mg QE value for aqueous extraction reported by Seo et al. [15]. Rattanachaikunsopon and Phumkhachorn [39] measured flavonoid contents of fresh and dry guava leaves by drying leaves for 72 h at 70 °C, extracting with methanol, and purifying using a chromatographic column. They found that flavonoid content was higher in dry leaves and that quercetin was the most abundant flavonoid.

Table 2. Total flavonoids in the aqueous, acetone and chloroform leaf extracts of the varieties Calvillo Siglo XXI and Hidrozac. The average values (±SD) are expressed as milligrams equivalent to quercetin per gram of extract (Mg QE/g).

Extracts	Total Flavonoids mg QE/g Extract
Water 2016 Calvillo Siglo XXI	180.77 ± 7.23 [d]
Hidrozac	152.61 ± 8.14 [c]
Water 2015 Calvillo Siglo XXI	108.54 ± 3.54 [b]
Hidrozac	77.83 ± 6.65 [a]
Acetone 2015 Calvillo Siglo XXI	239.45 ± 11.32 [e]
Hidrozac	135.88 ± 7.16 [c]
Chloroform 2015 Calvillo Siglo XXI	107.48 ± 13.30 [b]
Hidrozac	96.39 ± 4.57 [a,b]

Different letters indicate significant differences ($p < 0.05$).

3.2. *Radical Scavenging Ability In Vitro*

The assays for radical scavenging ability in vitro were conducted with aqueous, acetone, and chloroform leaf extracts of both guava varieties.

3.2.1. Hydroxyl Radicals

In general, the chloroform fraction had the lowest IC_{50}, followed by the aqueous fraction, and finally the acetone fraction (Table 3). Between the two varieties, chloroform or acetone showed no significant differences ($p < 0.05$), while the aqueous fraction did show significant differences ($p < 0.05$). The variety Calvillo Siglo XXI had a lower IC_{50} in both the aqueous and chloroform fractions, while the Hidrozac variety had the lowest IC_{50} in the acetone fraction. The IC_{50} values measured in the present work are up to 20 times higher than those values reported by Kim et al. [40] for aqueous extracts obtained by maceration for 24 h (110 μg/mL). A half maximal effective concentration (EC_{50}) of 5470–6700 for 50 μg/mL extracts was reported by Ademiluyi et al. [41], who used a mixture of MeOH and HCl for extraction of four different varieties of macerated guava.

Table 3. Hydroxyl radical scavenging ability in aqueous, acetone, and chloroform extracts of the leaves of Calvillo Siglo XXI and Calvillo. The average values (±SD) are expressed as half maximal inhibitory concentrations in micrograms per milliliter (IC_{50} μg/mL).

Extracts	Hydroxyl Radical Scavenging IC_{50} μg mL
Water 2016 Calvillo Siglo XXI	1607.81 ± 110.78 ^{b,c}
Hidrozac	2360.56 ± 104.80 ^{d}
Water 2015 Calvillo Siglo XXI	1726.51 ± 90.58 ^{c}
Hidrozac	2355.73 ± 60.07 ^{d}
Acetone 2015 Calvillo Siglo XXI	2416.04 ± 114.66 ^{d}
Hidrozac	2173.37 ± 108.42 ^{d}
Chloroform 2015 Calvillo Siglo XXI	1103.42 ± 28.62 ^{a}
Hidrozac	1355.08 ± 134.28 ^{b}

Different letters indicate significant differences ($p < 0.05$).

3.2.2. ABTS

The results of ABTS radical scavenging tests are described in Table 4. The results were expressed as the antioxidant capacity equivalent to a millimolar of trolox per milligram of extract (TEAC mM/mg). In general, the extracts with the greatest TEAC were obtained from acetone fractions, followed by the chloroform fractions, and finally the aqueous fractions. Between the two varieties, only the aqueous fraction showed significant differences ($p < 0.05$). In the study carried out by Díaz-De-Cerio et al. [42] with aqueous extracts of guava leaves obtained by sonication for 10 min and infusion at 3.5 and 7 min, TEAC values ranged from 0.18 to 1.13. The values from that study are two to four times lower than the aqueous fraction values measured in the present work.

Table 4. ABTS radical scavenging ability in the aqueous, acetone, and chloroform extracts of the leaves of Calvillo Siglo XXI and Hidrozac. The average values (±SD) are expressed as antioxidant capacity equivalent to a millimolar of trolox per milligram of extract (TEAC mM/mg).

Extracts	ABTS Radical Scavenging TEAC mM/mg
Water 2016 Calvillo Siglo XXI	2.64 ± 0.09 [b]
Hidrozac	3.34 ± 0.02 [c]
Water 2015 Calvillo Siglo XXI	2.37 ± 0.15 [a]
Hidrozac	4.10 ± 0.03 [d]
Acetone 2015 Calvillo Siglo XXI	5.28 ± 0.01 [f]
Hidrozac	5.24 ± 0.04 [f]
Chloroform 2015 Calvillo Siglo XXI	4.99 ± 0.02 [e]
Hidrozac	5.13 ± 0.02 [e,f]

Different letters indicate significant differences ($p < 0.05$); TEAC: trolox equivalent antioxidant capacity). ABTS: **2,2′-azino-bis(3-ethylbenzothiazoline-6-sulphonic acid).**

3.2.3. Radical DPPH

Table 5 shows the results of DPPH radical scavenging ability. The extracts with lower IC_{50} values were those obtained using acetone as a solvent. All the extracts in both varieties were significantly different ($p < 0.05$). The IC_{50} of the extracts of the acetone fraction obtained in this work was almost three times higher than IC_{50} values measured by You et al. [18] (34 μg/mL). The IC_{50} value of the aqueous fraction in the present work were also more than six times higher than the IC_{50} value measured from the aqueous fraction of guava leaves macerated for 24 h by Kim et al. [40] (120 μg/mL). IC_{50} values ranging from 730 to 910 μg/mL for extracts of four varieties of guava leaves macerated for 24 h using a mixture of MeOH/HCl have also been reported by Ademiluyi et al. [41], which are within the range measured in the present work.

Table 5. DPPH radical scavenging ability in the aqueous, acetone, and chloroform extracts of the leaves of Calvillo Siglo XXI and Hidrozac. The average values (±SD) are expressed as half maximal inhibitory concentration in micrograms per milliliter (IC_{50} μg/mL).

Extracts	DPP Radical Scavenging IC_{50} μg mL
Water 2016 Calvillo Siglo XXI	269.78 ± 12.89 [d]
Hidrozac	421.77 ± 13.17 [f]
Water 2015 Calvillo Siglo XXI	671.44 ± 16.36 [h]
Hidrozac	811.25 ± 7.74 [i]
Acetone 2015 Calvillo Siglo XXI	141.64 ± 1.66 [c]
Hidrozac	105.03 ± 1.70 [b]
Chloroform 2015 Calvillo Siglo XXI	385.15 ± 10.11 [e]
Hidrozac	608.32 ± 11.81 [g]
Ascorbic acid	78.60 ± 2.21 [a]

Different letters indicate significant differences ($p < 0.05$). DPP: 2,2-diphenyl-1-picrylhydrazyl radical.

3.2.4. ORAC-FL

The results of peroxyl scavenging ability were expressed as micromoles of trolox equivalents per microgram of extract (μm TE/μg) and are shown in Table 6. The extract with the greatest TE was the 2015 aqueous fraction of Calvillo Siglo XXI, with a value of 7.5 μM TE/μg. In general, the Calvillo Siglo XXI variety had larger values in water and acetone fractions than Hidrozac. In the chloroform fraction, no significant differences were observed ($p < 0.05$) for both varieties. It is worth mentioning that this is the first study reporting the use of ORAC to measure antioxidant capacity in extracts of guava leaves, obtaining interesting and complementary results to the measurement of antioxidant activity. This test can be recommended to study antioxidant capacity for both guava leaves and other extracts from different plant sources.

Table 6. Peroxyl radical scavenging ability in aqueous, acetone, and chloroform extracts of the leaves of Calvillo Siglo XXI and Hidrozac. The average values (±SD) are expressed as micromoles trolox equivalents per microgram of extract (μM TE/μg).

Extracts	Peroxyl Radical Scavenging μg TE/μg
Water 2016 Calvillo Siglo XXI	4.9 ± 0.75 ^{b,c}
Hidrozac	4.6 ± 0.80 ^{b,c}
Water 2015 Calvillo Siglo XXI	7.5 ± 0.73 ^{d}
Hidrozac	4.5 ± 0.87 ^{b}
Acetone 2015 Calvillo Siglo XXI	5.5 ± 0.65 ^{c}
Hidrozac	5.0 ± 0.25 ^{b,c}
Chloroform 2015 Calvillo Siglo XXI	2.1 ± 0.19 ^{a}
Hidrozac	2.1 ± 0.09 ^{a}

Different letters indicate significant differences ($p < 0.05$).

3.3. Correlation Analysis between Phenolic and Flavonoids Compounds and Radical Scavenging Ability

We observed a correlation between total phenolic compounds, total flavonoid compounds, ABTS, DPPH, radical hydroxyl, and ORAC test (Table 7). Comparing the correlation between the total flavonoids and the rest of the assays, the largest positive correlation was found with total phenolic compounds (0.61), followed by the hydroxyl radical test (0.38), and the ORAC value (0.31). The total flavonoids showed a strong negative correlation with the DPPH assay (−0.76). When total phenolic compounds were correlated with the rest of the assays, the greatest positive correlation was found against the ORAC assay (0.71), followed by the hydroxyl radical assay (0.69). Total phenolic compounds presented a strongly negative correlation with the DPPH assay (−0.59) and a weakly negative correlation with the ABTS assay (−0.15). Total phenolic compounds, ORAC value, and the hydroxyl radical (OH) assay had the highest positive correlations. This indicates that these assays are the most useful to measure antioxidant capacity in vitro from different extracts from leaves of *P. guajava* L. Chen et al. [43] reports a positive correlation between total polyphenols and other assays such as ABTS using guava leaf extracts. The negative correlation between the DPPH assay and total phenolics and total flavonoids found in this work also was reported by Ademiluyi et al. [41]. In addition, they reported a positive correlation between total phenolics and the ABTS assay, contrary to the data obtained in our research.

Table 7. Correlations between phenolic and flavonoid compounds and antioxidant properties of guava extracts.

	T.F.	T.P.	ABTS	DPPH	ORAC	OH
T.F.	1					
T.P.	0.61	1				
ABTS	0.06	−0.15	1			
DPPH	−0.76	−0.59	−0.35	1		
ORAC	0.31	0.71	−0.58	−0.04	1	
OH	0.38	0.69	0.01	−0.14	0.52	1

T.F. = Total flavonoids. T.P. = Total phenolics. OH = Hydroxyl radical. DPPH: 2,2-diphenyl-1-picrylhydrazyl; ORAC: Oxygen Radical Absorbance Capacity.

4. Conclusions

Significant differences in guava leaf extracts phenolic compound content and radical scavenging abilities were found between the varieties Calvillo Siglo XXI and Hidrozac. The phenolic and flavonoids contents as well as the ability to scavenging radicals were similar in both varieties, regardless of collection year. Extracts from guava leaves can donate electrons and hydrogen atoms, based on the results of the assays. Total polyphenol, hydroxyl radical, and ORAC assays are recommended for comparing differences between varieties. The novelty of this work is that there are no reports of tests with extracts of guava leaves from the varieties Hidrozac and Calvillo Siglo XXI. In addition, no work has been reported using the ORAC-FL trial with any variety of guava leaves. The results of this study will be complemented by a quantitative analysis of the phenolic compounds present in the different extracts by chromatographic methods. In addition, an in vivo test will be performed with rats in which aqueous extracts will be administered to evaluate their possible antihypertensive effect.

Acknowledgments: This work was supported by the Coordinación de la Investigación Científica Project 26.1 2016–2017 "Caracterización de un extracto de hojas de *Psidium guajava* L. y su efecto en los niveles de óxido nítrico y angiotensina ii en ratas espontáneamente hipertensas (SHR)". The team gratefully acknowledges the support of Consejo National de Ciencia y Tecnología (CONACYT) in the form of scholarship received for PhD studies. This research was partially supported with a nano spray-dryer acquired through project no. 253736 "Equipamiento para el fortalecimiento del grupo de investigación en caracterización de propiedades de los alimentos con impacto en los Programas Institucionales de Maestría y Doctorado en Ciencias Biológicas de la Universidad Michoacana de San Nicolás de Hidalgo—UMSNH", approved for author Héctor Eduardo Martínez-Flores in the program "Apoyo al Fortalecimiento y Desarrollo de la Infraestructura Científica y Tecnológica 2015" of the Consejo Nacional de Ciencia y Tecnología de México CONACYT. This project was also partially supported with a UV–vis spectrophotometer acquired through "Redes Temáticas de Colaboración Académica, Tercer año aprobado en la convocatoria 2011 (Marzo 2015), PRODEP", Red Materiales Nanoestructurados, Proyecto "Investigación y Desarrollo de Conductores Transparentes".

Author Contributions: Hector E. Martinez-Flores conceived and designed the experiments; Julio C. Camarena-Tello and Osvaldo Alvarez-Cortes performed the experiments; José S. Padilla-Ramírez contributed with the samples of the two varieties of *Psidium guajava* and discuss the data obtained during the experiments. Ma. G. Garnica-Romo contribute with the UV–vis equipment, reagents, materials, and analysis tools; Alfredo Saavedra-Molina, M. Carmen Bartolome-Camacho, and José O. Rodiles-López analyzed some of the results obtained in the experiments.

Conflicts of Interest: The authors declare no conflict of interest.

References

1. Lim, T.K. Psidium guajava. In *Edible Medicinal and Non-Medicinal Plants*; Springer Netherlands: New Delhi, India, 2012; Volume 3, pp. 684–727, ISBN 9789400725348.
2. SAGARPA. Aumenta 8.2 por ciento producción de guayaba en México en el último trienio. Available online: http://www.sagarpa.gob.mx/Delegaciones/distritofederal/boletines/Paginas/JAC_0006-3.aspx (accessed on 23 June 2017).
3. Pariona, A. Top Guava Producing Countries In The World—WorldAtlas.com. Available online: http://www.worldatlas.com/articles/top-guava-producing-countries-in-the-world.html (accessed on 11 October 2017).

4. Padilla Ramírez, J.S.; González-Gaona, E.; Perales de la Cruz, M.Á. Nuevas Variedades de Guayaba (*Psidium guajava*). Available online: http://biblioteca.inifap.gob.mx:8080/xmlui/handle/123456789/3454 (accessed on 14 June 2015).
5. Padilla-Ramírez, J.S.; González-Gaona, E.; Esquivel-Villagrana, F.; Mercado-Silva, E.; Hernández-Delgado, S.; Mayek-Pérez, N. Caracterización de germoplasma sobresaliente de guayabo de la región calvillo-cañones, méxico characterization. *Rev. Fitotécnica* **2002**, *25*, 393–399.
6. Martínez de Lara, J.; Barrientos-Lara, M.C.; Reyes de Anda, A.C.; Hernández-Delgado, S.; Padilla-Ramírez, J.S.; Mayek-Pérez, N. Diversidad fenotípica y genética en huertas de guayabo de calvillo, aguascalientes. *Rev. Fitotenica Mex.* **2004**, *27*, 243–249.
7. Tapia Pérez, D.; Porfirio Legaria, J.P. Variabilidad genética en cultivares de guayabo (*Psidium guajava* L.). *Rev. Fitotenica Mex.* **2007**, *30*, 391–401.
8. Pérez Gutierrez, R.M.; Mitchell, S.; Vargas Solis, R. *Psidium guajava*: A review of its traditional uses, phytochemistry and pharmacology. *J. Ethno-Pharmacol.* **2008**, *117*, 1–27. [CrossRef] [PubMed]
9. Díaz-De-Cerio, E.; Verardo, V.; Gómez-Caravaca, A.M.; Fernández-Gutiérrez, A.; Segura-Carretero, A. Exploratory characterization of phenolic compounds with demonstrated anti-diabetic activity in guava leaves at different Oxidation States. *Int. J. Mol. Sci.* **2016**, *17*, 699. [CrossRef] [PubMed]
10. Lozoya, X.; Reyes-Morales, H.; Chávez-Soto, M.A.; Martínez-García, M.D.C.; Soto-González, Y.; Doubova, S.V. Intestinal anti-spasmodic effect of a phytodrug of *Psidium guajava* folia in the treatment of acute diarrheic disease. *J. Ethnopharmacol.* **2002**, *83*, 19–24. [CrossRef]
11. Dai, J.; Mumper, R.J. Plant phenolics: Extraction, analysis and their antioxidant and anticancer properties. *Molecules* **2010**, *15*, 7313–7352. [CrossRef] [PubMed]
12. Brahmi, F.; Mechri, B.; Dabbou, S.; Dhibi, M.; Hammami, M. The efficacy of phenolics compounds with different polarities as antioxidants from olive leaves depending on seasonal variations. *Ind. Crops Prod.* **2012**, *38*, 146–152. [CrossRef]
13. DellaGreca, M.; Fiorentino, A.; Izzo, A.; Napoli, F.; Purcaro, R.; Zarrelli, A. Phytotoxicity of secondary metabolites from Aptenia cordifolia. *Chem. Biodivers.* **2007**, *4*, 118–128. [CrossRef] [PubMed]
14. Fiorentino, A.; DellaGreca, M.; D'Abrosca, B.; Oriano, P.; Golino, A.; Izzo, A.; Zarrelli, A.; Monaco, P. Lignans, neolignans and sesquilignans from Cestrum parqui l'Her. *Biochem. Syst. Ecol.* **2007**, *35*, 392–396. [CrossRef]
15. Seo, J.; Lee, S.; Elam, M.L.; Johnson, S.A.; Kang, J.; Arjmandi, B.H. Study to find the best extraction solvent for use with guava leaves (*Psidium guajava* L.) for high antioxidant efficacy. *Food Sci. Nutr.* **2014**, *2*, 174–180. [CrossRef] [PubMed]
16. Nantitanon, W.; Yotsawimonwat, S.; Okonogi, S. Factors influencing antioxidant activities and total phenolic content of guava leaf extract. *LWT Food Sci. Technol.* **2010**, *43*, 1095–1103. [CrossRef]
17. Barbalho, S.M.; Farinazzi-Machado, F.M.V.; Goulart, R.D.A.; Saad Brunnati, C.A.; Machado, A.M.; Ottoboni, B.; Teixeira, N. *Psidium guajava* (Guava): A Plant of Multipurpose Medicinal Applications. *Med. Aromat. Plants* **2012**, *1*, 1–6. [CrossRef]
18. You, D.-H.; Park, J.-W.; Yuk, H.-G.; Lee, S.-C. Antioxidant and tyrosinase inhibitory activities of different parts of guava (*Psidium guajava* L.). *Food Sci. Biotechnol.* **2011**, *20*, 1095–1100. [CrossRef]
19. Chen, H.-H. Hepatoprotective Effect of Guava (*Psidium guajava* L.) Leaf Extracts on Ethanol-Induced Injury on Clone 9 Rat Liver Cells. *Food Nutr. Sci.* **2011**, *2*, 983–988. [CrossRef]
20. Morais-Braga, M.F.B.; Carneiro, J.N.P.; Machado, A.J.T.; Sales, D.L.; dos Santos, A.T.L.; Boligon, A.A.; Athayde, M.L.; Menezes, I.R.A.; Souza, D.S.L.; Costa, J.G.M.; et al. Phenolic composition and medicinal usage of *Psidium guajava* Linn.: Antifungal activity or inhibition of virulence? *Saudi J. Biol. Sci.* **2017**, *24*, 302–313. [CrossRef] [PubMed]
21. Jeong, C.H.; Bae, Y.I.; Park, S.J.; Lee, S.K.; Hur, S.J. Antioxidant activities of aqueous extracts from three cultivars of guava leaf. *Food Sci. Biotechnol.* **2012**, *21*, 1557–1563. [CrossRef]
22. Siwarungson, N.; Ali, I.; Damsud, T. Comparative analysis of antioxidant and antimelanogenesis properties of three local guava (*Psidium guajava* L.) varieties of Thailand, via different extraction solvents. *J. Food Meas. Charact.* **2013**, *7*, 207–214. [CrossRef]
23. Prior, R.L. Oxygen radical absorbance capacity (ORAC): New horizons in relating dietary antioxidants/bioactives and health benefits. *J. Funct. Foods* **2015**, *18*, 797–810. [CrossRef]
24. Huang, D.; Ou, B.; Prior, R.L. The Chemistry behind Antioxidant Capacity Assays The Chemistry behind Antioxidant Capacity Assays. *J. Agric. Food Chem.* **2005**, *53*, 1841–1856. [CrossRef] [PubMed]

25. Barontini, M.; Bernini, R.; Carastro, I.; Gentili, P.; Romani, A. Synthesis and DPPH radical scavenging activity of novel compounds obtained from tyrosol and cinnamic acid derivates. *New J. Chem.* **2014**, *38*, 809–816. [CrossRef]
26. Bernini, R.; Barontini, M.; Cis, V.; Carastro, I.; Tofani, D.; Chiodo, R.A.; Lupattelli, P.; Incerpi, S. Synthesis and Evaluation of the Antioxidant Activity of Lipophilic Phenethyl Trifluoroacetate Esters by In Vitro ABTS, DPPH, and in Cell-Culture DCF Assays. *Molecules* **2018**, *23*, 208. [CrossRef] [PubMed]
27. Cortes-Penagos, C.J.; Cazares-Romero, A.; Flores-Alvarez, L.J.; Yahuaca-Juarez, B.; Padilla-Ramirez, J.S. Actividad antioxidante en cinco variedades de *Psidium guajava* L. *AGRO Product.* **2016**, *9*, 41–46.
28. Singleton, V.L.; Orthofer, R.; Lamuela-Raventos, R.M. Analysis of Total Phenols and Other Oxidation Substrates and Antioxidants by Means of Folin-Ciocalteu Reagent. *Methods Enzymol.* **1999**, *299*, 152–178.
29. Taga, M.S.; Miller, E.E.; Pratt, D.E. Chia seeds as a source of natural lipid antioxidants. *J. Am. Oil Chem. Soc.* **1984**, *61*, 928–931. [CrossRef]
30. Dewanto, V.; Wu, X.; Adom, K.K.; Liu, R.H. Thermal Processing Enhances the Nutritional Value of Tomatoes by Increasing Total Antioxidant Activity Thermal Processing Enhances the Nutritional Value of Tomatoes by Increasing Total Antioxidant Activity. *J. Agric. Food Chem.* **2002**, *50*, 3010–3014. [CrossRef] [PubMed]
31. Smirnoff, N.; Cumbes, Q. Hydroxyl radical scavenging activity of compatible solutes. *Phytochemistry* **1989**, *28*, 1057–1060. [CrossRef]
32. Zhang, D.; Wu, H.; Xia, Z.; Wang, C.; Cai, J.; Huang, Z.; Du, L.; Sun, P.; Xie, J. Partial characterization, antioxidant and antitumor activities of three sulfated polysaccharides purified from Bullacta exarata. *J. Funct. Foods* **2012**, *4*, 784–792. [CrossRef]
33. Fu, Z.F.; Tu, Z.C.; Zhang, L.; Wang, H.; Wen, Q.H.; Huang, T. Antioxidant activities and polyphenols of sweet potato (*Ipomoea batatas* L.) leaves extracted with solvents of various polarities. *Food Biosci.* **2016**, *15*, 11–18. [CrossRef]
34. Re, R.; Pellegrini, N.; Proteggente, A.; Pannala, A.; Yang, M.; Evans, C.R. Antioxidant Activity Applying an Improved Abts Radical. *Free Radic. Biol. Med.* **1999**, *26*, 1231–1237. [CrossRef]
35. Tachakittirungrod, S.; Ikegami, F.; Okonogi, S. Antioxidant active principles isolated from *Psidium guajava* grown in Thailand. *Sci. Pharm.* **2007**, *75*, 179–193. [CrossRef]
36. Brand-Williams, W.; Cuvelier, M.E.; Berset, C. Use of a free radical method to evaluate antioxidant activity. *LWT Food Sci. Technol.* **1995**, *28*, 25–30. [CrossRef]
37. Dávalos, A.; Gómez-Cordovés, C.; Bartolomé, B. Extending Applicability of the Oxygen Radical Absorbance Capacity (ORAC-Fluorescein) Assay. *J. Agric. Food Chem.* **2004**, *52*, 48–54. [CrossRef] [PubMed]
38. Ou, B.; Hampsch-woodill, M.; Prior, R.L. Development and Validation of an Improved Oxygen Radical Absorbance Capacity Assay Using Fluorescein as the Fluorescent Probe. Development and Validation of an Improved Oxygen Radical Absorbance Capacity Assay Using Fluorescein as the Fluorescent. *J. Agric. Food Chem.* **2001**, *49*, 4619–4626. [CrossRef] [PubMed]
39. Rattanachaikunsopon, P.; Phumkhachorn, P. Contents and antibacterial activity of flavonoids extracted from leaves of *Psidium guajava*. *J. Med. Plants Res.* **2010**, *4*, 393–396.
40. Kim, S.Y.; Kim, E.A.; Kim, Y.S.; Yu, S.K.; Choi, C.; Lee, J.S.; Kim, Y.T.; Nah, J.W.; Jeon, Y.J. Protective effects of polysaccharides from *Psidium guajava* leaves against oxidative stresses. *Int. J. Biol. Macromol.* **2016**, *91*, 804–811. [CrossRef] [PubMed]
41. Ademiluyi, A.O.; Oboh, G.; Ogunsuyi, O.B.; Oloruntoba, F.M. A comparative study on antihypertensive and antioxidant properties of phenolic extracts from fruit and leaf of some guava (*Psidium guajava* L.) varieties. *Comp. Clin. Path.* **2016**, *25*, 363–374. [CrossRef]
42. Díaz-De-Cerio, E.; Verardo, V.; Gómez-Caravaca, A.M.; Fernández-Gutiérrez, A.; Segura-Carretero, A. Determination of polar compounds in guava leaves infusions and ultrasound aqueous extract by HPLC-ESI-MS. *J. Chem.* **2015**, *2015*. [CrossRef]
43. Chen, H.Y.; Yen, G.C. Antioxidant activity and free radical-scavenging capacity of extracts from guava (*Psidium guajava* L.) leaves. *Food Chem.* **2007**, *101*, 686–694. [CrossRef]

5

Sex-Specificity of Oxidative Stress in Newborns Leading to a Personalized Antioxidant Nutritive Strategy

Jean-Claude Lavoie [1,*] and André Tremblay [2]

1 Department of Nutrition, Faculty of Medicine, Université de Montréal, Sainte-Justine Hospital, Montréal, QC H3T 1C5, Canada

2 Department Obstetrics & Gynecology, and department of Biochemistry and Molecular Medicine, Faculty of Medicine, University of Montreal, Sainte-Justine Hospital, Montréal, QC H3T 1C5, Canada; andre.tremblay@recherche-ste-justine.qc.ca

* Correspondence: jean-claude.lavoie@umontreal.ca

Abstract: Oxidative stress is a critical process that triggers several diseases observed in premature infants. Growing recognition of the detriment of oxidative stress in newborns warrants the use of an antioxidant strategy that is likely to be nutritional in order to restore redox homeostasis. It appears essential to have a personalized approach that will take into account the age of gestation at birth and the sex of the infant. However, the link between sex and oxidative stress remains unclear. The aim of this study was to find a common denominator explaining the discrepancy between studies related to sex-specific effects of oxidative stress. Results highlight a specificity of sex in the levels of oxidative stress markers linked to the metabolism of glutathione, as measured in the intracellular compartments. Levels of all sex-dependent oxidative stress markers are greater and markers associated to a better antioxidant defense are lower in boys compared to girls during the neonatal period. This sex-specific discrepancy is likely to be related to estrogen metabolism, which is more active in baby-girls and promotes the activation of glutathione metabolism. Conclusion: our observations suggest that nutritive antioxidant strategies need to target glutathione metabolism and, therefore, should be personalized considering, among others, the sex specificity.

Keywords: sex; gender; oxidative stress marker; newborn; prematurity; glutathione; personalized medicine; antioxidant nutrition

---

1. Introduction

Most newborn infants are at risk of oxidative injury following the swift exposure to an oxidant environment at the time of their first breaths, when the partial pressure of oxygen increases suddenly from 35 (umbilical vein) to 85 mmHg (arterial) [1–3]. However, this tremendous impulse stimulates several transcription factors (i.e., NFκB and Nrf2) favouring in hours or days, the elevation of endogenous antioxidant defense mechanisms [4,5]. Beyond this stimulation, the general antioxidant capacity [6,7] of preterm newborns remains lower than in term newborns, as suggested by higher levels of oxidative stress markers [8]. The oxidative stress in preterm neonates is frequently explained by a metabolic immaturity or by clinical treatments, such as oxygen supplementation and parenteral nutrition [9]. This situation has been a long-time concern to research teams since this stress is associated with several chronic diseases observed in this population, including bronchopulmonary dysplasia (BPD), necrotizing enterocolitis (NEC), retinopathy of prematurity (ROP) and cerebral haemorrhage [10,11]. Intense research is currently under progress to find ways to prevent oxidative stress in premature infants, and consequently to reduce the incidence of these pathologies. Eventually, an antioxidant therapy easily based on quality of nutrition will emerge. This would be likely performed under a personalized approach according to the age of gestation at birth or to the degree of oxidative stress. Should the sex of the newborn be considered in this definition of personalized antioxidant therapy? It is well known that the sex of the infant is a contributing factor to the incidence of these diseases [12]. For instance, the incidence of BPD [13,14], cerebral palsy and cognitive delay [15], ROP [10,15], among others, are reported to be higher in male infants.

The mathematical logic language suggests that if oxidative stress is at the base of these diseases and that sex of the infant is a contributing factor, then oxidative stress could be different according to the sex (defined here as biological value in contrast to "gender" that has a social value) of the newborn. The confirmation of this mathematical conclusion could influence future clinical personalised practice. Therefore, the purpose of this article is to review what it is known about oxidative stress in the newborn in respect to the sex. On this topic, scientific literature lacks consistency. The discrepancies may arise from the abundance of reported oxidative stress markers as well as biological compartments where they have been measured. The objective was to find a common denominator explaining why some studies document, and others not, differences between sex on oxidative stress markers during neonatal period of infants born at term or preterm.

2. Methods

In the present narrative review, literature assessment was undertaken in early 2018 on PubMed. The first search, including the filter "human", with the following keywords: oxidative stress AND (sex OR gender) AND newborn AND (preterm OR premature OR prematurity), has generated 17 articles. The term "sex or gender" was a great filter since without these two words, the search generated 496 articles. This first assessment, without limit of date of publication, suggested that "oxidative stress" was the first outcome of the investigations, and that the "sex" factor was very secondary. Another reason was that the investigators did not observe differences linked to the sex in their oxidative stress studies and they did not write "sex" or "gender" as keyword.

The search was enriched with the keyword "male OR female" in order to identify studies where the sex of the infants had been monitored. Thus, with the following keywords "oxidative stress AND (sex OR gender OR male OR female) AND newborn AND (preterm OR premature OR prematurity)" the search has generated 275 articles. From them, following reading of title or abstract, 38 were retained for the present article.

3. Results

Studies presented in Table 1 have been separated in three sections: studies with no reported comparison between sexes, studies of which the comparison did not reveal a statistical difference, and studies reporting a statistical difference between sexes. For each category, data were subsequently divided according to tissues where markers (of oxidative stress or antioxidant capacity or antioxidant defense) were measured.

A first observation was that difference according to the sex seemed to be linked to the studied tissues. Excepted for $F_2\alpha$-Isoprostane of which levels were reported to be sex dependent in two studies out of eight, data suggest that if sex-specific difference exists, it is not found in plasma, urine or bronchoalveolar fluids, which are considered extracellular compartments. In contrast, the difference according to the sex in oxidative stress markers was observed in tissues considered as intracellular compartments, such as erythrocytes, leukocytes, umbilical cord vein and placenta.

For the second observation, Table 1 has been redesigned (Table 2) to present data according to the character of the markers: radical (protein radical injury, lipid radical injury, DNA radical injury, global radical scavenging capacity, uric acid, vitamin A-C-E) or non-radical (glutathione metabolism, cellular uptake of cysteine, superoxide dismutase SOD). Among the 17 radical markers reported, only $F_2\alpha$-Isoprostane (reported by two studies out of eight), and protein radical markers and hydroperoxide content in placenta reported by one study, were found as sex-dependent. In contrast, items related to the metabolism of glutathione (glutathione, glutathione peroxidase (GPx), glutathione reductase (GSSG-R), glutathione S-transferase (GST), cellular uptake of cysteine) have been found as sex-dependent, and this in blood cells, placenta and in an umbilical cord vein model.

Finally, a third observation concerns the sex comparison by itself. Levels of all sex-dependent oxidative stress markers are greater and all markers associated to a better antioxidant defense are lower in boys compared to girls during the neonatal period of life.

Table 1. Studies in function of the type of comparisons reported between sexes.

Tissues: Markers	**Studies without Comparison between Sexes**	**No Statistically Difference between Sexes**	**Statistically Difference between Sexes**	
Plasma/serum:				
$F_{2\alpha}$-isoprostane	[16–18]		M > F	[19,20]
MDA/aldehydes	[21,22]	[20]		
TBARS	[23]	[24]		
Hydroperoxides	[25]	[20]		
Protein carbonyl	[18]			
Nitrotyrosine	[18]			
Ascorbyl radical	[26]			
DNA damage	[27]			
TOS	[28]	[24]		
TAC	[28]	[19,29]		
TAOC	[17,30]	[24]		
FRAP		[24]		
Glutathione	[31]			
SOD	[16,30]			
GPx	[30]			
Vitamin C	[32,33]			
Vitamins E, A	[32]			
Erythrocytes/cord blood/peripheral blood:				
TBARS	[23]			
Redox potential of glutathione	[8,9]			
Se		[34]		
GPx	[28]	[34,35]	M < F	[36]
GSSG-R		[35]	M < F	[36]
GST		[35]	M < F	[37]
CuZnSOD		[34]		
Urine:				
$F_{2\gamma}$-isoprostane	[8,16,38]			
8-OHdG	[38–42]			
Dityrosine	[8]			
Peroxides	[43]			
Bronchoalveolar lavage fluide/tracheobronchial aspirate fluid/airway aspirates:				
MDA	[13]			
Protein carbonyl	[44]			
TAA	[45]			
Vitamin C	[44]			
Acid uric	[44,45]			

Table 1. *Cont.*

Tissues: Markers	Studies without Comparison between Sexes	No Statistically Difference between Sexes	Statistically Difference between Sexes	
Umbilical cord vein:				
Glutathione			[a] Exposed to tBH: efflux M > F	[46]
Leukocytes isolated from tracheal aspirate:				
Glutathione			M < F	[6]
Glutathione synthesis		[47]		
GSSG-R			Exposed to $FiO_2 > 0.25$: M < F	[6]
γ-GT		[47]		
Cysteine uptake			M < F in Pre-term	[48]
Placenta:				
Protein carbonyl			M > F	[49]
Hydroperoxides			M > F	[49]
Nitrotyrosine			M > F	[49]
GPx			M < F	[49]

FRAP: Ferric reducing ability of plasma; GPx: glutathione peroxidase; GSSG-R: Disulfide glutathione reductase; GST: Glutathione S-transferase; γ-GT: gamma-glutamyltranspeptidase; MDA: malondialdehyde; 8-OHdG: 8-hydroydeoxy-guanosine; SOD: superoxide dismutase; TAA: Total antioxidant activity; TAC: Total antioxidant capacity; TAOC: Total antioxidant capacity; TBARS: thiobarbituric acid reactive substance; TOS: Total oxidant status; [a] Umbilical cord vein infused with *tert*-butylhydroxyperoxide, efflux of glutathione.

Table 2. Studied tissues in function of the type of oxidative stress markers (designed from Table 1).

Oxidative Stress Markers	Studied Tissues, Sex Effect Not Reported	Studied Tissues, Sex Effect Reported	Results
Radical injury/protein:			
Carbonyl	A.F.; [a] plasma	placenta	M > F
NitroTyrosine	plasma	placenta	M > F
Dityrosine	urine		
Radical injury/lipid:			
$F_2\alpha$-isoprostane	Urine [b] (3); plasma (3)	Plasma (2)	M > F
MDA/aldehydes	A.F.; plasma	Plasma	[c] =
TBARS	A.F.; plasma	Plasma	=
Radical injury/DNA:			
8-OHdG	Urine (5)		
Radical scavenging capacity/global:			
TOS	plasma	Plasma	=
TAC	plasma	Plasma (2)	=
TAOC	plasma	Plasma	=
TAA	A.F.		
FRAP		Plasma	=
Others radical markers:			
Vitamin C	A.F.; plasma		
Vitamin E, A	Plasma (2)		
Ascorbyl radical	Plasma		
Uric acid	A.F. (2)		

Table 2. *Cont.*

Oxidative Stress Markers	Studied Tissues, Sex Effect Not Reported	Studied Tissues, Sex Effect Reported	Results
Glutathione metabolism:			
Glutathione	Plasma	Umbilical cord vein	[d] loss: M > F
		Leukocytes	M < F
Redox	[e] Erythrocyte (2)		
Se		Erythrocyte	=
GPx	Erythrocyte; plasma	Erythrocyte (3);	M < F (2); = (1)
		Placenta	M < F
GSSG-R		Leukocyte	M < F
		Erythrocyte	M < F
GST		Erythrocyte (2)	M < F; =
γ-GT		Leukocyte	=
GSH synthesis		Leukocyte	=
Cysteine uptake		Leukocyte	M < F
Others non radical markers:			
CuZnSOD	Plasma (2)	Erythrocyte	=
[f] Peroxides	Plasma; Urine	Placenta	M > F

A.F.: Airway fluid, includes Bronchoalveolar lavage lavage or fluid/tracheobronchial aspirate fluid /airway aspirates fluid; FRAP: Ferric reducing ability of plasma; GPx: glutathione peroxidase; GSSG-R: Disulfide glutathione reductase; GST: Glutatione S-transferase; γ-GT: gamma-glutamyltranspeptidase; MDA: malondialdehyde; 8-OHdG: 8-hydroydeoxy-guanosine; SOD: superoxide dismutase; TAA: Total antioxidant activity; TAC: Total antioxidant capacity; TAOC: Total antioxidant capacity; TBARS: thiobarbituric acid reactive substance; TOS: Total oxidant status; [a] All-time, "Plasma" could include "serum"; [b] The number in parentheses indicates the number of studies when more than one; [c] =: no difference between F and M; [d] Umbilical cord vein infused with *tert*-butylhydroxyperoxide, efflux of glutathione; [e] "Erythrocyte" can include "red blood cell" and "whole blood"; [f] "Peroxide" could include "hydroperoxide" or "total peroxide".

4. Discussion

The principal outcome of the majority if not all assessed articles was to document the presence or not of oxidative stress in the neonatal population, which is not the purpose of the present article. Thus, experiments were not firstly designed to reach a sufficient statistical power to find a sex related difference. So, we must be careful in the fine interpretation of our observations. However, from the point of view of difference according to sex, the clear separation between extracellular and intracellular compartments as well as between radical versus non-radical markers of oxidative stress is remarkable. The few studies of sex-according differences observed in the extracellular compartments can be explained by the fact that these tissues represent a transit reservoir for waste cell products before their elimination, such as metabolites generated after a radical injury. These dynamic changes could not be enough sensitive to observe a difference between sexes. On the other hand, the most frequent observation of sex-according differences was done on glutathione and enzymes or systems in relation to glutathione. Glutathione metabolism is mainly an intracellular process. It controls the intracellular levels of peroxides (via GPx), aldehydes (via GST) and even radicals (via regeneration of oxidized vitamins C and E); thus, changes in glutathione metabolism could also explain the sex-specific differences reported for $F_2\alpha$-Isoprostane. The high significance between studies cited here on the difference between sexes suggests a different capacity of newborns to cope with an oxidative environment depending of their sex. Therefore, our suggestion from the mathematical logic conclusion outlined in the Introduction that the "oxidative stress could be different according to the sex" appears to be substantiated. Each data reporting a difference according to sex shows higher levels of oxidative stress markers and a lower antioxidant capacity (related to glutathione metabolism) in boys compared to girls. This observation, in line with the fact that the prevalence of diseases in baby boys is higher than in girls [12], suggest that an improvement of glutathione status could prevent or at least reduce prevalence of these diseases.

Glutathione defense is specialized in peroxide detoxification. Thus, with less effective glutathione metabolism, one can expect that males or cells from male infants are more susceptible to injury by peroxides. As part of the studies undertaken to understand the clinical impact of exposing newborn infants to an oxidant environment (such as the one occurring during specific clinical treatments), one was designed more than twenty years ago to assess the impact of peroxides on endothelial production of eicosanoids [46]; by this time the sex was already suspected to be an active factor. The experimental design was a 3.5 h perfusion of umbilical cord vein (from term infants born after repeated Cesarean sections) with a nutritive solution containing or not (control) organic peroxide (*tert*-butylhydroperoxide). Eluates were collected each hour. The pattern of release of the four eicosanoids and glutathione differed according to whether the umbilical cord vein derived from boys or girls. The glutathione release was not affected by peroxide in veins derived from girls, whereas the veins from boys were losing their glutathione content. This study revealed that the equilibrium between peroxides and glutathione differed between sexes. This difference according to the sex of the infants was also emphasized few years later by the demonstration that a short exposure (3–4 h) to *tert*-butylhydroperoxide induced the mortality of endothelial cells isolated from umbilical cord vein from infants born at term in primary culture; the mortality was higher when cells were derived from boys [6]. These two studies underline the relative fragility to an oxidative environment of cells from boys at time of birth.

Infant mortality is well known to be higher among boys. For instance, the World Health Organization reported that, in 2010, the prevalence rate was of 48 vs. 45/1000 births (M vs. F) in the world [50]; without China and India, the rates were 52 vs. 44/1000 births (M vs. F) [50]. The difference according to sex seems receded in function of time after birth in term infants. In situation reminiscent to the previous cited studies [6,46] concerning umbilical cord vein endothelial cells exposed to peroxides, infants born before 32 weeks of gestation are also routinely exposed to peroxides during the time of their parenteral nutrition. Indeed, parenteral nutrition is contaminated with high levels of peroxides [43,51,52]. These peroxides are strongly suspected to be at the origin of several diseases observed in this population. A recent meta-analysis [53] compared clinical outcomes of premature newborns according to whether or not their parenteral nutrition formula was photo-protected. Adequate protection against ambient light reduces by half the generation of peroxide in the parenteral nutrition [43,51,52]. The photo protection was associated to a 50% reduction in mortality at 36 weeks post-menstrual age. In girls, the reduction was from 11 to 4% whereas in boys, it was from 20 to 9%; note that the difference according to sex remained.

The literature has abundantly reported a high oxidative stress in preterm infants, and that stress is associated with several pathological complications observed in this population. Although the sex factor is well described for these diseases, the discrepancies between sex and oxidative stress cast doubt on the link between these parameters. Our observation reinforces the concept of the existence of a difference due to the sex of the newborn by specifying the type of markers to be monitored and in which biological compartment does it occur. The fact that the specific marker to follow is linked to glutathione metabolism suggests a role for estrogens to prevent or at least diminish undesired responses to oxidative stress. Indeed, circulating estrogen concentrations are very high during foetal development mostly due to the foetal adrenal contribution of precursor DHEA (dehydroepiandrostenedione) and subsequent placental conversion to estrogen [54]. As such, estrogens are clearly associated with embryogenesis and intrauterine sexual development. In addition, cellular effects to circulating estrogens are mainly dependent on the respective contribution of estrogen receptors ERα and ERβ, of which sex-specific differences in terms of their expression levels were reported [55–57]. Estrogen receptors have been shown to directly induce genes associated to cellular responses to oxidative stress, such as glutathione peroxidase, in foetal and adult tissues, strongly supporting a role of estrogen in the protection against oxidative stress [58–60]. Hormone activation of estrogen receptors also contributed to enhance the response of transcription factors Nrf2 and NFκB, resulting in induced expression of several genes encoding for antioxidant enzymes involved in glutathione metabolism [61–63].

Because there is increasing evidence on the importance of a fine regulation of homeostasis between oxidant and antioxidant molecules for a healthy development, the antioxidant strategies must be an essential part of clinical practice. This clinical approach should be personalized according, among others, to the sex of the newborn. Our observations suggest that these strategies should target glutathione metabolism. Certainly, one way to be favoured in the application of a personalized antioxidant strategy is enrichment of mother milk or parenteral nutrition, according to the mode of nutrition needed by the newborn. Human milk is known to have antioxidant properties since oxidative stress markers are lower in infants fed with human milk compared to infant formulas [64]. This property seems to depend, at least in part, from short peptides generated during digestion of milk by the baby. Thus, a promising approach would be to enrich the milk with specific hexapeptides as those generated following mimicking digestion of human milk [65]. These peptides have been demonstrated to have excellent antioxidant properties in vitro [65] and in vivo where they promote a glutathione increase [66]. However, further studies are needed to validate the benefit of such enrichment of milk formulas and possibly of human milk in order to improve antioxidant defense especially in preterm newborns. To reduce the incidence of bronchopulmonary dysplasia by improving glutathione status in premature infants (those on parenteral nutrition), several studies have tested the addition of cysteine (limiting amino acid for synthesis of glutathione) or N-acetylcysteine (precursor of cysteine). A meta-analysis underlined the failure of these approaches as much for glutathione level as for the chronic lung disease [67]. Others have proposed to infuse glutathione to prevent oxidative stress and lung damage in newborn animals exposed to high levels of oxygen [68]. Based on the fact that glutathione by itself has for a long-time been recognized to be a physiological pool of cysteine [69], a recent animal study has considered glutathione as a physiologic precursor of cysteine [70]. The enrichment of the intravenous solution with glutathione prevented the negative impacts of peroxides generated in parenteral nutrition on the oxidative stress, glutathione status, and lung integrity [70].

5. Conclusions

The importance of redox biology in health [71,72], as well as the increasing evidence for long-term influence of oxidative stress undergone early in life [73,74], supports the development of antioxidant approaches, especially during the neonatal period. The prevention of oxidative stress at this age is critical to warrant a healthy development throughout the whole life. Hence, the concept developed here strongly suggests that this approach should be personalized by including the sex specificity.

Acknowledgments: This work was supported by a grant from the Canadian Institutes of Health Research (PJT-148522).

Author Contributions: Jean-Claude Lavoie realized the conception of the research, article collection, and interpretation. André Tremblay contributed to completion of article collection, and interpretation of data. The two authors agree to ensuring that questions related to the accuracy or integrity of any part of the work, even ones in which the author was not personally involved, are appropriately investigated, resolved, and documented in the literature.

Conflicts of Interest: The authors declare no conflict of interest.

References

1. Murphy, P.J. The fetal circulation. Continuing Education in Anaesthesia. *Crit. Care Pain* **2005**, *5*, 107–112.
2. Dear, P.R. Monitoring oxygen in the newborn: Saturation of partial pressure? *Arch. Dis. Child.* **1987**, *62*, 879–881. [CrossRef] [PubMed]
3. Weisberg, H.F. Acid-Base Pathophysiology in the neonate and infant. *Ann. Clin. Lab. Sci.* **1982**, *12*, 245–253. [PubMed]

4. Pall, M.L.; Levine, S. Nrf2, a master regulator of detoxification and also antioxidant, anti-inflammatory and other cytoprotective mechanisms, is raised by health promoting factors. *Sheng Li Xue Bao* **2015**, *67*, 1–18. [PubMed]
5. Laughlin, M.H.; Simpson, T.; Sexton, W.L.; Brown, O.R.; Smith, J.K.; Korthuis, R.J. Skeletal muscle oxidative capacity, antioxidant enzymes, and exercise training. *J. Appl. Physiol.* **1985**, *6*, 2337–2343. [CrossRef] [PubMed]
6. Lavoie, J.C.; Chessex, P. Gender and maturation affect glutathione status in human neonatal tissues. *Free Radic. Biol. Med.* **1997**, *23*, 648–657. [CrossRef]
7. Rogers, S.; Witz, G.; Anwar, M.; Hiatt, M.; Hegyi, T. Antioxidant capacity and oxygen radical diseases in the preterm newborn. *Arch. Pediatr. Adolesc. Med.* **2000**, *154*, 544–548. [CrossRef] [PubMed]
8. Chessex, P.; Watson, C.; Kaczala, G.; Rouleau, T.; Lavoie, M.E.; Friel, J.; Lavoie, J.C. Determinants of oxidant stress in extremely low birth weight premature infants. *Free Radic. Biol. Med.* **2010**, *49*, 1380–1386. [CrossRef] [PubMed]
9. Mohamed, I.; Elremaly, W.; Rouleau, T.; Lavoie, J.C. Oxygen and parenteral nutrition—Two main oxidants—For extremely preterm infants: 'it all adds up. *J. Neonatal Perinatal Med.* **2015**, *8*, 189–197. [CrossRef] [PubMed]
10. Lee, J.W.; Davis, J.M. Future applications of antioxidants in premature infants. *Curr. Opin. Pediatr.* **2011**, *23*, 161–166. [CrossRef] [PubMed]
11. Perrone, S.; Tataranno, M.L.; Negro, S.; Cornacchione, S.; Longini, M.; Proietti, F.; Soubasi, V.; Benders, M.J.; Van Bel, F.; Buonocore, G. May oxidative stress biomarkers in cord blood predict the occurrence of necrotizing enterocolitis in preterm infants? *J. Matern. Fetal Neonatal Med.* **2012**, *25* (Suppl. 1), 128–131. [CrossRef] [PubMed]
12. Glass, H.C.; Costarino, A.T.; Stayer, S.A.; Brett, C.; Cladis, F.; Davis, P.J. Outcomes for extremely premature infants. *Anesth. Analg.* **2015**, *129*, 1337–1351. [CrossRef] [PubMed]
13. Madoglio, R.J.; Rugolo, L.M.S.S.; Kurokawa, C.S.; Sa, M.P.A.; Lyra, J.C.; Autunes, L.C.O. Inflammatory and oxidative stress airway markers in premature newborns of hypertensive mothers. *Braz. J. Med. Biol. Res.* **2016**, *49*, e5160. [CrossRef] [PubMed]
14. Kiciński, P.; Kęsiak, M.; Nowiczewski, M.; Gulczyńska, E. Bronchopulmonary dysplasia in very and extremely low birth weight infants - analysis of selected risk factors. *Pol. Merkur. Lekarski.* **2017**, *42*, 71–75. [PubMed]
15. Ludwig, C.A.; Chen, T.A.; Hernandez-Boussard, T.; Moshfeghi, A.A.; Moshfeghi, D.M. The Epidemiology of Retinopathy of Prematurity in the United States. *Ophthalmic Surg. Lasers Imaging Retina* **2017**, *48*, 553–562. [CrossRef] [PubMed]
16. Inayat, M.; Bany-Mohammed, F.; Valencia, A.; Tay, C.; Jacinto, J.; Aranda, J.V.; Beharry, K.D. Antioxidants and Biomarkers of Oxidative Stress in Preterm Infants with Symptomatic Patent Ductus Arteriosus. *Am. J. Perinatol.* **2015**, *32*, 895–904. [CrossRef] [PubMed]
17. Minghetti, L.; Suppiej, A.; Greco, A.; Franzoi, M.; Pascoli, I.; Zanardo, V. Oxidative stress in twin neonates is influenced by birth weight and weight discordance. *Clin. Biochem.* **2011**, *44*, 654–658. [CrossRef] [PubMed]
18. Ballard, P.L.; Truog, W.E.; Merrill, J.D.; Gow, A.; Posencheg, M.; Golombek, S.G.; Parton, L.A.; Luan, X.; Cnaan, A.; Ballard, R.A. Plasma biomarkers of oxidative stress: Relationship to lung disease and inhaled nitric oxide therapy in premature infants. *Pediatrics* **2008**, *121*, 555–561. [CrossRef] [PubMed]
19. Minghetti, L.; Greco, A.; Zanardo, V.; Suppiej, A. Early-life sex-dependent vulnerability to oxidative stress: The natural twining model. *J. Matern. Fetal Neonatal Med.* **2013**, *26*, 259–262. [CrossRef] [PubMed]
20. Qui, Y.; Wang, C.C.; Kuhn, H.; Rathmann, J.; Pang, C.P.; Rogers, M.C. Determinants of umbilical cord arterial 8-iso-prostaglandin F2alpha concentrations. *BJOG* **2000**, *107*, 973–981.
21. Ogihara, T.; Hirano, K.; Morinobu, T.; Kim, H.S.; Hiroi, M.; Ogihara, H.; Tamai, H. Raised concentrations of aldehyde lipid peroxidation products in premature infants with chronic lung disease. *Arch. Dis. Child. Fetal Neonatal Ed.* **1999**, *80*, F21–F25. [CrossRef] [PubMed]
22. Yiğit, S.; Yurdakök, M.; Kilinç, K.; Oran, O.; Erdem, G.; Tekinalp, G. Serum malondialdehyde concentration as a measure of oxygen free radical damage in preterm infants. *Turk. J. Pediatr.* **1998**, *40*, 177–183. [PubMed]
23. Gathwala, G.; Sharma, S. Phototherapy induces oxidative stress in premature neonates. *Indian J. Gastroenterol.* **2002**, *21*, 153–154. [PubMed]

24. Musilova, I.; Tothova, L.; Menon, R.; Vlkova, B.; Celec, P.; Hornychova, H.; Kutova, R.; Andrys, C.; Stepan, M.; Kacerovsky, M. Umbilical cord blood markers of oxidative stress in pregnancies complicated by preterm prelabor rupture of membranes. *J. Matern. Fetal Neonatal Med.* **2016**, *29*, 1900–1910. [CrossRef] [PubMed]
25. Buonocore, G.; Perrone, S.; Longini, M.; Vezzosi, P.; Marzocchi, B.; Paffetti, P.; Bracci, R. Oxidative stress in preterm neonates at birth and on the seventh day of life. *Pediatr. Res.* **2002**, *52*, 46–49. [CrossRef] [PubMed]
26. Ahola, T.; Fellman, V.; Kjellmer, I.; Raivio, K.O.; Lapatto, R. Plasma 8-isoprostane is increased in preterm infants who develop bronchopulmonary dysplasia or periventricular leukomalacia. *Pediatr. Res.* **2004**, *56*, 88–93. [CrossRef] [PubMed]
27. Norishadkam, M.; Andishmand, S.; Zavar Reza, J.; Zare Sakhvidi, M.J.; Hachesoo, V.R. Oxidative stress and DNA damage in the cord blood of preterm infants. *Mutat. Res.* **2017**, *824*, 20–24. [CrossRef] [PubMed]
28. Dizdar, E.A.; Uras, N.; Oguz, S.; Erdeve, O.; Sari, F.N.; Aydemir, C.; Dilmen, U. Total antioxidant capacity and total oxidant status after surfactant treatment in preterm infants with respiratory distress syndrome. *Ann. Clin. Biochem.* **2011**, *48*, 462–467. [CrossRef] [PubMed]
29. Akçay, A.; Tatar Aksoy, H.; Uras, N.; Dilmen, U. Reference values of oxidative stress biomarkers in healthy newborns. *Pediatr. Int.* **2013**, *55*, 604–607. [CrossRef] [PubMed]
30. Wang, Y.; Feng, Y.; Lu, L.N.; Wang, W.P.; He, Z.J.; Xie, L.J.; Hong, L.; Tang, Q.Y.; Cai, W. The effects of different lipid emulsions on the lipid profile, fatty acid composition, and antioxidant capacity of preterm infants: A double-blind, randomized clinical trial. *Clin. Nutr.* **2016**, *35*, 1023–1031. [CrossRef] [PubMed]
31. Mohamed, I.; Elremaly, W.; Rouleau, T.; Lavoie, J.C. Ascorbylperoxide contaminating parenteral nutrition is associated with bronchopulmonary dysplasia or death in extremely preterm infants. *JPEN J. Parenter. Enter. Nutr.* **2017**, *41*, 1023–1029. [CrossRef] [PubMed]
32. Baydas, G.; Karatas, F.; Gursu, M.F.; Bozkurt, H.A.; Ilhan, N.; Yasar, A.; Canatan, H. Antioxidant vitamin levels in term and preterm infants and their relation to maternal vitamin status. *Arch. Med. Res.* **2002**, *33*, 276–280. [CrossRef]
33. Guajardo, L.; Beharry, K.D.; Modanlou, H.D.; Aranda, J.V. Ascorbic acid concentrations in umbilical cord veins and arteries of preterm and term newborns. *Biol. Neonate* **1995**, *68*, 1–9. [CrossRef] [PubMed]
34. Tubman, T.R.; Halliday, H.L.; McMaster, D. Glutathione peroxidase and selenium levels in the preterm infant. *Biol. Neonate* **1990**, *58*, 305–310. [CrossRef] [PubMed]
35. Ceballos-Picot, I.; Trivier, J.M.; Nicole, A.; Sinet, P.M.; Thevenin, M. Age-correlated modifications of copper-zinc superoxide dismutase and glutahtione-related enzyme activities in human erythrocytes. *Clin. Chem.* **1992**, *38*, 66–70. [PubMed]
36. Hamon, I.; Valdes, V.; Frank, P.; Buchweiller, M.C.; Fresson, J.; Hascoet, J.M. Différences liées au sexe dans le métabolisme du glutathion (GSH) du grand prématuré/Gender-dependent differences in glutathione (GSH) metabolism in very preterm infants. *Arch. Pediatr.* **2011**, *18*, 247–252. [CrossRef] [PubMed]
37. Hunaiti, A.A. al-Shareef M.Interplay between glutathione-S-transferase and glucose-6-phosphate dehydrogenase in neonatal cord blood. *Biol. Neonate* **1997**, *72*, 273–278. [CrossRef] [PubMed]
38. Shoji, H.; Ikeda, N.; Hosozawa, M.; Ohkawa, N.; Matsunaga, N.; Suganuma, H.; Hisata, K.; Tanaka, K.; Shimizu, T. Oxidative stress early in infancy and neurodevelopmental outcome in very low-birthweight infants. *Pediatr. Int.* **2014**, *56*, 709–713. [CrossRef] [PubMed]
39. Kato, E.; Ibara, S.; Kumazawa, K.; Maruyama, Y.; Tokuhisa, T.; Matsui, T.; Shimono, R.; Maede, Y.; Minakami, H. Effects of supplemental oxygen on urinary 8-hydroxy-2′-deoxyguanosine levels in extremely low birth weight infants. *Free Radic. Res.* **2014**, *48*, 1285–1290. [CrossRef] [PubMed]
40. Joung, K.E.; Kim, H.S.; Lee, J.; Shim, G.H.; Choi, C.W.; Kim, E.K.; Kim, B.I.; Choi, J.H. Correlation of urinary inflammatory and oxidative stress markers in very low birth weight infants with subsequent development of bronchopulmonary dysplasia. *Free Radic. Res.* **2011**, *45*, 1024–1032. [CrossRef] [PubMed]
41. Ledo, A.; Arduini, A.; Asensi, M.A.; Sastre, J.; Escrig, R.; Brugada, M.; Aguar, M.; Saenz, P.; Vento, M. Human milk enhances antioxidant defenses against hydroxyl radical aggression in preterm infants. *Am. J. Clin. Nutr.* **2009**, *89*, 210–215. [CrossRef] [PubMed]
42. Matsubasa, T.; Uchino, T.; Karashima, S.; Kondo, Y.; Maruyama, K.; Tanimura, M.; Endo, F. Oxidative stress in very low birth weight infants as measured by urinary 8-OHdG. *Free Radic. Res.* **2002**, *36*, 189–193. [CrossRef] [PubMed]
43. Laborie, S.; Lavoie, J.C.; Chessex, P. Increased urinary peroxides in newborn infants receiving parenteral nutrition exposed to light. *J. Pediatr.* **2000**, *136*, 628–632. [CrossRef] [PubMed]

44. Schock, B.C.; Sweet, D.G.; Halliday, H.L.; Young, I.S.; Ennis, M. Oxidative stress in lavage fluid of preterm infants at risk of chronic lung disease. *Am. J. Physiol. Lung Cell Mol. Physiol.* **2001**, *281*, L1386–L1391. [CrossRef] [PubMed]
45. Vento, G.; Mele, M.C.; Mordente, A.; Romagnoli, C.; Matassa, P.G.; Zecca, E.; Zappacosta, B.; Persichilli, S. High total antioxidant activity and uric acid in tracheobronchial aspirate fluid of preterm infants during oxidative stress: An adaptive response to hyperoxia? *Acta Paediatr.* **2000**, *89*, 336–342. [CrossRef] [PubMed]
46. Lavoie, J.C.; Chessex, P. Gender-related response to a tert-butyl hydroperoxide-induced oxidation in human neonatal tissue. *Free Radic. Biol. Med.* **1994**, *16*, 307–313. [CrossRef]
47. Lavoie, J.C.; Chessex, P. Development of glutathione synthesis and gamma-glutamyltranspeptidase activities in tissues from newborn infants. *Free Radic. Biol. Med.* **1998**, *24*, 994–1001. [CrossRef]
48. Lavoie, J.C.; Rouleau, T.; Truttmann, A.C.; Chessex, P. Postnatal gender-dependent maturation of cellular cysteine uptake. *Free Radic Res* **2002**, *36*, 811–817. [CrossRef] [PubMed]
49. Stark, M.J.; Hodyl, N.A.; Wright, I.M.; Clifton, V.L. Influence of sex and glucocorticoid exposure on preterm placental pro-oxidant-antioxidant balance. *Placenta* **2011**, *32*, 865–870. [CrossRef] [PubMed]
50. World Health Organization. Sex Differentials in Infant Mortality (2001–2010). Available online: http://www.searo.who.int/entity/health_situation_trends/data/chi/sex-diff-imr/en/ (accessed on 2 March 2018).
51. Lavoie, J.C.; Bélanger, S.; Spalinger, M.; Chessex, P. Admixture of multivitamin preparation to parenteral nutrition: The major contributor to in vitro generation of peroxides. *Pediatr. Electr.* **1997**, *99*, e6. [CrossRef]
52. Lavoie, J.C.; Rouleau, T.; Tsopmo, A.; Friel, J.; Chessex, P. Influence of lung oxidant and antioxidant status on alveolarization: Role of light-exposed total parenteral nutrition. *Free Radic. Biol. Med.* **2008**, *45*, 572–577. [CrossRef] [PubMed]
53. Chessex, P.; Laborie, S.; Nasef, N.; Masse, B.; Lavoie, J.C. Shielding parenteral nutrition from light improves survival rate in premature infants: A meta-analysis. *JPEN J. Parenter. Enter. Nutr.* **2017**, *41*, 378–383. [CrossRef] [PubMed]
54. Kaludjerovic, J.; Ward, W.E. The Interplay between Estrogen and Fetal Adrenal Cortex. *J Nutr Metab* **2012**, *2012*, 837901. [CrossRef] [PubMed]
55. Vaskivuo, T.E.; Mäentausta, M.; Törn, S.; Oduwole, O.; Lönnberg, A.; Herva, R.; Isomaa, V.; Tapanainen, J.S. Estrogen receptors and estrogen-metabolizing enzymes in human ovaries during fetal development. *J. Clin. Endocrinol. Metab.* **2005**, *90*, 3752–3756. [CrossRef] [PubMed]
56. Pepe, G.J.; Billiar, R.B.; Albrecht, E.D. Regulation of baboon fetal ovarian folliculogenesis by estrogen. *Mol. Cell. Endocrinol.* **2006**, *247*, 41–46. [CrossRef] [PubMed]
57. Varshney, M.; Nalvarte, I. Genes, Gender, Environment, and Novel Functions of Estrogen Receptor Beta in the Susceptibility to Neurodevelopmental Disorders. *Brain Sci.* **2017**, *7*, 24. [CrossRef] [PubMed]
58. Lundholm, L.; Putnik, M.; Otsuki, M.; Andersson, S.; Ohlsson, C.; Gustafsson, J.A.; Dahlman-Wright, K. Effects of estrogen on gene expression profiles in mouse hypothalamus and white adipose tissue: Target genes include glutathione peroxidase 3 and cell death-inducing DNA fragmentation factor, alpha-subunit-like effector A. *J. Endocrinol.* **2008**, *196*, 547–557. [CrossRef] [PubMed]
59. Baek, I.J.; Jung, K.Y.; Yon, J.M.; Lee, S.R.; Lee, B.J.; Yun, Y.W.; Nam, S.Y. Phospholipid hydroperoxide glutathione peroxidase gene is regulated via an estrogen and estrogen receptor signaling in cultured mouse fetuses. *In Vitro Cell. Dev. Biol. Anim.* **2011**, *47*, 535–540. [CrossRef] [PubMed]
60. Lapointe, J.; Kimmins, S.; Maclaren, L.A.; Bilodeau, J.F. Estrogen selectively up-regulates the phospholipid hydroperoxide glutathione peroxidase in the oviducts. *Endocrinology* **2005**, *146*, 2583–2592. [CrossRef] [PubMed]
61. Wu, J.; Williams, D.; Walter, G.A.; Thompson, W.E.; Sidell, N. Estrogen increases Nrf2 activity through activation of the PI3K pathway in MCF-7 breast cancer cells. *Exp. Cell Res.* **2014**, *328*, 351–360. [CrossRef] [PubMed]
62. Vina, J.; Gambini, J.; Lopez-Grueso, R.; Abdelaziz, K.M.; Jove, M.; Borras, C. Females live longer than males: Role of oxidative stress. *Curr. Pharm. Des.* **2011**, *17*, 3959–3965. [CrossRef] [PubMed]
63. Zhu, C.; Wang, S.; Wang, B.; Du, F.; Hu, C.; Feng, Y.; Zhu, R.; Mo, M.; Cao, Y.; Li, A.; et al. 17β-Estradiol up-regulates Nrf2 via PI3/AKT and estrogen receptor signalling pathways to suppress light-induced degeneration in rat retina. *Neuroscience* **2015**, *304*, 328–339. [CrossRef] [PubMed]

64. Friel, J.K.; Martin, S.M.; Langdon, M.; Herzberg, G.R.; Buettner, G.R. Milk from mothers of both premature and full-term infants provides better antioxidant protection than does infant formula. *Pediatr. Res.* **2002**, *51*, 612–618. [CrossRef] [PubMed]
65. Tsopmo, A.; Romanowski, A.; Banda, L.; Lavoie, J.C.; Jenssen, H.; Friel, J. Novel anti-oxidative peptides from enzymatic digestion of human milk. *Food Chem.* **2011**, *126*, 1138–1143. [CrossRef]
66. Miloudi, K.; Tsopmo, A.; Friel, J.K.; Rouleau, T.; Comte, B.; Lavoie, J.C. Hexapeptides from human milk prevent the induction of oxidative stress from parenteral nutrition in the newborn guinea pig. *Pediatr. Res.* **2012**, *71*, 675–681. [CrossRef] [PubMed]
67. Soghier, L.M.; Brion, L.P. Cysteine, cystine or *N*-acetylcysteine supplementation in parenterally fed neonates. *Cochrane Database Syst. Rev.* **2006**, CD004869. [CrossRef]
68. Brown, L.A.; Perez, J.A.; Harris, F.L.; Clark, R.H. Glutathione supplements protect preterm rabbits from oxidative lung injury. *Am. J. Physiol.* **1996**, *270*, L446–L451. [CrossRef] [PubMed]
69. Meister, A.; Anderson, M.E.; Hwang, O. Intracellular cysteine and glutathione delivery systems. *J. Am. Coll. Nutr.* **1986**, *5*, 137–151. [CrossRef] [PubMed]
70. Elremaly, W.; Mohamed, I.; Rouleau, T.; Lavoie, J.C. Adding glutathione to parenteral nutrition prevents alveolar loss in newborn Guinea pig. *Free Radic. Biol. Med.* **2015**, *87*, 274–281. [CrossRef] [PubMed]
71. Jones, D.P.; Sies, H. The redox code. *Antioxid. Redox Signal.* **2015**, *23*, 734–746. [CrossRef] [PubMed]
72. Sies, H. Oxidative stress: A concept in redox biology and medicine. *Redox Biol.* **2015**, *4*, 180–183. [CrossRef] [PubMed]
73. Manti, S.; Marseglia, L.; D'Angelo, G.; Cuppari, C.; Cusumano, E.; Arrigo, T.; Gitto, E.; Salpietro, C. "Cumulative Stress": The Effects of Maternal and Neonatal Oxidative Stress and Oxidative Stress-Inducible Genes on Programming of Atopy. *Oxid. Med. Cell. Longev.* **2016**, *2016*, 8651820. [CrossRef] [PubMed]
74. Strakovsky, R.S.; Pan, Y.X. In utero oxidative stress epigenetically programs antioxidant defense capacity and adulthood diseases. *Antioxid. Redox Signal.* **2012**, *17*, 237–253. [CrossRef] [PubMed]

6

Natural Nanoparticles: A Particular Matter Inspired by Nature

Sharoon Griffin [1,2], Muhammad Irfan Masood [1,3], Muhammad Jawad Nasim [1], Muhammad Sarfraz [1], Azubuike Peter Ebokaiwe [4], Karl-Herbert Schäfer [3], Cornelia M. Keck [2] and Claus Jacob [1,*]

1 Division of Bioorganic Chemistry, School of Pharmacy, Saarland University, D-66123 Saarbruecken, Germany; sharoon.griffin@uni-saarland.de (S.G.); irfan_masood_79@yahoo.com (M.I.M.); jawad.nasim@uni-saarland.de (M.J.N.); s8musarf@stud.uni-saarland.de (M.S.)

2 Institute of Pharmaceutics and Biopharmaceutics, Philipps University of Marburg, 35037 Marburg, Germany; cornelia.keck@pharmazie.uni-marburg.de

3 Department of Biotechnology, University of Applied Sciences Kaiserslautern, 66482 Zweibruecken, Germany; karl-herbert.schaefer@hs-kl.de

4 Department of Chemistry/Biochemistry and Molecular Biology, Federal University, Ndufu-Alike Ikwo, 482131 Ndufu-Alike, Nigeria; azubike.ebokaiwe@funai.edu.ng

* Correspondence: c.jacob@mx.uni-saarland.de

Abstract: During the last couple of decades, the rapidly advancing field of nanotechnology has produced a wide palette of nanomaterials, most of which are considered as "synthetic" and, among the wider public, are often met with a certain suspicion. Despite the technological sophistication behind many of these materials, "nano" does not always equate with "artificial". Indeed, nature itself is an excellent nanotechnologist. It provides us with a range of fine particles, from inorganic ash, soot, sulfur and mineral particles found in the air or in wells, to sulfur and selenium nanoparticles produced by many bacteria and yeasts. These nanomaterials are entirely natural, and, not surprisingly, there is a growing interest in the development of natural nanoproducts, for instance in the emerging fields of phyto- and phyco-nanotechnology. This review will highlight some of the most recent—and sometimes unexpected—advances in this exciting and diverse field of research and development. Naturally occurring nanomaterials, artificially produced nanomaterials of natural products as well as naturally occurring or produced nanomaterials of natural products all show their own, particular chemical and physical properties, biological activities and promise for applications, especially in the fields of medicine, nutrition, cosmetics and agriculture. In the future, such natural nanoparticles will not only stimulate research and add a greener outlook to a traditionally high-tech field, they will also provide solutions—pardon—suspensions for a range of problems. Here, we may anticipate specific biogenic factories, valuable new materials based on waste, the effective removal of contaminants as part of nano-bioremediation, and the conversion of poorly soluble substances and materials to biologically available forms for practical uses.

Keywords: bioreduction; homogenization; microbes; nanoparticles; redox; selenium; sulfur; silver

---

1. Introduction

Today, nanotechnology and its diverse products are omnipresent and form an integral part of our products and lifestyle, from nanosilver in deodorants and nanoscopic particles with improved release properties in medicines all the way to "nanoimpregnations" of shower cabins, bath tubs and washing basins [1–3]. Whilst innovative materials containing particles with diameters in the one to one hundred nanometer range have emerged in many areas of our daily life, there has also been a feeling that such materials are "not quite natural". Not surprisingly, therefore, the field of nano-toxicology more recently has attracted a particular interest—and there has also been mounting concern regarding a possible toxic impact on humans and contamination of the environment with nanomaterials [4].

This concern is certainly not entirely unjustified, as some dramatic examples, for instance asbestos (average diameter ranging from three to five micrometers) and other, air-bound fine particle matter, such as the $PM_{2.5}$ fraction in exhaust gases, fumes and smoke illustrate [5–7]. Such critique, however, often ignores the fact that Nature itself is a skilled nanotechnologist, with numerous examples of common nanomaterials literally emanating from natural sources, such as volcanoes and mineral springs but also, in particular, from living organisms. Figure 1 provides a colorful reminder of such entirely natural sources of nanoscopic and microscopic particles. Indeed, life revolves around cells which themselves are microscopic in size (we do not account here for some rare and/or controversial nanobacteria) and metabolize molecules which are picoscopic, but also materials in between, which obviously are nanoscopic in their dimensions [8–10]. At the same time, nature also provides the inspiration and eventually also the ingredients—and even some of the methods—for natural nanomaterials.

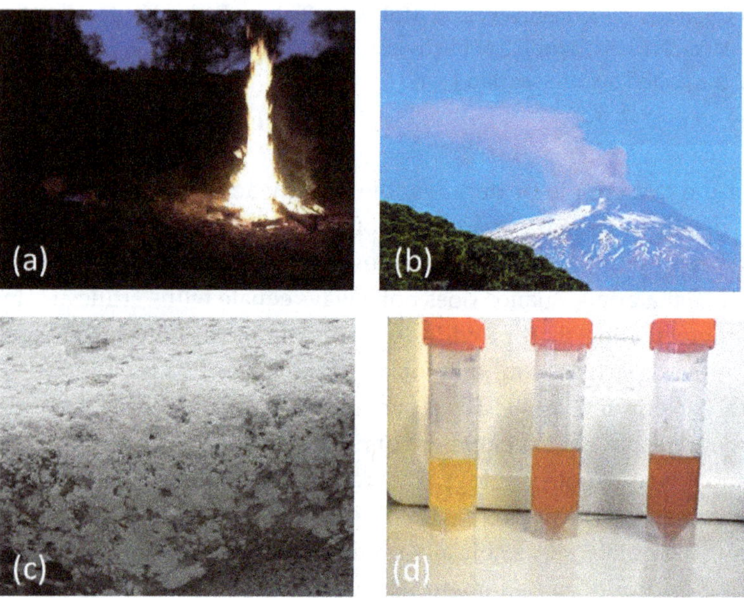

Figure 1. Nature itself is a skilled nanotechnologist. Microscopic and nanoscopic particles are formed, for instance, by combustion and are found: (**a**) near open fire; (**b**) as result of volcanic activity; (**c**) in form of precipitates; and (**d**) as bioreductively formed deposits of elements in certain bacteria. Photos provided by Marc Schäfer and Muhmmad Jawad Nasim.

Here, we will briefly consider the emerging field of natural nanoparticles. Before we start, we must, however, clarify what exactly is meant here. As any cunning linguist may have noted, the predicate "natural" may lead us into several directions. Indeed, there is a need for a distinction between nanomaterials which are, strictly speaking, natural, i.e., already present or formed in the environment without human intervention, and materials which are "nano" and also "bio". In the second case, the predicate "natural" equates with "biological", as in "natural products", which refers primarily to biological substances or materials [11–13]. Figure 2 illustrates this divide and provides a few selected examples of particularly interesting natural nanoparticles, nanoparticles of natural products and, eventually, naturally produced nanoparticles of natural products which we will discuss in more detail in the following sections. From the outset, we should emphasize that the field of natural nanotechnology is wide and diverse. Since we are unable to grasp it in its entirety, we will focus on a few highlights which we consider especially instructive, for instance in the fields of natural product-based nutrition, cosmetics, medicine or eco-friendly, "green" agriculture.

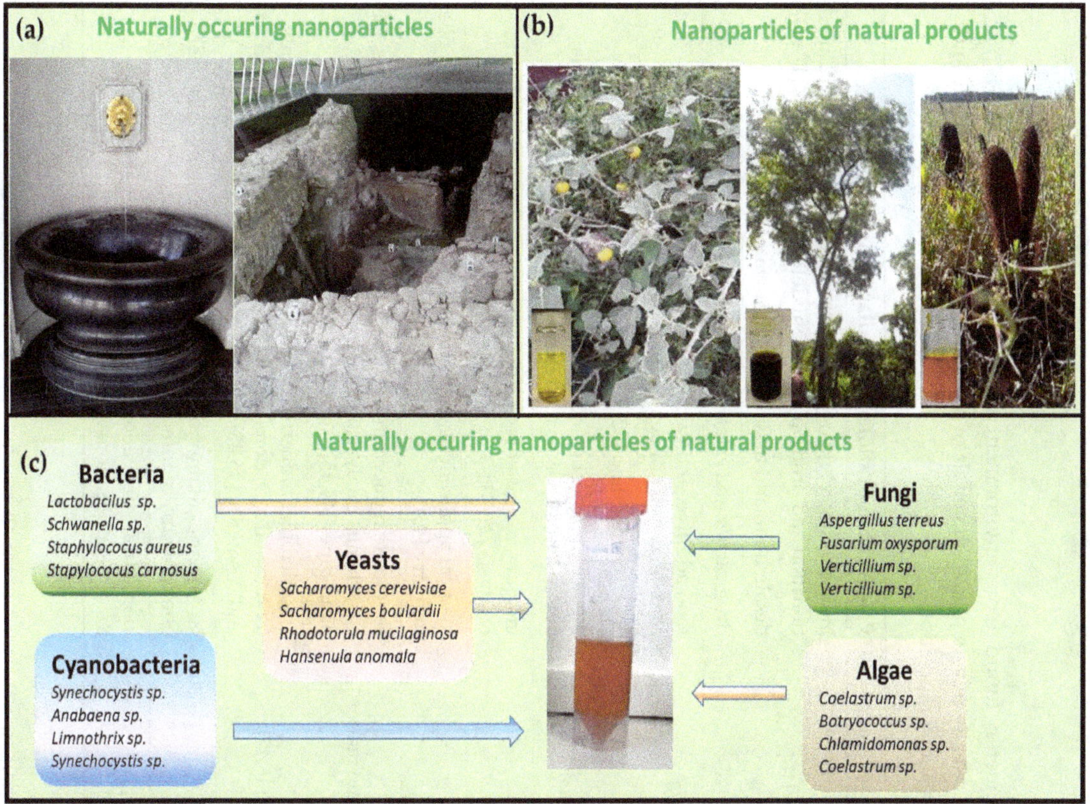

Figure 2. Examples of natural and biological materials which contain nanoscopic particles. (**a**) Naturally occurring nanoparticles of inorganic, elemental sulfur, for instance, are found at mineral wells rich in hydrogen sulfide, such as the Elisenbrunnen in Aachen. (**b**) In contrast, mechanically produced nanomaterials of natural products have been evaluated for medical and agricultural applications. (**c**) Eventually, there are also naturally produced nanomaterials of natural, biological products, such as nanoscopic particles of elemental selenium coated with microbial proteins which are formed by bioreductive or oxidative metabolism in bacteria and fungi.

2. Natural but Not Biological: The Free Flow of Inorganic Nanocomposites

Whilst hunting for nanoscopic materials in the environment, one soon realizes that a fair number of natural nanoparticles can be found outside the realm of life, for instance nanoscopic ash or soot particles as a result of volcanic activity, fires or other types of combustion. These particles are natural, yet usually not biological. Volcanic ash clouds contain a wide variety of polydisperse micro- and nanoparticles. These particles range from 100 to 200 nm in size and are chemically primarily composed of silicate and iron compounds. They are readily suspended in air and once inhaled may lead to serious respiratory disorders. Indeed, whilst particles of sizes in the lower micrometer range deposit in the upper respiratory tract, particles in the nanometer range penetrate deeply and deposit in tracheobronchial and alveolar regions where they can cause severe respiratory disorders [14]. "Carbon Nanotube" soot collected from the combustion of Texas Piñon Pine, for instance, contains multi-walled carbon nanotubes of 15 to 70 nm in size. These carbon-based objects readily become airborne and pose severe health hazards to animals and the human population [15].

Fire, however, is only one chemical process in the inorganic sphere which eventually may result in nanoscopic particles. Precipitation, oxidation and, to a lesser extent, reduction are also well suited to turn naturally occurring, inorganic materials into nanoparticles (Table 1).

Table 1. Selected examples of naturally occurring inorganic micro- and nanoparticles frequently found in our environment and associated with certain possible applications or biological implications. Please note that the practical applications mentioned usually rely on refined materials of particularly good particle quality and purity and not, or not yet, on the crude naturally occurring materials of similar constitution and composition.

Name	Chemical Formulae and Symbols	Natural Occurrence	Practical Implications (of Similar, Refined Materials)
Calcium Carbonate	$CaCO_3$	natural surface water [16]	industry, biotechnology, cancer therapy, drug delivery, plant nutrition and promotion of plant defense against pests [17–20]
Alumina	Al_2O_3		desalination and defluorination of water [21–23]
Silicate	SiO_4^{4-}		drug carrier and catalytic applications [24,25]
Silica	SiO_2	volcanic eruptions [26]	food additive, anti-caking agent, ultraviolet antireflection coating, cellular imaging and biomedical applications [27–30]
Bassanite (Calcium Sulfate)	$CaSO_4$	sea water [31]	bone regeneration [32]
Iron Oxide	Fe_3O_4	iceberg-hosted sediments [33]	medical diagnostics, controlled drug release, hyperthermia, biosensors, supercapacitor applications [34–37]
Manganese oxide	MnO_2	umber [38]	imaging, remediation of contaminated soil and ground water, catalysis [39–41]
Sulfur	S	mineral wells [42]	medical applications, (antimicrobial, cytotoxic), fertilizers, fiber industry [43]
Soot (in the form of carbon)	C	atmospheric particulate matter	composite reinforcements, nano-reactors, chemical sensors, gas adsorbents, catalyst supports, templates, actuators, probes, nano-pipes [44,45]
Silver	Ag	aquatic environment [46,47]	antimicrobial properties, nano-functionalized plastics, paints, food containers, domestic appliances, textiles, medical products and cosmetics [46,48]
Gold	Au	ore deposits [49]	biosensorics, immunoassays, medical applications and laser phototherapy of tumors [50]
Platinum	Pt	automobile exhausts [51]	biomedical applications, nano-biomedicine, catalytic and thermal applications [52–54]

Amazingly, our drinking water, once considered under the microscope, is full of polydisperse nanoscopic as well as microscopic solid materials, of irregular shape and chemically based primarily on $CaCO_3$ and $CaSO_4$, often laced with other elements, such as iron oxides. Figure 3 provides an example of such deposits found near a mineral well in Aachen, Germany, and a microscopic view of the particles found in this water. Admittedly, such particles are of a rather poor quality and cannot be compared to the perfectly shaped, well-defined and homogeneous nanomaterials achieved by modern nanotechnological processes. Nonetheless, chemical, as well as physical processes, such as weathering, the slow precipitation of iron oxide particles but also dissolution and precipitation of carbonates under the influence of CO_2 and the intermediate formation of hydrocarbonate (HCO_3^-), are able to generate such small-sized particle matter [55]. Abrasion, for instance, results in fine particle matter by scraping, cutting or grinding down larger lumps. There are numerous examples of natural nanomaterials formed this way, such as the $CaSO_4$ and silicate particles in spring water [16]. Indeed, such inorganic particles recently have inspired colleagues to synthesize a wide range of similar particles based on naturally occurring materials, such as—refined—nanoparticles of Fe_3O_4 and MnO_2 [56,57]. Concurrently, Nature, in cahoots with human activities, often unwillingly generates such "nanosized" particles from bulk materials, as the hot issue of microplastic in our oceans, fish and food highlights [58,59]. Nanoparticles generated by natural nanosizing are therefore not uncommon in our environment, and additional examples worth considering in earnest include the fine platinum particles released from millions of cars and their catalysts, as well as abrasion from tires, which are hardly "natural", yet slowly, but continuously, affect our environment and eventually also our health [60,61].

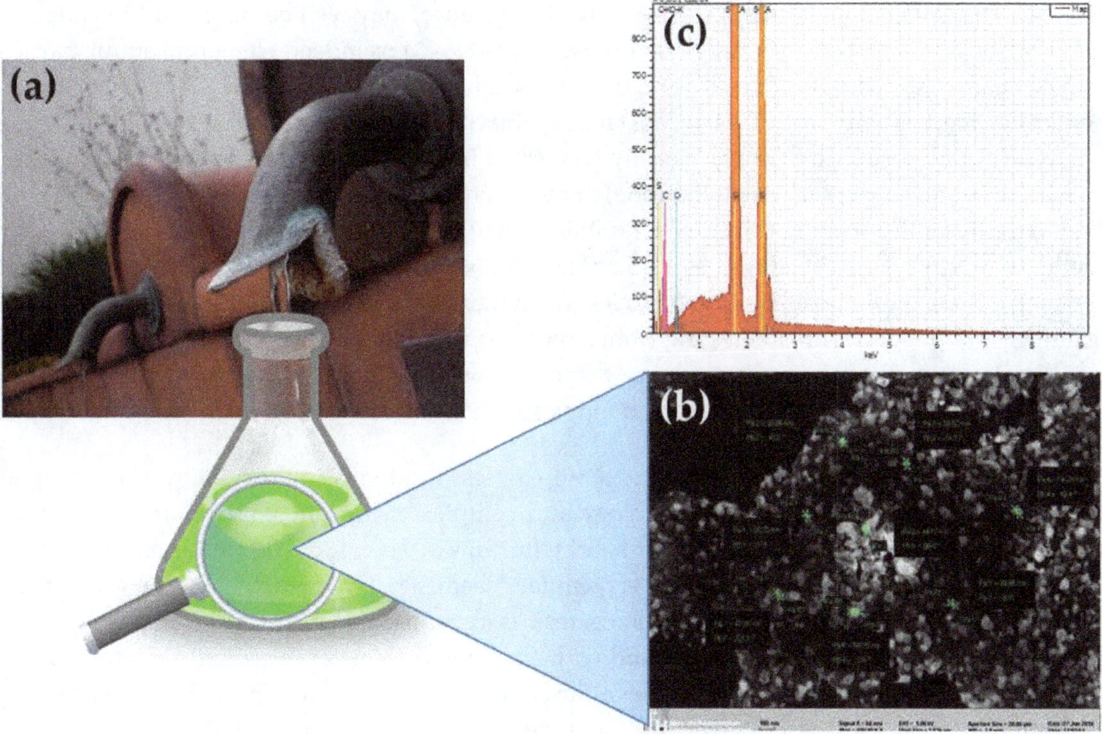

Figure 3. (**a**) The mineral wells in and near the town of Aachen in Germany are rich in sulfur, primarily in form of hydrogen sulfide (H_2S). Solid deposits of inorganic matter can therefore be found, for instance, at the Marktbrunnen in Burtscheid (image kindly provided by Roman Leontiev). (**b**) A microscopic investigation at 10,000-fold magnification reveals numerous microscopic and sub-microscopic particles and irregular agglomerates in this kind of water which (**c**) according to Energy Dispersion X-ray spectroscopy (EDX) consist of primarily of calcium salts and elemental sulfur [42].

Besides such "simple" physical and chemical events, there are similar, albeit more controlled particle generating processes, often based on spontaneous oxidation. One frequently observed example is the oxidation of hydrogen sulfide (H_2S) gas or hydrogen sulfide ions (HS^-) dissolved in waters of volcanic origin, such as volcanic lakes or mineral springs and wells which are common in many regions of the planet [62,63]. Here, the sulfide present in the water is oxidized by oxygen in the air to small particles of or containing elemental sulfur which can be found in the water itself, as in the Elisenbrunnen or Marktbrunnen in Aachen and, eventually, as part of larger sulfur deposits at or near the sulfide source. As before, Nature's inorganic chemistry is not the best nanotechnologist, and those particles are of a rather poor quality, polydisperse and also not entirely pure either. Still, they are already quite well defined—at least regarding chemical composition—and represent an interesting nanomaterial which is formed entirely naturally and can be obtained in considerable amounts and concentrations. From the perspective of resources, the flow of sulfur nanoparticles from volcanic sources is both, sustainable and virtually free of any costs. In the future, such natural sulfur nanoparticles from mineral wells may well be "harvested" or employed directly, for instance as a substitute for colloidal sulfur in agriculture, or may require some "maturation" in form of spontaneous or controlled oxidation of the hydrogen sulfide contained within the water. Nonetheless, simple medical applications, for instance on skin, also appear feasible. Indeed, many of the mineral wells particularly rich in sulfide, such as Bad Nenndorf or Bad Wiessee in Germany, offer bathing—rather than drinking—as part of therapy [64].

From a more scientific perspective, there are also still issues in the water which may need to be resolved. The active ingredient(s) in these wells, for instance, may well be simple sulfide (HS^-), as traditionally assumed, but also inorganic polysulfides (HS_x^-) or indeed elemental sulfur particles (S_8) [42]. Curiously, as these three classes of species exhibit their own, characteristic physical and chemical properties and reactivities, for instance in the context of the "cellular thiolstat" [65]. These Reactive Sulfur Species (RSS) are also easily converted into each other in the presence of oxidants (such as air), reductants (such as glutathione) or even spontaneously by mutual interactions in form of an extensive sulfur-centered "redox scrambling" [66]. Similarly, selenite (SeO_3^{2-}) often occurs together with sulfur and, if reduced by H_2S or HS^-, is able to form a wide range of elemental sulfur, selenium and mixed selenosulfur nanoparticles. As in the case of the sulfur particles in mineral wells, such selenosulfur species are interesting from a more applied, biological point of view. Selenosulfur compounds are well established and widely known, for instance, as active ingredients of certain anti-dandruff shampoos and even feature in movies such as "Evolution" [67,68].

Most of these nanocomposites generated more or less randomly in the wild by crude chemical processes are of an equally crude morphology and complex chemical composition. Good quality nanoparticles of elemental sulfur, selenium and tellurium can be produced under more controlled conditions in the laboratory employing a very similar "chemistry". The redox comproportionation of sulfide (HS^-) and sulfite (SO_3^{2-}), for instance, results in nanoscopic sulfur monodisperse particles of almost uniform size and round shape, and with an average diameter of around 150 nm. Similarly, the reduction of selenite (SeO_3^{2-}) with the sulfur-containing amino acid L-cysteine yields spherical selenium nanoparticles with diameters in the range of 50 nm. Reduction of tellurite (TeO_3^{2-}) with hydrazine (N_2H_4) even enables the generation of tellurium particles in the form of nanoscopic needles [69].

Inspiration for this kind of simple redox chemistry does not stop at the chalcogens. There are many other examples of spontaneous chemical (redox) transformations which eventually lead to small particles, such as the reduction of silver (Ag^+) or gold (Au^{3+}) cations to elemental silver or gold particles, respectively. In the following sections, we will therefore consider such reduction and oxidation reactions also in the context of other natural, biological agents.

3. Bioreductive Formation of Nanoparticles

Whilst volcanoes and mineral springs rely on simple chemical transformations to generate nanoparticles, living cells can recruit an entire arsenal of biotransformations to eventually produce such composites. Indeed, the living cell is mostly dealing with "nanotechnology", i.e., with objects of a nanoscopic size. Just to get a feeling for dimensions: A strand of DNA is 2.5 nm in diameter, a typical virus is around 100 nm wide and a typical bacterium is ten times bigger, i.e., in the range of 1–3 μm. Mammalian and plant cells are comparably large, occasionally reaching 50 μm in diameter [70,71]. It is therefore not surprising that cells, and here microbial cells in particular, engage in some sort of "nanotechnology". Still, in the context of nanoparticles, there is one major caveat: Living cells normally do not prefer "the solid state", as any deposits formed intracellularly may stress and eventually kill them in a suicide-like process. The expulsion of such particles requires a more sophisticated machinery, effort and energy for excretion. Hence the formation of deposits inside cells is not that common—but also not entirely unknown either. When exposed to inorganic salts (e.g., containing S^{2-}, SeO_3^{2-}, Ag^+ and Au^{3+}), certain bacteria such as *Pseudomonas aeruginosa*, *Thiobacillus*, *Serratia*, and *Stenotrophomonas* species employ a reductive or oxidizing pathway of detoxification which eventually leads to the formation of elemental particles [72–77]. Such processes are rather well established and studied in the context of sulfur and selenium as well as silver nanoparticles, but also seem to apply to nanoparticles of gold and even platinum [78]. The particles produced by such biogenic factories are often of a surprisingly good quality, for instance small spherical shapes of an almost uniform size (Figure 4).

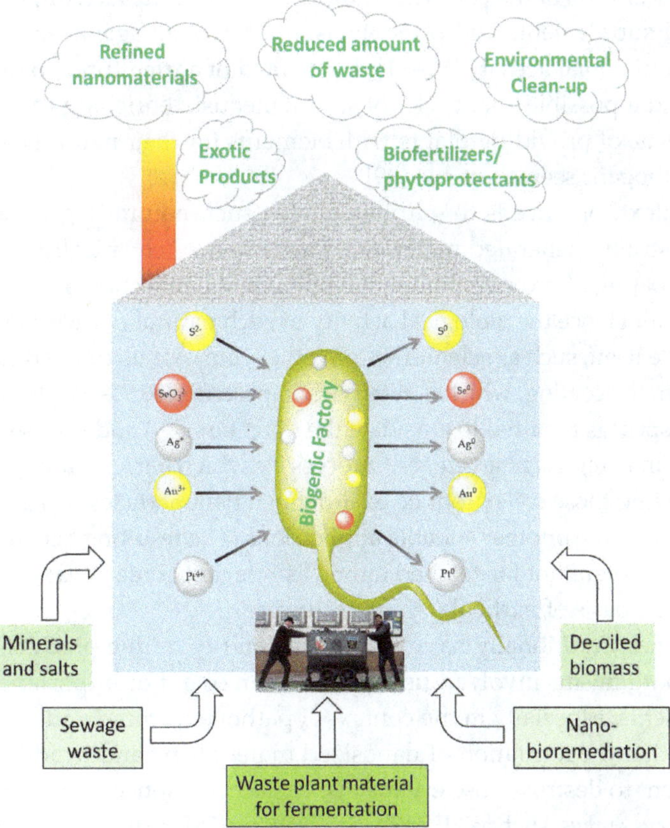

Figure 4. Schematic illustration of the biogenic factory which is able to turn biological substances, extracts, plants, algae and even waste biomass into amazing new products and nanomaterials. A particular interest resides on the added value resulting from the use and "up-cycling" of by-products and waste, such as de-oiled herbs, spent grains and coffee grounds, as these materials initially are not only food-grade but otherwise would go to waste and hence impact negatively on the environment. Photo taken at Hassel (Saar) and kindly provided by Elizabeth Jacob.

Not surprisingly, such biological processes may be exploited in practice to produce such particles of good quality and yield. This is the case, for instance, for selenium nanoparticles in dairy products produced by bacteria such as *Shewanella* sp. and *Lactobacillus* sp. Here, microorganisms which ferment the milk are also able to reduce selenite to elemental selenium for an additional "kick" [79,80]. Such processes are also of interest in the context of bioremediation and decontamination of soils enriched in certain toxic metals or semi-metals. Indeed, the removal of environmental contaminants (such as heavy metals, organic and inorganic pollutants) from contaminated sites using nanoparticles or nanomaterials formed by or in plants, fungi and bacteria with the assistance of nanotechnology, often referred to as nanobioremediation (NBR), is an emerging, environmentally friendly and economical alternative to traditional chemical methods [81,82]. Here, the three main strategies of modern bioremediation include the use of plants, microbes and isolated enzymes, for instance, laccase or nitrate reductase [83,84].

Whilst bioremediation is clearly an emerging topic related to microbially formed natural nanoparticles, it aims primarily at the removal of contaminants. Even so, there is also a more positive side to this approach. Here, the nanoparticles generated by such organisms are no longer seen as contaminants but actually as valuable nanomaterials of a more or less natural origin (Figure 4). Within this context, several of these bioreductively formed "natural" nanoparticles have been explored recently with sight on potential medical and agricultural applications [85–88].

It is possible, for instance, to recruit harmless microorganisms, such as *Saccharomyces cerevisiae* and *Staphylococcus carnosus* to generate fairly homogeneous selenium nanoparticles from SeO_3^{2-} with average diameters of 60 nm and 80 nm, respectively [89,90]. These particles can be harvested from the yeasts and bacteria after lysis of the cell. The authors of such studies have speculated about possible applications as food supplements and possibly as antimicrobial agents as some of these particles exhibit a certain antimicrobial activity [89–91]. In the field of agriculture, possible applications have even more facets, and a possible "hat trick" of simultaneously enriching the soil with selenium for fortified food products, of providing plants with elements for their natural defense systems and of eradicating plant pathogens seems feasible [89].

Within this context, one needs to emphasize that such naturally generated particles are not comparable to industrially generated materials. They are not "chemically pure", and usually also contain a "natural" coating of proteins whose composition is a reflection of the yeasts or bacteria they have been produced in. Hence the biological activity of such natural particles may stem from the bulk material of the particle itself, such as selenium, from other compounds trapped or contained within the particle, and also from the coating, which is often rich in proteins [89,92–94]. In such cases an extensive "intracellular diagnostics" is required to elucidate the exact target(s) and precise mode(s) of action [95].

Eventually, one may envisage an elegant process by which bacteria are grown on contaminated soils, and by remediating those soils produce well-defined nanoparticles which may be harvested and used in medicine, agriculture or other suitable applications. The resulting benefits of such an approach may be substantial—and are not far-fetched either, as relevant contaminants, such as heavy metals, often also represent the basis of particularly interesting particles.

As these strategies traditionally have focused primarily on the production of nanomaterials, the fate of the microorganisms involved usually has been of minor importance. Still, there may be some additional benefits, especially in the context of pathogenic fungi and bacteria. Several studies have demonstrated that the formation of nanosized materials by and inside pathogenic bacteria is an effective instrument to destroy those organisms. It has been noticed, for instance, that pathogenic strains of *Staphyllococcus aureus*, such as HEMSA and HEMSA 5M, reduce SeO_3^{2-} to elemental selenium when confronted with exceptionally high concentrations of this anion (around 2 mM) in an apparent attempt to deal with this exposure [96]. Eventually, this protective strategy fails and the deposits of selenium formed inside the bacteria kill these cells. This kind of "suicidal natural nanotechnology" is found among many bacteria and fungi, including pathogenic ones [89]. It partially explains in part the antimicrobial action often associated with SeO_3^{2-} and SeO_4^{2-} and other Reactive Selenium Species (RSeS), as well as with TeO_3^{2-} and TeO_4^{2-} [89]. Such activities may be specific for certain organisms, endowing these agents and associated processes with certain "sensor/effector" properties. In the future, this kind of natural nanotechnology therefore may provide an interesting avenue to compromise, weaken, damage or perhaps even kill such pathogenic organisms [89].

4. Redox Chemistry with Natural Products

Just as many bacteria and fungi are able to produce nanoparticles of fairly good quality, this approach requires a certain effort in form of culturing and harvesting. It frequently also results in contamination with microbial biomolecules. Not surprisingly, alternative strategies have been developed which employ specific, isolated cellular components instead of whole cells to achieve the kind of—mostly bioreductive—chemistry which is usually required for the biological production of nanoparticles. As mentioned above, enzymes, such as laccase and nitrate reductase, are already employed in NBR, and similar avenues, based on isolated enzymes and simple natural reductants (or oxidants) have recently been explored as a means to generate nanoparticles [97–100]. Ascorbic acid, L-cysteine, reduced glutathione (GSH), flavonoids and a couple of other natural reducing agents are rather abundant in Nature and easy to obtain. Not surprisingly, these agents have been investigated already to produce nanoparticles of sulfur, selenium and silver, to name just a few [101–105]. Other redox active secondary metabolites, such as terpeniods (e.g., eugenol), flavonoids (e.g., luteolin and quercetin), sugars (e.g., glucose and sucrose) and certain amino acids (e.g., aspartate) have also been employed successfully to generate metal nanoparticles [101]. Besides simple plant metabolites, peptides have been considered, for example oligopeptides containing tryptophan residues. These peptides reduce metal ions to peptide-functionalized silver and gold nanoparticles [106]. Larger molecules, including redox active proteins, can also—chemically—produce nanoparticles, for instance particles of elemental platinum [107]. There are also reports that proteins from natural sources, such as whole cow milk, reduce metal cations, and generate, for instance, good quality nanoparticles of silver [108].

These few selected examples demarcate a particularly promising field of natural, biological nanotechnology, whereby isolated natural compounds, mixtures or even entire articles, such as whole milk, are used to produce nanomaterials. In practice, Nature provides a plethora of such reducing agents in form of compounds, peptides, proteins and enzymes. Indeed, certain microorganisms, plants and plant extracts are rich in antioxidants, with millimolar concentrations of ascorbic acid and thiols present therein [109–112]. As any lover of marmite will know, such extracts can be acquired rather easily, often as left-overs or by-products, such as yeast extracts from breweries. From an ecological and economical perspective, extracts are often superior to whole organisms and plants but also to isolated and extensively purified substances. Not surprisingly, therefore, such extracts are not only interesting from the prospect of being natural and fit for human consumption, but also since they are widely available and cheap [113,114]. Within this context, one rather noteworthy study has employed aqueous extracts of the fungus *Amylomyces rouxii* (strain KSU-09 isolated from the roots of *Phoenix dactylifera*) to generate silver nanoparticles [115].

In the context of plants, in particular, extracts are common and readily available. Not surprisingly, aqueous extracts of *Nelumbo nucifera* (root), *Embelia ribes* (seed), *Rosmarinus officinalis, Ocimum basilicum, Petroselinum crispum* (leaf and root), *Citrus limon* (peel), *Vitis vinifera* (peel), *Cucumis sativus* (peel), *Mimusops elengi* Linn. (leaf), *Acalypha indica* (leaf), *Zingiber officinalis* and *Capsicum frutescens*, among others, are frequently used to produce nanoparticles of Ag, Au, Fe_3O_4 and ZnO [116–124]. Indeed, this emerging field of "phyto-nanotechnology" provides numerous advantages (Figure 5). The materials employed, such as extracts of herbs, are often available as cheap by-products, yet still rich in active ingredients, and therefore of value for further processing. One should also remember that some of these plant products are "food grade", and hence entail possible applications in nutrition and cosmetics [125]. Together with other "readily available" biomass, such as microalgae, such materials are well suited for the controlled synthesis of good quality nanoparticles [126]. Indeed, the emerging field of "phyco-nanotechnology" relies explicitly on algae for bio-nanomanufacture as these organisms are not only highly interesting from a scientific point of view, but also readily available, easy to culture and environmentally friendly to use [127].

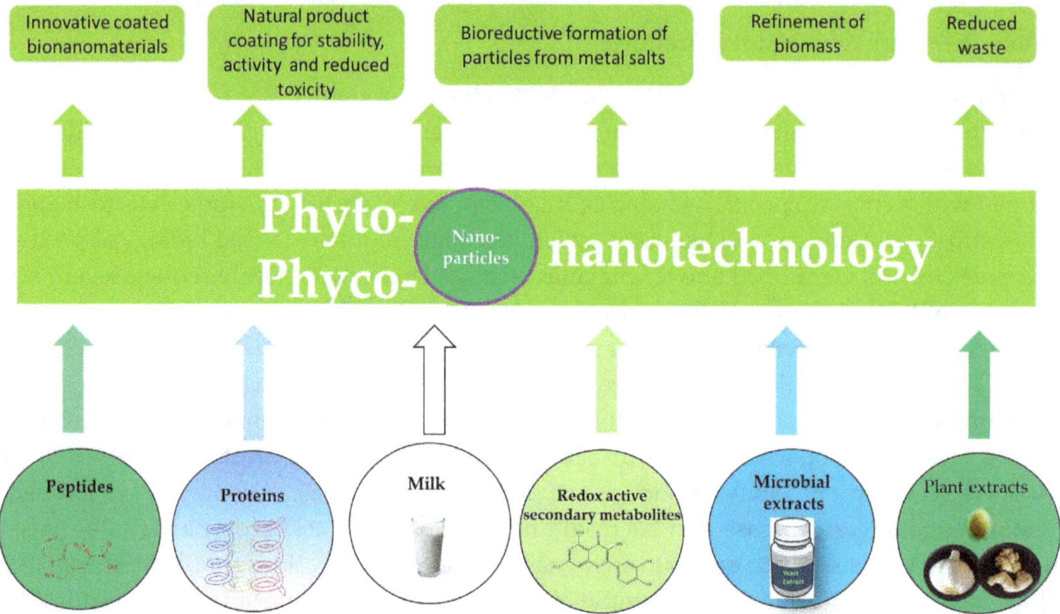

Figure 5. The emerging field of phyto-nanotechnology employs isolated biological components and substances to form, modify or coat nanoparticles. These particles often exhibit interesting properties, such as pronounced biological activity, and may therefore be employed in medicine or agriculture. Phyto-nanotechnology also offers new and innovative uses for plant materials and biomass, which otherwise may have been wasted. Here, the field of phyco-nanotechnology, which is centered around algae, for many biological, manufacturing, ecological and economical reasons today represents a particularly interesting area of research and development.

Besides these more obvious applications of extracts and by-products in phyto-nanotechnology, one should also briefly mention two additional applications in this field. One is the use of such "waste" biomass as feedstock for bacteria and fungi able to generate nanoparticles in vivo [101,128]. In this case, the biomass is not used directly as reducing material, as above, but rather indirectly—and probably more extensively—to promote the growth of suitable bacteria able to perform this kind of bioreduction. The second application concerns the coating of nanoparticles. As mentioned above, nanomaterials produced by bacteria are often coated with proteins, and this coating may endow such particles with improved stability, further features and especially also additional biological activities. It is therefore not surprising that natural substances, such as extracts of Darjeeling tea, have been investigated as coatings for silver nanoparticles to provide stability against agglomeration and also to reduce toxicity [129].

In general, these materials—literally—provide a fertile ground for future research and development, especially in the context of turning biomass waste into (nanomaterial) value (Figure 5).

5. Milling Vanilla

Thus far, natural products have been employed primarily to generate, cover or coat nanoparticles. This raises the question if such biological materials themselves may not be converted into nanoparticles. Similar to naturally occurring abrasion mentioned earlier, methods such as grinding, milling and (high pressure) homogenization provide a wide and colorful arsenal of methods able to "mill down" almost any material, including chemical elements in their solid state, sparingly soluble food supplements and medications, and, actually, also plant parts and even entire trees [130]. The resulting particles of such natural products are of a unique nature, as they are still natural products, yet have been transformed into an unusual, unnatural size and shape.

It is therefore hardly surprising that many natural products have been nanosized (or "nanonized") during the last couple of years. Antioxidants such as rutin, for instance, have been turned into so-called "nanocrystals" using an eloquent technique which involves wet bead milling (WBM) and high-pressure homogenization (HPH) [131,132]. Here, nanotechnology can be used to produce nanoparticles with a dramatically improved solubility, excellent release kinetics and hence a good bioavailability and biological activity. This approach is particularly attractive in the field of—often sparingly soluble—antioxidants and plant products rich in such antioxidants, i.e., substances and materials which originally have poor release kinetics on the lipid/aqueous surface of the skin but thanks to the new technology can nowadays be used easily, for instance in cosmetics.

The basic physical principles behind this approach of nanosizing natural products are illustrated in Figure 6. Indeed, the principle of nanosizing coarse materials to improve their biological activity is very simple and is mainly based on the Noyes–Whitney equation, one of the major equations in biopharmacy (Equation (1)).

$$\frac{dc}{dt} = D \cdot A \cdot \frac{(c_S - c_0)}{h} \tag{1}$$

where dc/dt is the dissolution rate, D the diffusion coefficient, A the total surface area of the particles, c_S the saturation solubility of the active ingredient, c_0 the concentration of dissolved active ingredient in the solvent and h the diffusional distance.

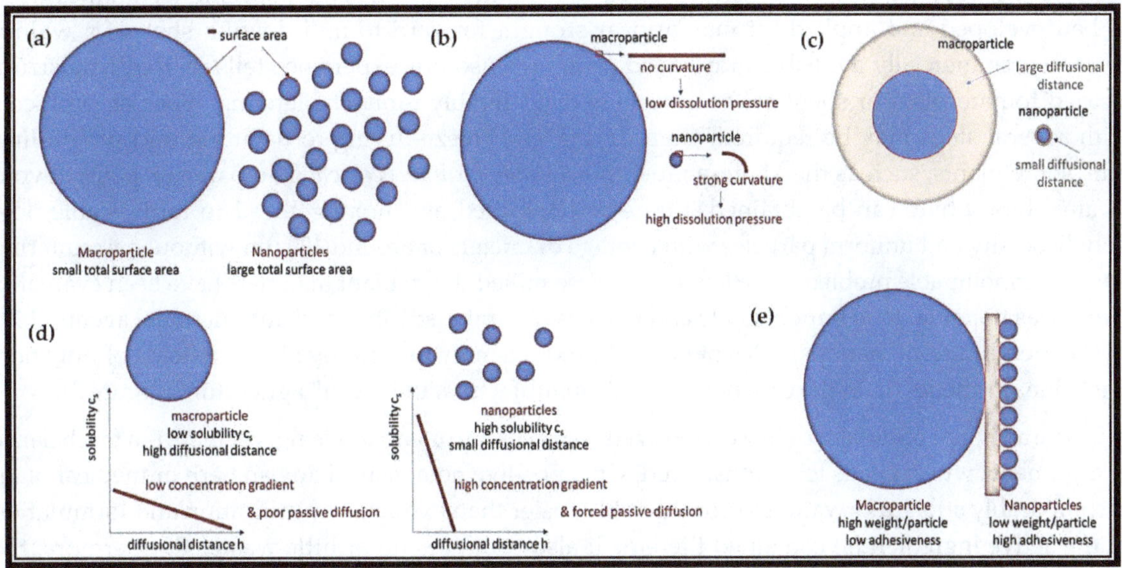

Figure 6. Properties of nanoparticles: (**a**) increased rate of dissolution; (**b**) enhanced saturation solubility; (**c**) decreased diffusional distance; (**d**) higher concentration gradient; and (**e**) improved adhesiveness.

When nanosizing coarse material the rate of dissolution dc/dt increases, because the total surface area of the particles involved increases (Figure 6a). In this case, the saturation solubility increases due to a higher dissolution pressure, which is explained by a higher curvature of the particles (Kelvin equation, Figure 6b) and the diffusional distance is also decreased (Prantl equation, Figure 6c). Eventually, nanosizing leads to a significant increase in the overall velocity of dissolution, which is especially interesting if active ingredients dissolve slowly or are even poorly soluble in water. Furthermore, nanosizing improves the bioactivity of poorly soluble active ingredients. As a result of the increase in solubility the concentration gradient, when compared to larger sized materials, is increased [133]. If the active ingredient is taken up by the body (or the plant) via passive diffusion, the concentration gradient is the driving force for uptake or permeation. Hence the higher the concentration gradient, the faster and more efficient the uptake will be (Figure 6d). Eventually, the smaller the size of a particle, the faster it will dissolve and the higher its bioactivity will be [134].

There are also additional benefits. Nanosized materials possess a much higher adhesiveness to surfaces than coarse materials. This is due to the much larger surface to volume ratio of nanoparticles, which translates into considerably more attaching points per volume and therefore to less forces needed to stick to a surface (Figure 6e). Hence, after administration or application, nanoparticles tend to adhere much tighter and longer to surfaces, the time to dissolve and to penetrate is prolonged, therefore further increasing the bioactivity of active ingredients. Due to these superior features and the ease of production, nanosizing, i.e., the production of nanocrystals, has become a major formulation principle in pharmaceutics to improve the bioactivity of pharmaceutically active ingredients [135–137].

In the field of natural products, nanosizing has opened up a promising avenue to augment further their potential. It is possible, for instance, to convert simple, intrinsically "insoluble" materials, such as elemental sulfur, selenium and tellurium—and, of course, many of the other solid elements of the Periodic Table—into nanosuspenions with interesting biological activities [69]. In the case of the three chalcogens, a pronounced biological activity, for instance against *Steinernema feltiae*, *Escherichia coli* and *Saccaromyces cerevisiae* has been observed which compares well with the one of the corresponding elemental particles obtained by redox chemistry or bioreduction in *S. carnosus* [89].

Nanosizing chemically pure substances or mixtures is comparably straight forward, yet the matter literally becomes more complicated once natural samples such as barks, shells, seeds or even dried fruits, roots or entire plants are milled and homogenized. Here, specific techniques need to be developed and applied. It may appear straight forward to mill down a shell of a walnut or some commercially available grape seed flour, even so our experience tells us that nanosizing a dried tomato plant or spent coffee ground is considerably more challenging. Specific protocols with several steps may be required, from drying and freeze-drying to defatting and pre-milling. Still, some plants, such as the Maltese mushroom *Cynomorium coccinem* L., a parasitic plant devoid of any chlorophyll, can be obtained, freeze-dried, milled and homogenized to fairly stable, low polydispersity and uniform particles with average diameters of around 400 nm without encountering any unsurmountable problems [138]. Some of these milled down plant materials have been evaluated already as potential food supplements and even as natural medicines and antimicrobial agents [130]. In the medium term, nanoparticles of natural products may be employed in the fields of nutrition, medicine, cosmetics or, in the case of large scale manufacture, in "green" agriculture (Figure 7).

The activities observed for those nanosized materials are often promising, yet there is a fine balance of arguments which needs to be considered. On a positive note, nanosizing an herb or medical plant is comparably straightforward and considerably easier than extraction, purification and formulation of the active ingredient(s) contained therein. It also produces no or little waste. Furthermore, the nanoparticles essentially are still "natural", at least as far as their chemical composition is concerned, contain all the ingredients of the plant, have not undergone any extensive modifications and, notably, have not been treated with any organic solvents. Ideally, they even represent a natural slow release system of bioavailable and biologically active ingredients. In the case of HPH, such materials initially are also sterile and, as more recent studies have confirmed, can also be lyophilized and resuspended without loss of physical properties or activity once a simple stabilizer such as mannitol is added [139–141].

Eventually, some caution is required as such materials are intrinsically ill defined chemically, often contain fibrous materials, are prone to fouling if contaminated with microorganisms and also require certain stabilizers so not to aggregate in nanosuspension or as a result of freeze-drying. In analogy to the 1980s German pop band "Milli Vanilli", milling vanilla is clearly exciting, fancy, hot and full of potential, yet some care must be taken and there is still considerable need for further investigation and improvement, especially once the power fails and the chips are down [142].

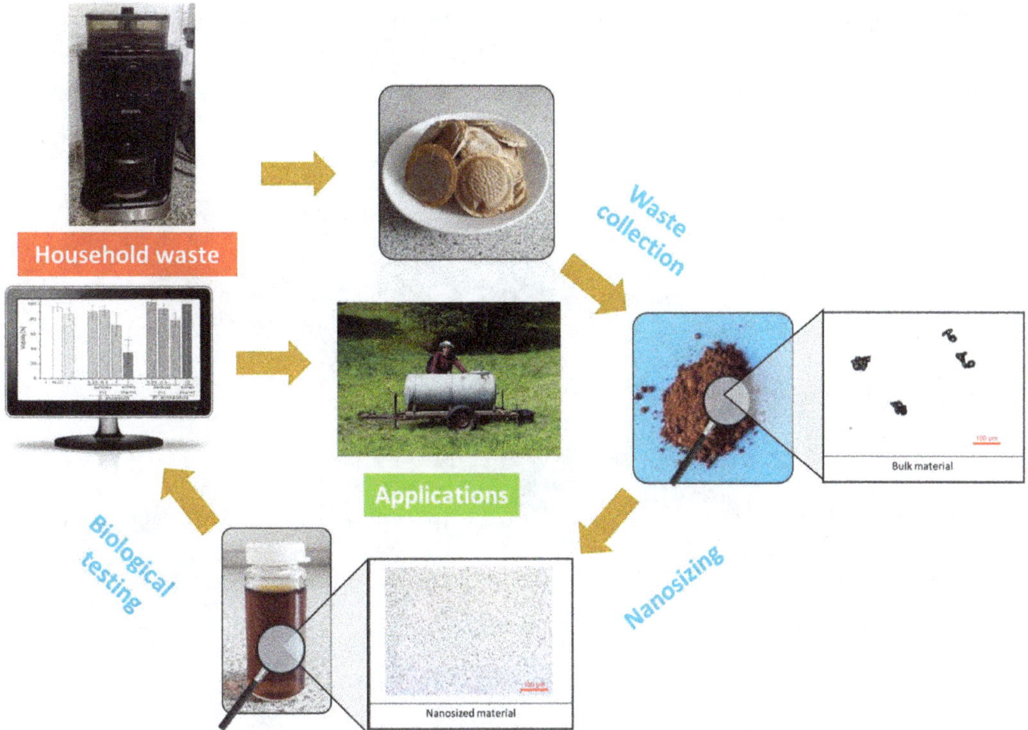

Figure 7. A schematic overview of theutilization of nanosizing techniques for turning waste into value.

6. Conclusions

The previous sections have highlighted just a few selected recent developments at the interface of nanotechnology and natural products research. We have seen that nature itself is well suited to produce a repertoire of nanomaterials by processes such as combustion, abrasion, precipitation and oxidation, and, if the biosphere is included, by bioreduction and related processes. Some of the natural nanoparticles obtained in this way may be useful in medicine, agriculture or other fields of technology and engineering. Not surprisingly, this has stimulated research into these native materials and processes, and has also inspired strategies to generate biological and biologically active materials using similar materials and methods. It is now time to take stock and to anticipate some of the most exciting developments which the next couple of years may bring (Figure 8).

First, it seems plausible that some freely flowing inorganic substances, such as H_2S, which hitherto have "only" been used in spa towns to pickle and macerate affluent pensioners or have been wasted entirely, may be reconsidered as valuable precursors of fine chemicals, including certain nanoparticles. Here, some "hat tricks" may also be feasible, such as the reaction of H_2S from mineral springs with fumes rich in SO_2 as part of an elegant sulfur redox comproportionation, or a reaction of H_2S with NO_2. Such "waste chemistry" may not only be employed to produce the desired nanoparticles—in this case of sulfur, but also to detoxify two individual environmental hazards simultaneously [42]. Those ideas are still speculative, however, early studies into this direction are marred by issues, such as adequate concentrations and how to bring the hazards—literally—under one roof. It seems to us that crucial but manageable research is required to define the correct ingredients and conditions for such manufacture and large-scale production of particles of sulfur and related elements, such as selenium.

Secondly, natural nanotechnology employing organisms such as yeasts and certain harmless bacteria, but also isolated enzymes, may in future be recruited to generate a variety of particular particle matter, starting with selenium and embracing large parts of the Periodic Table, but also other inorganic materials, such as insoluble metal oxides. Indeed, it seems today that a wide palette of insoluble matter may be generated inside bacteria. Whilst traditionally harvesting of such particles has involved lysis of cells, some organisms also release their particles into the supernatant, as has been demonstrated for resveratrol-conjugated gold nanoparticles produced by the *Delftia* sp. strain KCM-006 [143]. Such in vivo generation of nanoparticles may provide further impetus for bioremediation and inspire new avenues to tackle some pathogenic organisms unable to release their particles with undesired intracellular deposits.

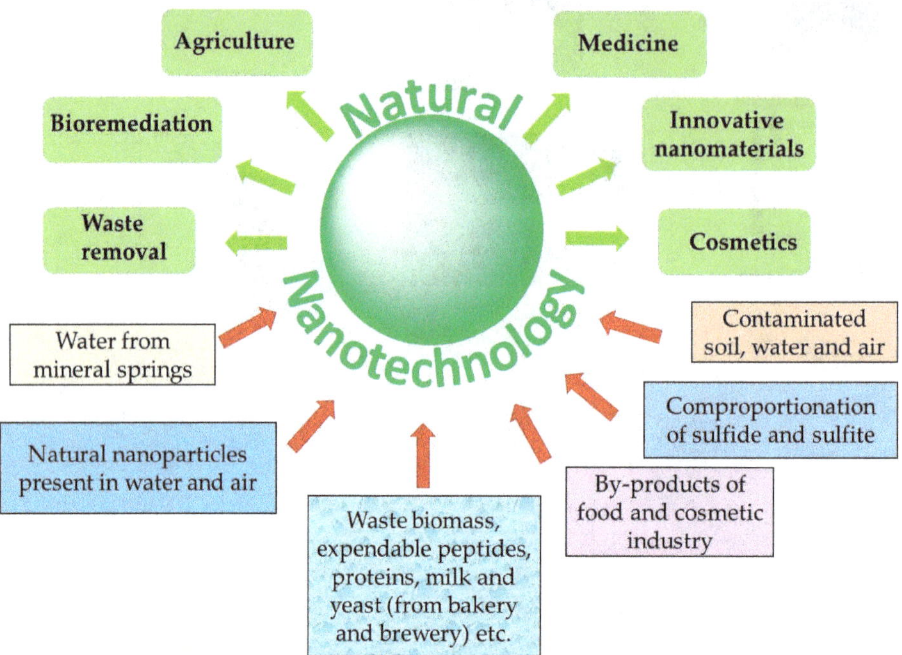

Figure 8. Natural nanotechnology with its various inorganic and biological aspects provides a wide range of opportunities and applications, not only in medicine and cosmetics, but also in less obvious areas such as agriculture and waste removal.

Thirdly, the use of certain plant products, such as de-oiled herbs, as reagents in nano-manufacture may be considered more widely, especially in the context of waste management and "up-cycling". Here, plant waste from harvests or processes such as baking or brewing may provide an interesting alternative to pure chemicals, as they are natural and readily available in large quantities and at low cost. As mentioned already, these materials may either be employed directly as reducing agents or coatings or, more indirectly, as feedstock for bacteria able to generate nanoparticles via a bioreductive avenue. From an ecological perspective, it would be especially intriguing to employ nanosized waste as feedstock for bacteria naturally producing natural nanoparticles.

Fourthly, milling and homogenization of plants may unlock a whole treasure chest of new products, as it can be employed to render hitherto insoluble materials into nanosuspensions with interesting release properties. Many of these products originate in agriculture and, once processed, may be used there as well, hence providing the basis for interesting production and application cycles. This field is still in its early stages of research and development and most certainly will lead to many obstacles and pitfalls, but also to some truly innovative ideas, methods and products.

Eventually, we are likely to witness a rapidly growing interest in various fields of bio-nanotechnology, such as phyto- and phyco-nanotechnology, not only with sight on product development, but also in many areas of basic research which accompany such developments. In the longer run, it may even be possible to explore some of these leads to generate nanoparticles of natural products, such as active ingredients of plants, using natural processes, including bacterial or fungal fermentation, in vitro bioreduction or abrasion. Here, the two meanings of natural, i.e., in form of the material or as part of the method, may eventually meet and merge. Most of this is obviously still speculative today, and time will tell which of these leads are green, fruitful inspirations and which are more the kind of red herring which will stay in the fishbowl of the laboratory.

Acknowledgments: The authors would like to acknowledge their respective Universities for financial support: The University of Saarland, University of Applied Sciences Kaiserslautern, Federal University of Ndufu-Alike Ikwo and the Philipps University of Marburg. The authors would also like to acknowledge the financial support provided by Higher Education Commission of Pakistan and TWAS-DFG. Special thanks go to the members of the "Academiacs International" network for their helpful discussions and advice.

Author Contributions: Sharoon Griffin, Muhammad Irfan Masood, Muhammad Jawad Nasim, Muhammad Sarfraz, Azubuike Peter Ebokaiwe, Karl-Herbert Schäfer, Cornelia M. Keck and Claus Jacob wrote the manuscript.

Conflicts of Interest: The authors declare no conflict of interest.

References

1. Kettler, K.; Krystek, P.; Giannakou, C.; Hendriks, A.J.; de Jong, W.H. Exploring the effect of silver nanoparticle size and medium composition on uptake into pulmonary epithelial 16HBE14o-cells. *J. Nanopart. Res.* **2016**, *18*, 1–11. [CrossRef] [PubMed]
2. Moss, D.M.; Siccardi, M. Optimizing nanomedicine pharmacokinetics using physiologically based pharmacokinetics modelling. *Br. J. Pharmacol.* **2014**, *171*, 3963–3979. [CrossRef] [PubMed]
3. Vincent, B.B.; Loeve, S. Metaphors in nanomedicine: The case of targeted drug delivery. *NanoEthics* **2014**, *8*, 1–17. [CrossRef]
4. Roy, D.N.; Goswami, R.; Pal, A. Nanomaterial and toxicity: What can proteomics tell us about the nanotoxicology? *Xenobiotica* **2017**, *47*, 632–643.
5. Brunner, T.J.; Wick, P.; Manser, P.; Spohn, P.; Grass, R.N.; Limbach, L.K.; Bruinink, A.; Stark, W.J. In vitro cytotoxicity of oxide nanoparticles: Comparison to asbestos, silica, and the effect of particle solubility. *Environ. Sci. Technol.* **2006**, *40*, 4374–4381. [CrossRef] [PubMed]
6. Cassee, F.R.; Heroux, M.E.; Gerlofs-Nijland, M.E.; Kelly, F.J. Particulate matter beyond mass: Recent health evidence on the role of fractions, chemical constituents and sources of emission. *Inhal. Toxicol.* **2013**, *25*, 802–812. [CrossRef] [PubMed]
7. Kukkonen, J.; Bozó, L.; Palmgren, F.; Sokhi, R.S. Particulate matter in urban air. In *Air Quality in Cities: Saturn Eurotrac-2 Subproject Final Report*; Moussiopoulos, N., Ed.; Springer: Berlin/Heidelberg, Germany, 2003; pp. 91–120.
8. Urbano, P.; Urbano, F. Nanobacteria: Facts or fancies? *PLoS Pathog.* **2007**, *3*, 567–570. [CrossRef] [PubMed]
9. Kajander, E.O.; Ciftcioglu, N.; Miller-Hjelle, M.A.; Hjelle, J.T. Nanobacteria: Controversial pathogens in nephrolithiasis and polycystic kidney disease. *Curr. Opin. Nephrol. Hypertens.* **2001**, *10*, 445–452. [CrossRef] [PubMed]
10. Ciftcioglu, N.; Mckay, D.S.; Mathew, G.; Kajander, E.O. Nanobacteria: Fact or fiction? Characteristics, detection, and medical importance of novel self-replicating, calcifying nanoparticles. *J. Investig. Med.* **2006**, *54*, 385–394. [CrossRef] [PubMed]
11. Pasula, R.R.; Lim, S. Engineering nanoparticle synthesis using microbial factories. In *Engineering Biology*; Institution of Engineering and Technology: Stevenage, UK, 2017; Volume 1, pp. 12–17.
12. Patel, V.; Berthold, D.; Puranik, P.; Gantar, M. Screening of cyanobacteria and microalgae for their ability to synthesize silver nanoparticles with antibacterial activity. *Biotechnol. Rep.* **2015**, *5*, 112–119. [CrossRef] [PubMed]
13. Mukherjee, P.; Ahmad, A.; Mandal, D.; Senapati, S.; Sainkar, S.R.; Khan, M.I.; Ramani, R.; Parischa, R.; Ajayakumar, P.V.; Alam, M.; et al. Bioreduction of $AuCl_4^-$ ions by the fungus, *Verticillium* sp. and surface trapping of the gold nanoparticles formed. *Angew. Chem. Int. Ed.* **2001**, *40*, 3585–3588. [CrossRef]
14. Lahde, A.; Gudmundsdottir, S.S.; Joutsensaari, J.; Tapper, U.; Ruusunen, J.; Ihalainen, M.; Karhunen, T.; Torvela, T.; Jokiniemi, J.; Jarvinen, K.; et al. In vitro evaluation of pulmonary deposition of airborne volcanic ash. *Atmos. Environ.* **2013**, *70*, 18–27. [CrossRef]
15. Murr, L.E.; Guerrero, P.A. Carbon nanotubes in wood soot. *Atmos. Sci. Lett.* **2006**, *7*, 93–95. [CrossRef]
16. Wu, C.Y.; Martel, J.; Wong, T.Y.; Young, D.; Liu, C.C.; Lin, C.W.; Young, J.D. Formation and characteristics of biomimetic mineralo-organic particles in natural surface water. *Sci. Rep.* **2016**, *6*. [CrossRef] [PubMed]
17. Boyjoo, Y.; Pareek, V.K.; Liu, J. Synthesis of micro and nano-sized calcium carbonate particles and their applications. *J. Mater. Chem. A* **2014**, *2*, 14270–14288. [CrossRef]

18. Koo, A.N.; Min, K.H.; Lee, H.J.; Jegal, J.H.; Lee, J.W.; Lee, S.C. Calcium carbonate mineralized nanoparticles as an intracellular transporter of cytochromec for cancer therapy. *Chem. Asian J.* **2015**, *10*, 2380–2387. [CrossRef] [PubMed]
19. Dizaj, S.M.; Barzegar-Jalali, M.; Zarrintan, M.H.; Adibkia, K.; Lotfipour, F. Calcium carbonate nanoparticles as cancer drug delivery system. *Expert Opin. Drug Deliv.* **2015**, *12*, 1649–1660. [CrossRef] [PubMed]
20. Hua, K.H.; Wang, H.C.; Chung, R.S.; Hsu, J.C. Calcium carbonate nanoparticles can enhance plant nutrition and insect pest tolerance. *J. Pestic. Sci.* **2015**, *40*, 208–213. [CrossRef]
21. Setiawan, H.; Khairani, R.; Rahman, M.A.; Septawendar, R.; Mukti, R.R.; Dipojono, H.K.; Purwasasmita, B.S. Synthesis of zeolite and gamma-alumina nanoparticles as ceramic membranes for desalination applications. *J. Aust. Ceram. Soc.* **2017**, *53*, 531–538. [CrossRef]
22. Singh, I.B.; Gupta, A.; Dubey, S.; Shafeeq, M.; Banerjee, P.; Sinha, A.S.K. Sol-gel synthesis of nanoparticles of gamma alumina and their application in defluoridation of water. *J. Sol-Gel Sci. Technol.* **2016**, *77*, 416–422. [CrossRef]
23. Nazari, A.; Sanjayan, J.G. Hybrid effects of alumina and silica nanoparticles on water absorption of geopolymers: Application of Taguchi approach. *Measurement* **2015**, *60*, 240–246. [CrossRef]
24. Palaniraja, J.; Arunachalam, P.; Vijayalakshmi, U.; Ghanem, M.A.; Roopan, S.M. Synthesis of calcium silicate nanoparticles and its catalytic application in Friedlander reaction. *Inorg. Nano-Met. Chem.* **2017**, *47*, 946–949. [CrossRef]
25. Wu, J.; Zhu, Y.J.; Chen, F.; Zhao, X.Y.; Zhao, J.; Qi, C. Amorphous calcium silicate hydrate/block copolymer hybrid nanoparticles: Synthesis and application as drug carriers. *Dalton Trans.* **2013**, *42*, 7032–7040. [CrossRef] [PubMed]
26. Strambeanu, N.; Demetrovici, L.; Dragos, D. Natural sources of nanoparticles. In *Nanoparticles' Promises and Risks: Characterization, Manipulation, and Potential Hazards to Humanity and the Environment*; Lungu, M., Neculae, A., Bunoiu, M., Biris, C., Eds.; Springer International Publishing: Cham, Switzerland, 2015; pp. 9–19.
27. Sun, R.; Yin, L.; Zhang, S.H.; He, L.; Cheng, X.J.; Wang, A.N.; Xia, H.W.; Shi, H.B. Simple light-triggered fluorescent labeling of silica nanoparticles for cellular imaging applications. *Chem. Eur. J.* **2017**, *23*, 13893–13896. [CrossRef] [PubMed]
28. Xu, Z.G.; Ma, X.Q.; Gao, Y.E.; Hou, M.L.; Xue, P.; Li, C.M.; Kang, Y.J. Multifunctional silica nanoparticles as a promising theranostic platform for biomedical applications. *Mater. Chem. Front.* **2017**, *1*, 1257–1272. [CrossRef]
29. Liu, X.N.; Lu, X.R.; Wen, P.; Shu, X.Y.; Chi, F.T. Synthesis of ultrasmall silica nanoparticles for application as deep-ultraviolet antireflection coatings. *Appl. Surf. Sci.* **2017**, *420*, 180–185. [CrossRef]
30. Bergin, I.L.; Witzmann, F.A. Nanoparticle toxicity by the gastrointestinal route: Evidence and knowledge gaps. *Int. J. Biomed. Nanosci. Nanotechnol.* **2013**, *3*, 163–210. [CrossRef] [PubMed]
31. Stawski, T.M.; Van Driessche, A.E.S.; Ossorio, M.; Rodriguez-Blanco, J.D.; Besselink, R.; Benning, L.G. Formation of calcium sulfate through the aggregation of sub-3 nanometre primary species. *Nat. Commun.* **2016**, *7*. [CrossRef] [PubMed]
32. Park, Y.B.; Mohan, K.; Al-Sanousi, A.; Almaghrabi, B.; Genco, R.J.; Swihart, M.T.; Dziak, R. Synthesis and characterization of nanocrystalline calcium sulfate for use in osseous regeneration. *Biomed. Mater.* **2011**, *6*. [CrossRef] [PubMed]
33. Guo, H.B.; Barnard, A.S. Naturally occurring iron oxide nanoparticles: Morphology, surface chemistry and environmental stability. *J. Mater. Chem. A* **2013**, *1*, 27–42. [CrossRef]
34. Groult, H.; Poupard, N.; Herranz, F.; Conforto, E.; Bridiau, N.; Sannier, F.; Bordenave, S.; Piot, J.M.; Ruiz-Cabello, J.; Fruitier-Arnaudin, I.; et al. Family of bioactive heparin-coated iron oxide nanoparticles with positive contrast in magnetic resonance imaging for specific biomedical applications. *Biomacromolecules* **2017**, *18*, 3156–3167. [CrossRef] [PubMed]
35. Saeedi, M.; Vahidi, O.; Bonakdar, S. Synthesis and characterization of glycyrrhizic acid coated iron oxide nanoparticles for hyperthermia applications. *Mater. Sci. Eng. C* **2017**, *77*, 1060–1067. [CrossRef] [PubMed]
36. Elrouby, M.; Abdel-Mawgoud, A.M.; Abd El-Rahman, R. Synthesis of iron oxides nanoparticles with very high saturation magnetization form TEA-Fe(III) complex via electrochemical deposition for supercapacitor applications. *J. Mol. Struct.* **2017**, *1147*, 84–95. [CrossRef]
37. Perez, J.M. Iron oxide nanoparticles—Hidden talent. *Nat. Nanotechnol.* **2007**, *2*, 535–536. [CrossRef] [PubMed]
38. Wikipedia. Umber. Available online: https://en.wikipedia.org/wiki/Umber (accessed on 19 December 2017).

39. Yuan, J.K.; Yang, J.; Suib, S.L. Synthesis of microporous manganese oxide nanoparticles and their catalysis applications. *Abstr. Pap. Am. Chem. Soc.* **2004**, *227*, U1310.
40. Zhao, D.Y.; Han, B.; Xie, W.B.; An, B. Applications of stabilized manganese oxide and Fe-Mn binary oxides nanoparticles for in situ remediation of contaminated soil and groundwater. *Abstr. Pap. Am. Chem. Soc.* **2014**, *247*. [CrossRef]
41. Luo, Y.; Yang, J.; Li, J.C.; Yu, Z.B.; Zhang, G.X.; Shi, X.Y.; Shen, M.W. Facile synthesis and functionalization of manganese oxide nanoparticles for targeted T_1-weighted tumor MR imaging. *Colloid Surf. B* **2015**, *136*, 506–513. [CrossRef] [PubMed]
42. Faulstich, L.; Griffin, S.; Nasim, M.J.; Masood, M.I.; Ali, W.; Alhamound, S.; Omran, Y.; Kim, H.; Kharma, A.; Schafer, K.H.; et al. Nature's hat-trick: Can we use sulfur springs as ecological source for materials with agricultural and medical applications? *Int. Biodeterior. Biodegrad.* **2017**, *119*, 678–686. [CrossRef]
43. Suleiman, M.; Al Ali, A.; Hussein, A.; Hammouti, B.; Hadda, T.B.; Warad, I. Sulfur nanoparticles: Synthesis, characterizations and their applications. *J. Mater. Environ. Sci.* **2013**, *4*, 1029–1033.
44. Terrones, M. Carbon nanotubes: Synthesis and properties, electronic devices and other emerging applications. *Int. Mater. Rev.* **2004**, *49*, 325–377. [CrossRef]
45. Popov, V.N. Carbon nanotubes: Properties and application. *Mater. Sci. Eng. R* **2004**, *43*, 61–102. [CrossRef]
46. McGillicuddy, E.; Murray, I.; Kavanagh, S.; Morrison, L.; Fogarty, A.; Cormican, M.; Dockery, P.; Prendergast, M.; Rowan, N.; Morris, D. Silver nanoparticles in the environment: Sources, detection and ecotoxicology. *Sci. Total Environ.* **2017**, *575*, 231–246. [CrossRef] [PubMed]
47. Zhang, C.Q.; Hu, Z.Q.; Deng, B.L. Silver nanoparticles in aquatic environments: Physiochemical behavior and antimicrobial mechanisms. *Water Res.* **2016**, *88*, 403–427. [CrossRef] [PubMed]
48. Rai, M.; Ingle, A.P.; Paralikar, P. Sulfur and sulfur nanoparticles as potential antimicrobials: From traditional medicine to nanomedicine. *Expert Rev. Anti-Infect.* **2016**, *14*, 969–978. [CrossRef] [PubMed]
49. Hough, R.M.; Noble, R.R.P.; Reich, M. Natural gold nanoparticles. *Ore Geol. Rev.* **2011**, *42*, 55–61. [CrossRef]
50. Dykman, L.A.; Khlebtsov, N.G. Gold nanoparticles in biology and medicine: Recent advances and prospects. *Acta Nat.* **2011**, *3*, 34–55.
51. Rauch, S.; Hemond, H.F.; Barbante, C.; Owari, M.; Morrison, G.M.; Peucker-Ehrenbrink, B.; Wass, U. Importance of automobile exhaust catalyst emissions for the deposition of platinum, palladium, and rhodium in the northern hemisphere. *Environ. Sci. Technol.* **2005**, *39*, 8156–8162. [CrossRef] [PubMed]
52. Cheng, Q.; Liu, Y. Multifunctional platinum-based nanoparticles for biomedical applications. *Wiley Interdiscip. Rev. Nanomed. Nanobiotechnol.* **2017**, *9*. [CrossRef] [PubMed]
53. Sheny, D.S.; Philip, D.; Mathew, J. Synthesis of platinum nanoparticles using dried anacardium occidentale leaf and its catalytic and thermal applications. *Spectrochim. Acta Part A* **2013**, *114*, 267–271. [CrossRef] [PubMed]
54. Pedone, D.; Moglianetti, M.; De Luca, E.; Bardi, G.; Pompa, P.P. Platinum nanoparticles in nanobiomedicine. *Chem. Soc. Rev.* **2017**, *46*, 4951–4975. [CrossRef] [PubMed]
55. Blanco-Andujar, C.; Ortega, D.; Pankhurst, Q.A.; Thanh, N.T.K. Elucidating the morphological and structural evolution of iron oxide nanoparticles formed by sodium carbonate in aqueous medium. *J. Mater. Chem.* **2012**, *22*, 12498–12506. [CrossRef]
56. Cho, M.H.; Choi, E.-S.; Kim, S.; Goh, S.-H.; Choi, Y. Redox-responsive manganese dioxide nanoparticles for enhanced MR imaging and radiotherapy of lung cancer. *Front. Chem.* **2017**, *5*. [CrossRef] [PubMed]
57. Song, S.Q.; Rao, R.C.; Yang, H.X.; Liu, H.D.; Zhang, A.M. Facile synthesis of Fe_3O_4/MWCNTs by spontaneous redox and their catalytic performance. *Nanotechnology* **2010**, *21*. [CrossRef] [PubMed]
58. Santillo, D.; Miller, K.; Johnston, P. Microplastics as contaminants in commercially important seafood species. *Integr. Environ. Assess.* **2017**, *13*, 516–521. [CrossRef] [PubMed]
59. Cole, M.; Lindeque, P.; Halsband, C.; Galloway, T.S. Microplastics as contaminants in the marine environment: A review. *Mar. Pollut. Bull.* **2011**, *62*, 2588–2597. [CrossRef] [PubMed]
60. Pawlak, J.; Lodyga-Chrucinska, E.; Chrustowicz, J. Fate of platinum metals in the environment. *J. Trace Elem. Med. Biol.* **2014**, *28*, 247–254. [CrossRef] [PubMed]
61. Zimmermann, S.; Sures, B. Significance of platinum group metals emitted from automobile exhaust gas converters for the biosphere. *Environ. Sci. Pollut. Res.* **2004**, *11*, 194–199. [CrossRef]
62. Ezoe, Y.; Lin, C.H.; Noto, M.; Watanabe, Y.; Yoshimura, K. Evolution of water chemistry in natural acidic environments in Yangmingshan, Taiwan. *J. Environ. Monit.* **2002**, *4*, 533–540. [CrossRef] [PubMed]

63. Berlo, K.; van Hinsberg, V.J.; Vigouroux, N.; Gagnon, J.E.; Williams-Jones, A.E. Sulfide breakdown controls metal signature in volcanic gas at Kawah Ijen volcano, Indonesia. *Chem. Geol.* **2014**, *371*, 115–127. [CrossRef]
64. Mitchell, S.C.; Waring, R.H. Sulphate absorption across biological membranes. *Xenobiotica* **2016**, *46*, 184–191. [CrossRef] [PubMed]
65. Jacob, C. Redox signalling via the cellular thiolstat. *Biochem. Soc. Trans.* **2011**, *39*, 1247–1253. [CrossRef] [PubMed]
66. Giles, G.; Nasim, M.; Ali, W.; Jacob, C. The reactive sulfur species concept: 15 years on. *Antioxidants* **2017**, *6*. [CrossRef] [PubMed]
67. Cummins, L.M.; Kimura, E.T. Safety evaluation of selenium sulfide antidandruff shampoos. *Toxicol. Appl. Pharmacol.* **1971**, *20*, 89–96. [CrossRef]
68. Evolution. Available online: https://en.Wikipedia.Org/wiki/evolution_(2001_film) (accessed on 20 December 2017).
69. Schneider, T.; Baldauf, A.; Ba, L.A.; Jamier, V.; Khairan, K.; Sarakbi, M.B.; Reum, N.; Schneider, M.; Roseler, A.; Becker, K.; et al. Selective antimicrobial activity associated with sulfur nanoparticles. *J. Biomed. Nanotechnol.* **2011**, *7*, 395–405. [CrossRef] [PubMed]
70. Brown, T. The human genome. In *Genomes*, 2nd ed.; Wiley: Oxford, UK, 2002.
71. Shors, T. Virus architecture and nomenclature. In *Understanding Viruses*, 2nd ed.; Jones & Bartlett Learning: Burlington, MA, USA, 2011.
72. Janssen, A.; de Keizer, A.; van Aelst, A.; Fokkink, R.; Yangling, H.; Lettinga, G. Surface characteristics and aggregation of microbiologically produced sulphur particles in relation to the process conditions. *Colloid Surf. B* **1996**, *6*, 115–129. [CrossRef]
73. Mishra, S.; Singh, B.R.; Naqvi, A.H.; Singh, H.B. Potential of biosynthesized silver nanoparticles using *Stenotrophomonas* sp. BHU-S7 (MTCC 5978) for management of soil-borne and foliar phytopathogens. *Sci. Rep.* **2017**, *7*. [CrossRef] [PubMed]
74. Mishra, S.; Singh, B.R.; Singh, A.; Keswani, C.; Naqvi, A.H.; Singh, H.B. Biofabricated silver nanoparticles act as a strong fungicide against *Bipolaris sorokiniana* causing spot blotch disease in wheat. *PLoS ONE* **2014**, *9*, e97881. [CrossRef] [PubMed]
75. Malhotra, A.; Dolma, K.; Kaur, N.; Rathore, Y.S.; Ashish; Mayilraj, S.; Choudhury, A.R. Biosynthesis of gold and silver nanoparticles using a novel marine strain of *Stenotrophomonas*. *Bioresour. Technol.* **2013**, *142*, 727–731. [CrossRef] [PubMed]
76. Singh, P.K.; Kundu, S. Biosynthesis of gold nanoparticles using bacteria. *Proc. Natl. Acad. Sci. India Sect. B* **2014**, *84*, 331–336. [CrossRef]
77. Stefess, G.C.; Torremans, R.A.M.; DeSchrijver, R.; Robertson, L.A.; Kuenen, J.G. Quantitative measurement of sulphur formation by steady state and transient state continuous cultures of autotrophic thiobacillus species. *Appl. Microbiol. Biot.* **1996**, *45*, 169–175. [CrossRef]
78. Kuppusamy, P.; Yusoff, M.M.; Maniam, G.P.; Govindan, N. Biosynthesis of metallic nanoparticles using plant derivatives and their new avenues in pharmacological applications—An updated report. *Saudi Pharm. J.* **2016**, *24*, 473–484. [CrossRef] [PubMed]
79. Wright, M.H.; Farooqui, S.M.; White, A.R.; Greene, A.C. Production of manganese oxide nanoparticles by *Shewanella* species. *Appl. Environ. Microbiol.* **2016**, *82*, 5402–5409. [CrossRef] [PubMed]
80. Garmasheva, I.; Kovalenko, N.; Voychuk, S.; Ostapchuk, A.; Livins'ka, O.; Oleschenko, L. Lactobacillus species mediated synthesis of silver nanoparticles and their antibacterial activity against opportunistic pathogens in vitro. *Bioimpacts* **2016**, *6*, 219–223. [CrossRef] [PubMed]
81. Singh, B.K.; Walker, A. Microbial degradation of organophosphorus compounds. *FEMS Microbiol. Rev.* **2006**, *30*, 428–471. [CrossRef] [PubMed]
82. Yadav, K.K.; Singh, J.K.; Gupta, N.; Kumar, V. A review of nanobioremediation technologies for environmental cleanup: A novel biological approach. *J. Mater. Environ. Sci.* **2017**, *8*, 740–757.
83. Sanghi, R.; Verma, P.; Puri, S. Enzymatic formation of gold nanoparticles using phanerochaete chrysosporium. *Adv. Chem. Eng. Sci.* **2011**, *1*, 1–8. [CrossRef]
84. Durán, N.; Marcato, P.D.; Alves, O.L.; De Souza, G.I.H.; Esposito, E. Mechanistic aspects of biosynthesis of silver nanoparticles by several *Fusarium oxysporum* strains. *J. Nanobiotechnol.* **2005**, *3*. [CrossRef] [PubMed]
85. Duhan, J.S.; Kumar, R.; Kumar, N.; Kaur, P.; Nehra, K.; Duhan, S. Nanotechnology: The new perspective in precision agriculture. *Biotechnol. Rep.* **2017**, *15*, 11–23. [CrossRef] [PubMed]

86. Iavicoli, I.; Leso, V.; Beezhold, D.H.; Shvedova, A.A. Nanotechnology in agriculture: Opportunities, toxicological implications, and occupational risks. *Toxicol. Appl. Pharmacol.* **2017**, *329*, 96–111. [CrossRef] [PubMed]
87. Salata, O. Applications of nanoparticles in biology and medicine. *J. Nanobiotechnol.* **2004**, 2. [CrossRef] [PubMed]
88. Li, X.Q.; Xu, H.Z.; Chen, Z.S.; Chen, G.F. Biosynthesis of nanoparticles by microorganisms and their applications. *J. Nanomater.* **2011**. [CrossRef]
89. Estevam, E.C.; Griffin, S.; Nasim, M.J.; Denezhkin, P.; Schneider, R.; Lilischkis, R.; Dominguez-Alvarez, E.; Witek, K.; Latacz, G.; Keck, C.; et al. Natural selenium particles from *Staphylococcus carnosus*: Hazards or particles with particular promise? *J. Hazard. Mater.* **2017**, *324*, 22–30. [CrossRef] [PubMed]
90. Zhang, L.; Li, D.P.; Gao, P. Expulsion of selenium/protein nanoparticles through vesicle-like structures by saccharomyces cerevisiae under microaerophilic environment. *World J. Microbiol. Biotechnol.* **2012**, *28*, 3381–3386. [CrossRef] [PubMed]
91. Skalickova, S.; Milosavljevic, V.; Cihalova, K.; Horky, P.; Richtera, L.; Adam, V. Selenium nanoparticles as a nutritional supplement. *Nutrition* **2017**, *33*, 83–90. [CrossRef] [PubMed]
92. Wang, T.T.; Yang, L.B.; Zhang, B.C.; Liu, J.H. Extracellular biosynthesis and transformation of selenium nanoparticles and application in H_2O_2 biosensor. *Colloid Surf. B* **2010**, *80*, 94–102. [CrossRef] [PubMed]
93. Yazdi, M.H.; Mahdavi, M.; Varastehmoradi, B.; Faramarzi, M.A.; Shahverdi, A.R. The immunostimulatory effect of biogenic selenium nanoparticles on the 4T1 breast cancer model: An in vivo study. *Biol. Trace Elem. Res.* **2012**, *149*, 22–28. [CrossRef] [PubMed]
94. Prakash, N.T.; Sharma, N.; Prakash, R.; Raina, K.K.; Fellowes, J.; Pearce, C.I.; Lloyd, J.R.; Pattrick, R.A.D. Aerobic microbial manufacture of nanoscale selenium: Exploiting nature's bio-nanomineralization potential. *Biotechnol. Lett.* **2009**, *31*, 1857–1862. [CrossRef] [PubMed]
95. Manikova, D.; Letavayova, L.M.; Vlasakova, D.; Kosik, P.; Estevam, E.C.; Nasim, M.J.; Gruhlke, M.; Slusarenko, A.; Burkholz, T.; Jacob, C.; et al. Intracellular diagnostics: Hunting for the mode of action of redox-modulating selenium compounds in selected model systems. *Molecules* **2014**, *19*, 12258–12279. [CrossRef] [PubMed]
96. Castellucci Estevam, E.; Witek, K.; Faulstich, L.; Nasim, M.J.; Latacz, G.; Dominguez-Alvarez, E.; Kiec-Kononowicz, K.; Demasi, M.; Handzlik, J.; Jacob, C. Aspects of a distinct cytotoxicity of selenium salts and organic selenides in living cells with possible implications for drug design. *Molecules* **2015**, *20*, 13894–13912. [CrossRef] [PubMed]
97. Reddy, C.A.; Mathew, Z. Bioremediation potential of white rot fungi. In *British Mycological Society Symposium Series*; Cambridge University Press: Cambridge, UK, 2001; pp. 52–78.
98. Padhi, S.K.; Tripathy, S.; Sen, R.; Mahapatra, A.S.; Mohanty, S.; Maiti, N.K. Characterisation of heterotrophic nitrifying and aerobic denitrifying *Klebsiella pneumoniae* CF-S9 strain for bioremediation of wastewater. *Int. Biodeterior. Biodegrad.* **2013**, *78*, 67–73. [CrossRef]
99. Duran, N.; Cuevas, R.; Cordi, L.; Rubilar, O.; Diez, M.C. Biogenic silver nanoparticles associated with silver chloride nanoparticles (Ag@AgCl) produced by laccase from *Trametes versicolor*. *SpringerPlus* **2014**, *3*. [CrossRef] [PubMed]
100. Anil Kumar, S.; Abyaneh, M.K.; Gosavi, S.W.; Kulkarni, S.K.; Pasricha, R.; Ahmad, A.; Khan, M.I. Nitrate reductase-mediated synthesis of silver nanoparticles from $AgNO_3$. *Biotechnol. Lett.* **2007**, *29*, 439–445. [CrossRef] [PubMed]
101. Makarov, V.V.; Love, A.J.; Sinitsyna, O.V.; Makarova, S.S.; Yaminsky, I.V.; Taliansky, M.E.; Kalinina, N.O. "Green" nanotechnologies: Synthesis of metal nanoparticles using plants. *Acta Nat.* **2014**, *6*, 35–44.
102. Khodashenas, B.; Ghorbani, H.R. Synthesis of silver nanoparticles with different shapes. *Arab. J. Chem.* **2015**. [CrossRef]
103. Singh, A.K.; Kanchanapally, R.; Fan, Z.; Senapati, D.; Ray, P.C. Synthesis of highly fluorescent water-soluble silver nanoparticles for selective detection of Pb(II) at the parts per quadrillion (PPQ) level. *Chem. Commun.* **2012**, *48*, 9047–9049. [CrossRef] [PubMed]
104. Zhou, T.; Rong, M.; Cai, Z.; Yang, C.J.; Chen, X. Sonochemical synthesis of highly fluorescent glutathione-stabilized Ag nanoclusters and S^{2-} sensing. *Nanoscale* **2012**, *4*, 4103–4106. [CrossRef] [PubMed]
105. Jain, S.; Mehata, M.S. Medicinal plant leaf extract and pure flavonoid mediated green synthesis of silver nanoparticles and their enhanced antibacterial property. *Sci. Rep.* **2017**, *7*. [CrossRef] [PubMed]

106. Si, S.; Mandal, T.K. Tryptophan-based peptides to synthesize gold and silver nanoparticles: A mechanistic and kinetic study. *Chem. Eur. J.* **2007**, *13*, 3160–3168. [CrossRef] [PubMed]
107. Brodin, J.D.; Carr, J.R.; Sontz, P.A.; Tezcan, F.A. Exceptionally stable, redox-active supramolecular protein assemblies with emergent properties. *Proc. Natl. Acad. Sci. USA* **2014**, *111*, 2897–2902. [CrossRef] [PubMed]
108. Lee, K.J.; Park, S.H.; Govarthanan, M.; Hwang, P.H.; Seo, Y.S.; Cho, M.; Lee, W.H.; Lee, J.Y.; Kamala-Kannan, S.; Oh, B.T. Synthesis of silver nanoparticles using cow milk and their antifungal activity against phytopathogens. *Mater. Lett.* **2013**, *105*, 128–131. [CrossRef]
109. Arrigoni, O.; De Tullio, M.C. Ascorbic acid: Much more than just an antioxidant. *Biochim. Biophys. Acta Gen. Subj.* **2002**, *1569*, 1–9. [CrossRef]
110. Yamada, C.; Kawai, H.; Yoshida, K. Improving ascorbic acid content of tomato fruits by the oxidized yeast extract. In *Plant Nutrition for Sustainable Food Production and Environment, Proceedings of the XIII International Plant Nutrition Colloquium, Tokyo, Japan, 13–19 September 1997*; Ando, T., Fujita, K., Mae, T., Matsumoto, H., Mori, S., Sekiya, J., Eds.; Springer: Dordrecht, The Netherlands, 1997; pp. 973–974.
111. Balcerczyk, A.; Grzelak, A.; Janaszewska, A.; Jakubowski, W.; Koziol, S.; Marszalek, M.; Rychlik, B.; Soszynski, M.; Bilinski, T.; Bartosz, G. Thiols as major determinants of the total antioxidant capacity (reprinted from thiol metabolism and redox regulation of cellular functions). *Biofactors* **2003**, *17*, 75–82. [CrossRef] [PubMed]
112. Swiegers, J.H.; Capone, D.L.; Pardon, K.H.; Elsey, G.M.; Sefton, M.A.; Francis, I.L.; Pretorius, I.S. Engineering volatile thiol release in *Saccharomyces cerevisiae* for improved wine aroma. *Yeast* **2007**, *24*, 561–574. [CrossRef] [PubMed]
113. Kerr, E.D.; Schulz, B.L. Vegemite beer: Yeast extract spreads as nutrient supplements to promote fermentation. *PeerJ* **2016**, *4*, e2271. [CrossRef] [PubMed]
114. Shulman, K.I.; Walker, S.E.; Mackenzie, S.; Knowles, S. Dietary restriction, tyramine, and the use of monoamine-oxidase inhibitors. *J. Clin. Psychopharmacol.* **1989**, *9*, 397–402. [CrossRef] [PubMed]
115. Musarrat, J.; Dwivedi, S.; Singh, B.R.; Al-Khedhairy, A.A.; Azam, A.; Naqvi, A. Production of antimicrobial silver nanoparticles in water extracts of the fungus *Amylomyces rouxii* strain KSU-09. *Bioresour. Technol.* **2010**, *101*, 8772–8776. [CrossRef] [PubMed]
116. Sreekanth, T.V.; Ravikumar, S.; Eom, I.Y. Green synthesized silver nanoparticles using nelumbonucifera root extract for efficient protein binding, antioxidant and cytotoxicity activities. *J. Photochem. Photobiol. B* **2014**, *141*, 100–105. [CrossRef] [PubMed]
117. Ravikumar, S.; Sreekanth, T.V.M.; Eom, I.Y. Interaction studies of greenly synthesized gold nanoparticles with bovine serum albumin (BSA) using fluorescence spectroscopy. *J. Nanosci. Nanotechnol.* **2015**, *15*, 9617–9623. [CrossRef] [PubMed]
118. Dhayalan, M.; Denison, M.I.J.; Jegadeeshwari, L.A.; Krishnan, K.; Gandhi, N.N. In vitro antioxidant, antimicrobial, cytotoxic potential of gold and silver nanoparticles prepared using *Embelia ribes*. *Nat. Prod. Res.* **2017**, *31*, 465–468. [CrossRef] [PubMed]
119. Stan, M.; Popa, A.; Toloman, D.; Silipas, T.D.; Vodnar, D.C. Antibacterial and antioxidant activities of ZnO nanoparticles synthesized using extracts of *Allium Sativum*, *Rosmarinus officinalis* and *Ocimum basilicum*. *Acta Metall Sin. Engl.* **2016**, *29*, 228–236. [CrossRef]
120. Stan, M.; Popa, A.; Toloman, D.; Silipas, T.-D.; Vodnar, D.C.; Katona, G. Enhanced antibacterial activity of zinc oxide nanoparticles synthesized using *Petroselinum crispum* extracts. In *AIP Conference Proceedings*; AIP Publishing: College Park, MD, USA, 2015; Volume 1700.
121. Stan, M.; Lung, I.; Soran, M.L.; Leostean, C.; Popa, A.; Stefan, M.; Lazar, M.D.; Opris, O.; Silipas, T.D.; Porav, A.S. Removal of antibiotics from aqueous solutions by green synthesized magnetite nanoparticles with selected agro-waste extracts. *Process Saf. Environ.* **2017**, *107*, 357–372. [CrossRef]
122. Prakash, P.; Gnanaprakasam, P.; Emmanuel, R.; Arokiyaraj, S.; Saravanan, M. Green synthesis of silver nanoparticles from leaf extract of *Mimusops elengi*, Linn. for enhanced antibacterial activity against multi drug resistant clinical isolates. *Colloid Surf. B* **2013**, *108*, 255–259. [CrossRef] [PubMed]
123. Krishnaraj, C.; Ramachandran, R.; Mohan, K.; Kalaichelvan, P.T. Optimization for rapid synthesis of silver nanoparticles and its effect on phytopathogenic fungi. *Spectrochim. Acta Part A* **2012**, *93*, 95–99. [CrossRef] [PubMed]

124. Otunola, G.A.; Afolayan, A.J.; Ajayi, E.O.; Odeyemi, S.W. Characterization, antibacterial and antioxidant properties of silver nanoparticles synthesized from aqueous extracts of *Allium sativum*, *Zingiber officinale*, and *Capsicum frutescens*. *Pharmacogn. Mag.* **2017**, *13*, S201–S208. [CrossRef] [PubMed]
125. Barbulova, A.; Colucci, G.; Apone, F. New trends in cosmetics: By-products of plant origin and their potential use as cosmetic active ingredients. *Cosmetics* **2015**, *2*, 82–92. [CrossRef]
126. Chokshi, K.; Pancha, I.; Ghosh, T.; Paliwal, C.; Maurya, R.; Ghosh, A.; Mishra, S. Green synthesis, characterization and antioxidant potential of silver nanoparticles biosynthesized from de-oiled biomass of thermotolerant oleaginous microalgae acutodesmus dimorphus. *RSC Adv.* **2016**, *6*, 72269–72274. [CrossRef]
127. Harish, S.P. Phyco-nanotechnology: New horizons of gold nano-factories. *Proc. Natl. Acad. Sci. India Sect. B* **2016**. [CrossRef]
128. Shankar, S.S.; Rai, A.; Ahmad, A.; Sastry, M. Rapid synthesis of Au, Ag, and bimetallic Au core-Ag shell nanoparticles using neem (*Azadirachta indica*) leaf broth. *J. Colloid Interface Sci.* **2004**, *275*, 496–502. [CrossRef] [PubMed]
129. Nune, S.K.; Chanda, N.; Shukla, R.; Katti, K.; Kulkarni, R.R.; Thilakavathy, S.; Mekapothula, S.; Kannan, R.; Katti, K.V. Green nanotechnology from tea: Phytochemicals in tea as building blocks for production of biocompatible gold nanoparticles. *J. Mater. Chem* **2009**, *19*, 2912–2920. [CrossRef] [PubMed]
130. Griffin, S.; Tittikpina, N.K.; Al-Marby, A.; Alkhayer, R.; Denezhkin, P.; Witek, K.; Gbogbo, K.A.; Batawila, K.; Duval, R.E.; Nasim, M.J.; et al. Turning waste into value: Nanosized natural plant materials of *Solanum incanum* L. and *Pterocarpus erinaceus* poir with promising antimicrobial activities. *Pharmaceutics* **2016**, *8*. [CrossRef] [PubMed]
131. Mauludin, R.; Müller, R.H.; Keck, C.M. Development of an oral rutin nanocrystal formulation. *Int. J. Pharm.* **2009**, *370*, 202–209. [CrossRef] [PubMed]
132. Mueller, R.H.; Keck, C.M. Second generation of drug nanocrystals for delivery of poorly soluble drugs: smartCrystal technology. *Eur. J. Pharm. Sci.* **2008**, *34*, S20–S21. [CrossRef]
133. Keck, C.M.; Muller, R.H. Drug nanocrystals of poorly soluble drugs produced by high pressure homogenisation. *Eur. J. Pharm. Biopharm.* **2006**, *62*, 3–16. [CrossRef] [PubMed]
134. Muller, R.H.; Gohla, S.; Keck, C.M. State of the art of nanocrystals—Special features, production, nanotoxicology aspects and intracellular delivery. *Eur. J. Pharm. Biopharm.* **2011**, *78*, 1–9. [CrossRef] [PubMed]
135. Muller, R.H.; Keck, C.M. Challenges and solutions for the delivery of biotech drugs—A review of drug nanocrystal technology and lipid nanoparticles. *J. Biotechnol.* **2004**, *113*, 151–170. [CrossRef] [PubMed]
136. Muller, R.H.; Keck, C.M. Twenty years of drug nanocrystals: Where are we, and where do we go? *Eur. J. Pharm. Biopharm.* **2012**, *80*, 1–3. [CrossRef] [PubMed]
137. Scholz, P.; Keck, C.M. Nanocrystals: From raw material to the final formulated oral dosage form—A review. *Curr. Pharm. Des.* **2015**, *21*, 4217–4228. [CrossRef] [PubMed]
138. Griffin, S.; Alkhayer, R.; Mirzoyan, S.; Turabyan, A.; Zucca, P.; Sarfraz, M.; Nasim, M.; Trchounian, A.; Rescigno, A.; Keck, C.; et al. Nanosizing *Cynomorium*: Thumbs up for potential antifungal applications. *Inventions* **2017**, *2*. [CrossRef]
139. Abdelwahed, W.; Degobert, G.; Stainmesse, S.; Fessi, H. Freeze-drying of nanoparticles: Formulation, process and storage considerations. *Adv. Drug Deliv. Rev.* **2006**, *58*, 1688–1713. [CrossRef] [PubMed]
140. Alihosseini, F.; Ghaffari, S.; Dabirsiaghi, A.R.; Haghighat, S. Freeze-drying of ampicillin solid lipid nanoparticles using mannitol as cryoprotectant. *Braz. J. Pharm. Sci.* **2015**, *51*, 797–802. [CrossRef]
141. Patrignani, F.; Lanciotti, R. Applications of high and ultra high pressure homogenization for food safety. *Front. Microbiol.* **2016**, *7*. [CrossRef] [PubMed]
142. Wikipedia. Milli Vanilli. Available online: https://en.wikipedia.org/wiki/Milli_Vanilli (accessed on 20 December 2017).
143. Ganesh Kumar, C.; Poornachandra, Y.; Mamidyala, S.K. Green synthesis of bacterial gold nanoparticles conjugated to resveratrol as delivery vehicles. *Colloids Surf. B* **2014**, *123*, 311–317. [CrossRef] [PubMed]

7

High Vitamin C Status is Associated with Elevated Mood in Male Tertiary Students

Juliet M. Pullar *, Anitra C. Carr, Stephanie M. Bozonet and Margreet C. M. Vissers

Centre for Free Radical Research, Department of Pathology and Biomedical Science, University of Otago, Christchurch, P.O. Box 4345, Christchurch 8140, New Zealand; anitra.carr@otago.ac.nz (A.C.C.); stephanie.bozonet@otago.ac.nz (S.M.B.); margreet.vissers@otago.ac.nz (M.C.M.V.)

* Correspondence: juliet.pullar@otago.ac.nz

Abstract: Micronutrient status is thought to impact on psychological mood due to the role of nutrients in brain structure and function. The aim of the current study was to investigate the association of vitamin C status with mood state in a sample of male tertiary students. We measured fasting plasma vitamin C levels as an indicator of vitamin C status, and subjective mood was determined using the Profile of Mood States (POMS) questionnaire. One hundred and thirty-nine male students aged 18 to 35 years were recruited from local tertiary institutes in Christchurch, New Zealand. The average plasma vitamin C concentration was 58.2 ± 18.6 (SD) μmol/L and the average total mood disturbance score was 25.5 ± 26.6 (possible score −32 to 200 measuring low to high mood disturbance, respectively). Plasma vitamin C concentration was inversely correlated with total mood disturbance as assessed by POMS ($r = -0.181$, $p < 0.05$). Examination of the individual POMS subscales also showed inverse associations of vitamin C status with depression, confusion, and anger. These findings suggest that high vitamin C status may be associated with improved overall mood in young adult males.

Keywords: vitamin C; ascorbate; plasma; mood; total mood disturbance; POMS

---

1. Introduction

Evidence is accumulating that increased consumption of fruit and vegetables is associated with enhanced mood and psychological well-being [1–5]. While it is possible that fruit and vegetable intake is simply a marker of a "healthier" lifestyle, fruit and vegetables are rich in micronutrients, and there are a number of these that may contribute to an effect on mood [6,7]. Fatigue and depression are known to closely precede the physical symptoms of scurvy—a disease caused by vitamin C deficiency [8,9]—suggesting that vitamin C may also be a moderator of mood. Although known for its antioxidant properties, vitamin C (ascorbate) is also a cofactor for a family of biosynthetic and regulatory enzymes with important functions throughout the body. Critically, it is required for the synthesis of the monoamine neurotransmitters dopamine, noradrenaline, and possibly serotonin [10], deficiencies and dysregulation of which have been hypothesised to contribute to depression [11]. Vitamin C is also a cofactor for enzymes involved in the synthesis of carnitine, which is required for the generation of metabolic energy and has been implicated in the fatigue and lethargy associated with scurvy [10,12]. Furthermore, vitamin C regulates the epigenome; it is a cofactor for enzymes involved in both DNA and histone demethylation [13,14]. Epigenetic modifications provide a mechanism by which environmental signals, such as stress, can alter gene expression and neural function and thereby affect behaviour, cognition, and mental health [15].

Vitamin C levels are tightly regulated throughout the body, and its distribution is generally thought to reflect a functional requirement [16]. Concentrations are highest in the brain and other neuroendocrine tissues such as the pituitary and adrenal glands [17]. Indeed, animal models have shown that the brain is the last organ to be depleted of vitamin C during prolonged deficiency, suggesting a vital role in this tissue [18,19].

Several observational studies have suggested a relationship between vitamin C status—typically measured by dietary intake—and mood [20–22]. These are further supported by a number of small intervention trials in which participants were supplemented with oral vitamin C [23–27]. Hoffer and co-workers found that supplementation with 1 g/day reduced mood disturbance and psychological distress in acutely hospitalised patients [24]. Similarly, a reduction in anxiety was observed in high school students given 500 mg/day of vitamin C compared to a placebo [23]. We have shown an improvement in subjective mood in a group of male tertiary students supplemented with two gold kiwifruit per day, a food source particularly high in vitamin C (~130 mg vitamin C per kiwifruit). A significant effect was observed in those individuals with higher total mood disturbance at baseline [25]. In addition to a decrease in total mood disturbance, a decrease in fatigue, an increase in vigour, and a trend towards a decrease in depression were demonstrated.

The aim of the current study was to investigate the association of vitamin C status with subjective mood. We measured fasting plasma vitamin C levels as an indicator of vitamin C status in a sample of male tertiary students, and subjective mood was determined using a Profile of Mood States (POMS) questionnaire. This test has been validated and shown to be reliable for assessing mood states [28].

2. Materials and Methods

2.1. Study Design

This cross-sectional survey was undertaken between April and September 2012. Sample size calculations based on our previous vitamin C studies [29,30] with a standard deviation of 16 μmol/L at 5% type I error indicated 140 participants were required. When sample size was calculated based on the POMS total mood disturbance (TMD) score, a standard deviation of 25 units (as per our previous study [25]) and precision of 5 units at 5% type I error indicated 96 participants were required. A total of 139 male tertiary-level students aged 18 to 35 years and residing in Christchurch, New Zealand at the time of the study were recruited. Recruitment was through verbal or visual/electronic advertisements at local tertiary institutes. The study received ethical approval from the Upper South B Regional Ethics Committee, Christchurch (ethics reference URB/11/12/048). Informed consent was obtained prior to interview and sampling. At the interview, the participants completed a mood questionnaire, a health and lifestyle questionnaire, and blood samples were taken. Participants' height and weight were recorded by the study interviewer, and the body mass index (BMI) was calculated (kg/m^2).

2.2. Vitamin C Analysis

Fasting peripheral blood was collected by venipuncture into 4 mL K_3-EDTA vacutainer tubes (Becton Dickinson, Auckland, New Zealand) and immediately placed on ice. Samples were centrifuged at 4 °C to separate plasma, and this was mixed with an equal volume of ice-cold 0.54 mol/L perchloric acid solution containing the metal chelator diethylene-triamine-penta-acetic acid (DTPA) [29]. After centrifugation, the deproteinated plasma samples were stored at −80 °C prior to analysis by HPLC with electrochemical detection, as described previously [29]. Plasma vitamin C concentration is expressed as μmol/L.

2.3. Analysis of Mood

The Profile of Mood States (POMS) questionnaire was used to determine the participants' mood during the previous week. Scores were calculated using a POMS standard scoring grid (Psychological Assessments, Australia). The form comprises 65 mood-related adjectives, which are rated on a 5-point Likert-type scale ranging from 0 (not at all) to 4 (extremely) and then categorised into six mood subscales: tension-anxiety, depression-dejection, anger-hostility, vigour-activity, fatigue-inertia, and confusion-bewilderment. A TMD score is calculated by adding the depression, fatigue, tension, anger, and confusion sub-scores and then subtracting the vigour score. TMD scores range from −32 to 200; a higher score indicates more severe mood disturbance [28].

2.4. Statistical Analysis

Data are represented as mean ± SD and 95% confidence intervals. Correlations were tested using Pearson's Correlation Coefficient with SPSS software (version 22, IBM Corp. Armonk, NY, USA) and differences between nonparametric independent samples used the Mann–Whitney U test; p values ≤ 0.05 were considered significant.

3. Results

One hundred and thirty-nine male students aged 18 to 35 years were recruited from local tertiary institutes in Christchurch, New Zealand. No exclusion criteria were applied. The baseline characteristics of the study participants are presented in Table 1. The range of plasma levels was 5 μmol/L to 101 μmol/L, with a mean fasting plasma vitamin C concentration of 58 μmol/L. These are normal fasting values. The majority of the cohort had adequate vitamin C concentrations of 50 μmol/L or greater (71%). Roughly one quarter of participants had inadequate vitamin C status of 23–50 μmol/L [31], 2% were marginal (i.e., 11–23 μmol/L), and 0.7% had actual vitamin C deficiency (i.e., <11 μmol/L). The average TMD score of the participants was 25.5, which is similar to values obtained for male college students in the United States [28].

Table 1. Characteristics of individuals who completed the study.

Participant Characteristics	Mean ± SD	95% CI	n (%)
Age (years)	21.2 ± 2.5	20.8, 21.6	-
Ethnicity	-	-	-
Maori	-	-	13 (9)
NZ European	-	-	106 (76)
Weight (kg)	81.6 ± 15.9	78.9, 84.3	-
Height (cm)	180 ± 7.3	178.8, 181.3	-
BMI (kg/m^2)	25.1 ± 4.3	24.4, 25.8	-
Vitamin C (μmol/L)	58.2 ± 18.6	55.1, 61.3	-
Adequate	-	-	99 (71)
Inadequate	-	-	36 (26)
Marginal	-	-	3 (2)
Deficient	-	-	1 (0.7)
TMD score	25.5 ± 26.6	21.0, 30.0	-

TMD score was n = 138, otherwise data are for n = 139. Plasma vitamin C was classified as deficient <11 μmol/L, marginal 11–23 μmol/L, inadequate 23–50 μmol/L, or adequate >50 μmol/L. TMD, total mood disturbance; CI, confidence interval; NZ, New Zealand; BMI, body mass index.

We investigated the relationship between vitamin C status, as assessed by plasma vitamin C concentration, and subjective mood (Table 2). Plasma vitamin C concentration was inversely correlated with total mood disturbance, as assessed by POMS ($r = -0.181$, $p < 0.05$). Examination of the individual POMS subscales also showed inverse associations of vitamin C status with depression and anger.

Furthermore, when participants were split into two groups around either the average plasma vitamin C concentration of 58.2 μmol/L or the adequacy of their vitamin C status (50 μmol/L cut-off), higher total mood disturbance, as assessed by POMS, was associated with lower plasma vitamin C concentration (Figure 1A,B). When participants were divided around the mean plasma vitamin C concentration, median TMD scores were 25 (IQR 4-52) in the low vitamin C group and 17 (IQR 4-36) in the high vitamin C group. Similarly, participants split around the adequacy of vitamin C status had a median TMD score of 27 (IQR 13-53) in the inadequate group and 17.5 (IQR 3-37) in the adequate group. In addition, those with adequate vitamin C status had significantly lower POMS subscores for depression and confusion as compared to those with inadequate status (Table 3).

Table 2. Pearson linear correlations of plasma vitamin C with mood.

POMS Subscore	r	*p* Value
Total mood disturbance	−0.181	0.034
Depression	−0.192	0.024
Fatigue	−0.061	0.480
Tension	−0.098	0.255
Anger	−0.172	0.044
Vigour	0.100	0.245
Confusion	−0.148	0.084

Total mood disturbance is the sum of the depression, fatigue, tension, anger, and confusion subscores minus the vigour score; $n = 138$.

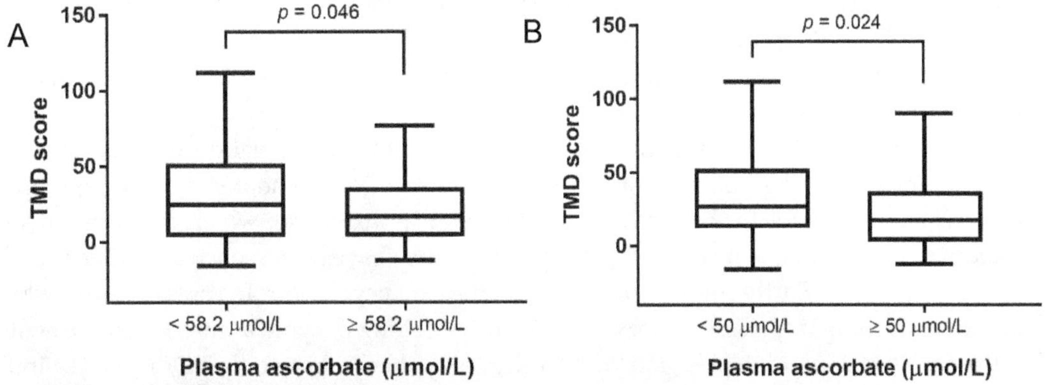

Figure 1. Relationship between total mood disturbance (TMD) score and plasma vitamin C concentration. (**A**) Participants were divided around the mean plasma vitamin C concentration of 58.2 μmol/L. (**B**) Participants were divided around adequacy of vitamin C status (a plasma concentration of 50 μmol/L indicates adequacy). Box plots show median TMD score with the 25th and 75th percentiles as boundaries; whiskers indicate the minimum and maximum of all the data. The TMD score was significantly different between the two groups for each graph (Mann–Whitney U test on ranks).

Table 3. Association of plasma vitamin C adequacy with Profile of Mood States (POMS) mood subscales.

POMS Subscore	*p* Value
Total mood disturbance	0.024
Depression	0.012
Fatigue	0.235
Tension	0.195
Anger	0.131
Vigour	0.453
Confusion	0.022

Participants were divided into two groups based on the adequacy of their vitamin C status (50 μmol/L cut-off). Differences in the TMD subscores were tested using the Mann–Whitney U test on ranks.

4. Discussion

The brain and central nervous system have a requirement for specific dietary nutrients [32,33]. Supplementation studies have shown an improvement in symptoms for certain mental health disorders with intake of nutrient formulations [34–38]; however, nutrients are also likely to be vital for normal psychological functioning and well-being in healthy individuals. The specific nutrients that are important for brain health are still being investigated. In the present study, we found a significant association between vitamin C status and current mood state in a sample of young adult males. Those individuals with the highest plasma vitamin C concentrations were more likely to have elevated mood.

Mood refers to a positive or negative emotional state of varying intensity that changes in response to life circumstances [39]. Mood is considered long-lasting in contrast to the more acutely experienced emotions. In our study, we used the POMS questionnaire to measure mood state during the previous week. As well as providing a total mood score, POMS gives five different measures of negative mood (depression, fatigue, tension, anger, and confusion) and a single measure of positive mood (vigour). In addition to the relationship observed with overall mood, we have shown significant inverse correlations of vitamin C status with the depression, anger, and confusion subscores in the young men studied. No relationship was observed with the positive mood state vigour despite our previous studies showing an increase in feelings of vigour with a food-based intervention that markedly elevated vitamin C levels [25] and despite emerging evidence for the association of dietary factors with positive well-being [1]. It should be noted that in the study cohort, there were only a few individuals with low vitamin C status of <23 μmol/L, meaning we were unable to investigate the mood state of this group. Rather, our results have shown that those with adequate vitamin C status (>50 μmol/L) tended to have an elevated mood.

One of the best-established functions of vitamin C is in the regulation of neurotransmitter biosynthesis, including that of catecholamines dopamine, norepinephrine, and epinephrine. Vitamin C acts as a cofactor for the enzyme dopamine β-hydroxylase, which converts dopamine to norepinephrine [40]. Animal models of vitamin C deficiency have shown decreased norepinephrine concentrations [41–43]. Furthermore, vitamin C can also recycle tetrahydrobiopterin, which is necessary for activation of tyrosine hydroxylase, the rate-limiting enzyme in catecholamine synthesis that synthesizes the dopamine precursor L-3,4-dihydroxyphenylalanine (L-DOPA) [44]. Similarly, tetrahydrobiopterin is a cofactor for tryptophan hydroxylase [45], the initial and rate-limiting enzyme in the synthesis of the neurotransmitter serotonin. There is also evidence emerging that vitamin C is involved in neuronal maturation and functioning [46]. Indeed, brain neurons contain some of the highest levels of vitamin C observed in any mammalian tissue [46]; glial ascorbate concentrations are much lower by comparison.

While the underlying pathophysiology of depression is not yet fully understood, these effects of vitamin C on neurochemistry may provide a mechanism by which it can affect this disorder. An early hypothesis suggested that deficiencies in dopamine, noradrenaline, and serotonin were responsible for major depressive symptoms [11], with some antidepressants elevating levels of these neurotransmitters in the central nervous system. However, it is now apparent that the molecular basis of depression is significantly more complex. Disturbances in dopamine, noradrenaline, and serotonin neurotransmission itself may contribute to the disorder. A more recent hypothesis suggests that low-grade inflammation and immune dysregulation, possibly as a result of psychosocial stressors, may trigger the development and persistence of depression [47]. For example, cytokines are known to induce depressive-type behaviours, and abnormal expressions of proinflammatory cytokines have been shown in patients with depression [48–50]. Oxidative stress markers are also elevated in patients with depression [51]. Vitamin C has a number of anti-inflammatory activities as well as being an excellent antioxidant and reducing agent, and it may be able to modulate some of these responses [12,52,53].

A limitation of the current study is that the data is cross-sectional and does not take into account potential confounders of the relationship between vitamin C status and mood, for example, socioeconomic status or other health behaviours. We did not determine the potential impact of any major recent life events that may affect mood in our cohort. Other unmeasured confounders may also have occurred simultaneously in our participants, such as deficiency in another micronutrient or a lower level of physical activity. Thus, we cannot definitively determine whether the relationship between vitamin C status is direct or, as influenced by the confounders above, indirect or parallel. Additionally, it may be that those with better mental health eat more fruits and vegetables causing higher vitamin C status, that is, higher vitamin C status is a consequence of better mood and mental health. In order to provide evidence of a direct relationship between plasma vitamin C status and mood, well-conducted randomized controlled trials are required. This will allow the direction of the relationship to be firmly established and will also allow the effect of any confounders to be eliminated as these should be evenly distributed between the two groups.

Levels of vitamin C in our cohort were generally higher than has been reported in other similar populations [54–56]. For example, a recent study in a cohort from Poland showed 7% of participants were marginally deficient in vitamin C [55], while a United States sample found 12–16% were marginally deficient [54]. Dietary information from our cohort indicated that there were a significant number of individuals who regularly used dietary supplements or consumed fruit juice containing vitamin C. It was our estimation that these dietary vitamin C sources contributed significantly to the high mean plasma status of our cohort. Apparent differences between the study populations may also reflect shortcomings in the sample handling and processing used in the studies described above, as inadequate processing can, and commonly does, increase the proportion of samples which are vitamin C deficient [57].

5. Conclusions

In conclusion, our findings suggest a possible relationship between vitamin C status and mood state in young adult male students in New Zealand. The current study is cross-sectional and further well-conducted intervention trials are required for proof of causality. There are a number of biological justifications for a positive effect of vitamin C on mood, particularly owing to its role in brain homeostasis and function.

Author Contributions: M.C.M.V. and J.M.P. conceived the study; J.M.P., A.C.C., and M.C.M.V. contributed to the study design; J.M.P. coordinated the study; J.M.P. and A.C.C. conducted the interviews; and S.M.B. measured vitamin C status. J.M.P. analysed the data and wrote the paper. All authors edited the paper.

Funding: This research received no external funding.

Acknowledgments: We express our gratitude to the young men who participated in this study. We acknowledge Jo Kepple for the use of Primorus Clinical Trials Unit, Susan Woods for the use of the Ara Institute of Canterbury Health Centre, and Joan Allardyce for the use of University of Canterbury Health Centre. We acknowledge John Pearson for statistical advice and Maria Webb for assistance with recruitment.

Conflicts of Interest: The authors declare no conflict of interest.

References

1. Blanchflower, D.G.; Oswald, A.J.; Stewart-Brown, S. Is Psychological Well-Being Linked to the Consumption of Fruit and Vegetables? *Soc. Indic. Res.* **2013**, *114*, 785–801. [CrossRef]
2. Conner, T.S.; Brookie, K.L.; Richardson, A.C.; Polak, M.A. On carrots and curiosity: Eating fruit and vegetables is associated with greater flourishing in daily life. *Br. J. Health Psychol.* **2015**, *20*, 413–427. [CrossRef] [PubMed]
3. Tsai, A.C.; Chang, T.L.; Chi, S.H. Frequent consumption of vegetables predicts lower risk of depression in older Taiwanese—Results of a prospective population-based study. *Public Health Nutr.* **2012**, *15*, 1087–1092. [CrossRef] [PubMed]
4. Bishwajit, G.; O'Leary, D.P.; Ghosh, S.; Sanni, Y.; Shangfeng, T.; Zhanchun, F. Association between depression and fruit and vegetable consumption among adults in South Asia. *BMC Psychiatry* **2017**, *17*, 15. [CrossRef] [PubMed]
5. Mujcic, R.; Oswald, J. Evolution of Well-Being and Happiness After Increases in Consumption of Fruit and Vegetables. *Am. J. Public Health* **2016**, *106*, 1504–1510. [CrossRef] [PubMed]

6. Rooney, C.; McKinley, M.C.; Woodside, J.V. The potential role of fruit and vegetables in aspects of psychological well-being: A review of the literature and future directions. *Proc. Nutr. Soc.* **2013**, *72*, 420–432. [CrossRef] [PubMed]
7. Kaplan, B.J.; Crawford, S.G.; Field, C.J.; Simpson, J.S. Vitamins, minerals, and mood. *Psychol. Bull.* **2007**, *133*, 747–760. [CrossRef] [PubMed]
8. Levine, M.; Conry-Cantilena, C.; Wang, Y.; Welch, R.W.; Washko, P.W.; Dhariwal, K.R.; Park, J.B.; Lazarev, A.; Graumlich, J.F.; King, J.; et al. Vitamin C pharmacokinetics in healthy volunteers: Evidence for a recommended dietary allowance. *Proc. Natl. Acad. Sci. USA* **1996**, *93*, 3704–3709. [CrossRef] [PubMed]
9. Crandon, J.H.; Lund, C.C.; Dill, D.B. Experimental human scurvy. *N. Engl. J. Med.* **1940**, *223*, 353–369. [CrossRef]
10. Englard, S.; Seifter, S. The biochemical functions of ascorbic acid. *Annu. Rev. Nutr.* **1986**, *6*, 365–406. [CrossRef] [PubMed]
11. Delgado, P.L. Depression: The case for a monoamine deficiency. *J. Clin. Psychiatry* **2000**, *61*, 7–11. [PubMed]
12. Du, J.; Cullen, J.J.; Buettner, G.R. Ascorbic acid: Chemistry, biology and the treatment of cancer. *Biochim. Biophys. Acta* **2012**, *1826*, 443–457. [CrossRef] [PubMed]
13. Minor, E.A.; Court, B.L.; Young, J.I.; Wang, G. Ascorbate induces ten-eleven translocation (Tet) methylcytosine dioxygenase-mediated generation of 5-hydroxymethylcytosine. *J. Biol. Chem.* **2013**, *288*, 13669–13674. [CrossRef] [PubMed]
14. Blaschke, K.; Ebata, K.T.; Karimi, M.M.; Zepeda-Martinez, J.A.; Goyal, P.; Mahapatra, S.; Tam, A.; Laird, D.J.; Rao, A.; Lorincz, M.C.; et al. Vitamin C induces Tet-dependent DNA demethylation and a blastocyst-like state in ES cells. *Nature* **2013**, *500*, 222–226. [CrossRef] [PubMed]
15. Zhang, T.Y.; Meaney, M.J. Epigenetics and the environmental regulation of the genome and its function. *Annu. Rev. Psychol.* **2010**, *61*, 439–466. [CrossRef] [PubMed]
16. Lindblad, M.; Tveden-Nyborg, P.; Lykkesfeldt, J. Regulation of vitamin C homeostasis during deficiency. *Nutrients* **2013**, *5*, 2860–2879. [CrossRef] [PubMed]
17. Hornig, D. Distribution of ascorbic acid, metabolites and analogues in man and animals. *Ann. N. Y. Acad. Sci.* **1975**, *258*, 103–118. [CrossRef] [PubMed]
18. Hughes, R.E.; Hurley, R.J.; Jones, P.R. The retention of ascorbic acid by guinea-pig tissues. *Br. J. Nutr.* **1971**, *6*, 433–438. [CrossRef]
19. Vissers, M.C.; Bozonet, S.M.; Pearson, J.F.; Braithwaite, L.J. Dietary ascorbate intake affects steady state tissue concentrations in vitamin C-deficient mice: Tissue deficiency after suboptimal intake and superior bioavailability from a food source (kiwifruit). *Am. J. Clin. Nutr.* **2011**, *93*, 292–301. [CrossRef] [PubMed]
20. Gariballa, S. Poor vitamin C status is associated with increased depression symptoms following acute illness in older people. *Int. J. Vitam. Nutr. Res.* **2014**, *84*, 12–17. [CrossRef] [PubMed]
21. Cheraskin, E.; Ringsdorf, W.M., Jr.; Medford, F.H. Daily vitamin C consumption and fatigability. *J. Am. Geriatr. Soc.* **1976**, *24*, 136–137. [CrossRef] [PubMed]
22. Prohan, M.; Amani, R.; Nematpour, S.; Jomehzadeh, N.; Haghighizadeh, M.H. Total antioxidant capacity of diet and serum, dietary antioxidant vitamins intake, and serum hs-CRP levels in relation to depression scales in university male students. *Redox Rep.* **2014**, *19*, 133–139. [CrossRef] [PubMed]
23. De Oliveira, I.J.; de Souza, V.V.; Motta, V.; Da-Silva, S.L. Effects of Oral Vitamin C Supplementation on Anxiety in Students: A Double-Blind, Randomized, Placebo-Controlled Trial. *Pak. J. Biol. Sci.* **2015**, *18*, 11–18. [CrossRef] [PubMed]
24. Wang, Y.; Liu, X.J.; Robitaille, L.; Eintracht, S.; MacNamara, E.; Hoffer, L.J. Effects of vitamin C and vitamin D administration on mood and distress in acutely hospitalized patients. *Am. J. Clin. Nutr.* **2013**, *98*, 705–711. [CrossRef] [PubMed]
25. Carr, A.C.; Bozonet, S.M.; Pullar, J.M.; Vissers, M.C. Mood improvement in young adult males following supplementation with gold kiwifruit, a high-vitamin C food. *J. Nutr. Sci.* **2013**, *2*, e24. [CrossRef] [PubMed]
26. Huck, C.J.; Johnston, C.S.; Beezhold, B.L.; Swan, P.D. Vitamin C status and perception of effort during exercise in obese adults adhering to a calorie-reduced diet. *Nutrition* **2013**, *29*, 42–45. [CrossRef] [PubMed]
27. Zhang, M.; Robitaille, L.; Eintracht, S.; Hoffer, L.J. Vitamin C provision improves mood in acutely hospitalized patients. *Nutrition* **2011**, *27*, 530–533. [CrossRef] [PubMed]
28. McNair, D.; MaH, J.W.P. *Profile of Mood States Technical Update*; North Tonawnada: New York, NY, USA, 2005.

29. Carr, A.C.; Pullar, J.M.; Moran, S.; Vissers, M.C. Bioavailability of vitamin C from kiwifruit in non-smoking males: Determination of 'healthy' and 'optimal' intakes. *J. Nutr. Sci.* **2012**, *1*, e14. [CrossRef] [PubMed]
30. Carr, A.C.; Bozonet, S.M.; Pullar, J.M.; Simcock, J.W.; Vissers, M.C. A randomized steady-state bioavailability study of synthetic versus natural (kiwifruit-derived) vitamin C. *Nutrients* **2013**, *5*, 3684–3695. [CrossRef] [PubMed]
31. Lykkesfeldt, J.; Poulsen, H.E. Is vitamin C supplementation beneficial? Lessons learned from randomised controlled trials. *Br. J. Nutr.* **2010**, *103*, 1251–1259. [CrossRef] [PubMed]
32. Bourre, J.M. Effects of nutrients (in food) on the structure and function of the nervous system: Update on dietary requirements for brain. Part 1: Micronutrients. *J. Nutr. Health Aging* **2006**, *10*, 377–385. [PubMed]
33. Gomez-Pinilla, F. Brain foods: The effects of nutrients on brain function. *Nat. Rev. Neurosci.* **2008**, *9*, 568–578. [CrossRef] [PubMed]
34. Kaplan, B.J.; Fisher, J.E.; Crawford, S.G.; Field, C.J.; Kolb, B. Improved mood and behavior during treatment with a mineral-vitamin supplement: An open-label case series of children. *J. Child Adolesc. Psychopharmacol.* **2004**, *14*, 115–122. [CrossRef] [PubMed]
35. Rucklidge, J.J.; Eggleston, M.J.F.; Johnstone, J.M.; Darling, K.; Frampton, C.M. Vitamin-mineral treatment improves aggression and emotional regulation in children with ADHD: A fully blinded, randomized, placebo-controlled trial. *J. Child Psychol. Psychiatry* **2018**, *59*, 232–246. [CrossRef] [PubMed]
36. Rucklidge, J.; Taylor, M.; Whitehead, K. Effect of micronutrients on behavior and mood in adults With ADHD: Evidence from an 8-week open label trial with natural extension. *J. Atten. Disord.* **2011**, *15*, 79–91. [CrossRef] [PubMed]
37. Sarris, J.; Logan, A.C.; Akbaraly, T.N.; Amminger, G.P.; Balanza-Martinez, V.; Freeman, M.P.; Hibbeln, J.; Matsuoka, Y.; Mischoulon, D.; Mizoue, T.; et al. Nutritional medicine as mainstream in psychiatry. *Lancet Psychiatry* **2015**, *2*, 271–274. [CrossRef]
38. Mischoulon, D.; Freeman, M.P. Omega-3 fatty acids in psychiatry. *Psychiatr. Clin. N. Am.* **2013**, *36*, 15–23. [CrossRef] [PubMed]
39. Polak, M.A.; Richardson, A.C.; Flett, J.A.M.; Brookie, K.L.; Conner, T.S. Measuring Mood: Considerations and Innovations for Nutrition Science. In *Nutrition for Brain Health and Cognitive Performance*; Dye, L., Best, T., Eds.; Taylor Japan and Francis: London, UK, 2015; pp. 93–119.
40. Diliberto, E.J.; Daniels, A.J., Jr.; Viveros, O.H. Multicompartmental secretion of ascorbate and its dual role in dopamine beta-hydroxylation. *Am. J. Clin. Nutr.* **1991**, *54*, 1163S–1172S. [CrossRef] [PubMed]
41. Hoehn, S.K.; Kanfer, J.N. Effects of chronic ascorbic acid deficiency on guinea pig lysosomal hydrolase activities. *J. Nutr.* **1980**, *110*, 2085–2094. [CrossRef] [PubMed]
42. Deana, R.; Bharaj, B.S.; Verjee, Z.H.; Galzigna, L. Changes relevant to catecholamine metabolism in liver and brain of ascorbic acid deficient guinea-pigs. *Int. J. Vitam. Nutr. Res.* **1975**, *45*, 175–182. [PubMed]
43. Bornstein, S.R.; Yoshida-Hiroi, M.; Sotiriou, S.; Levine, M.; Hartwig, H.G.; Nussbaum, R.L.; Eisenhofer, G. Impaired adrenal catecholamine system function in mice with deficiency of the ascorbic acid transporter (SVCT2). *FASEB J.* **2003**, *17*, 1928–1930. [CrossRef] [PubMed]
44. May, J.M.; Qu, Z.C.; Meredith, M.E. Mechanisms of ascorbic acid stimulation of norepinephrine synthesis in neuronal cells. *Biochem. Biophys. Res. Commun.* **2012**, *426*, 148–152. [CrossRef] [PubMed]
45. Kuzkaya, N.; Weissmann, N.; Harrison, D.G.; Dikalov, S. Interactions of peroxynitrite, tetrahydrobiopterin, ascorbic acid, and thiols: Implications for uncoupling endothelial nitric-oxide synthase. *J. Biol. Chem.* **2003**, *278*, 22546–22554. [CrossRef] [PubMed]
46. May, J.M. Vitamin C transport and its role in the central nervous system. *Subcell. Biochem.* **2012**, *56*, 85–103. [PubMed]
47. Berk, M.; Williams, L.J.; Jacka, F.N.; O'Neil, A.; Pasco, J.A.; Moylan, S.; Allen, N.B.; Stuart, A.L.; Hayley, A.C.; Byrne, M.L.; et al. So depression is an inflammatory disease, but where does the inflammation come from? *BMC Med.* **2013**, *11*, 200. [CrossRef] [PubMed]
48. Udina, M.; Castellvi, P.; Moreno-Espana, J.; Navines, R.; Valdes, M.; Forns, X.; Langohr, K.; Sola, R.; Vieta, E.; Martin-Santos, R. Interferon-induced depression in chronic hepatitis C: A systematic review and meta-analysis. *J. Clin. Psychiatry* **2012**, *73*, 1128–1138. [CrossRef] [PubMed]
49. Zou, W.; Feng, R.; Yang, Y. Changes in the serum levels of inflammatory cytokines in antidepressant drug-naive patients with major depression. *PLoS ONE* **2018**, *13*, e0197267. [CrossRef] [PubMed]

50. Jeon, S.W.; Kim, Y.K. The role of neuroinflammation and neurovascular dysfunction in major depressive disorder. *J. Inflamm. Res.* **2018**, *11*, 179–192. [CrossRef] [PubMed]
51. Liu, T.; Zhong, S.; Liao, X.; Chen, J.; He, T.; Lai, S.; Jia, Y. A Meta-Analysis of Oxidative Stress Markers in Depression. *PLoS ONE* **2015**, *10*, e0138904. [CrossRef] [PubMed]
52. Carr, A.C.; Rosengrave, P.C.; Bayer, S.; Chambers, S.; Mehrtens, J.; Shaw, G.M. Hypovitaminosis C and vitamin C deficiency in critically ill patients despite recommended enteral and parenteral intakes. *Crit Care* **2017**, *21*, 300. [CrossRef] [PubMed]
53. Carr, A.C.; Maggini, S. Vitamin C and Immune Function. *Nutrients* **2017**, *9*, e1211. [CrossRef] [PubMed]
54. Johnston, C.S.; Solomon, R.E.; Corte, C. Vitamin C status of a campus population: College students get a C minus. *J. Am. Coll. Health* **1998**, *46*, 209–213. [CrossRef] [PubMed]
55. Szczuko, M.; Seidler, T.; Stachowska, E.; Safranow, K.; Olszewska, M.; Jakubowska, K.; Gutowska, I.; Chlubek, D. Influence of daily diet on ascorbic acid supply to students. *Roczniki Państwowego Zakładu Higieny* **2014**, *65*, 213–220. [PubMed]
56. Cahill, L.; Corey, P.N.; El-Sohemy, A. Vitamin C deficiency in a population of young Canadian adults. *Am. J. Epidemiol.* **2009**, *170*, 464–471. [CrossRef] [PubMed]
57. Pullar, J.M.; Bayer, S.; Carr, A.C. Appropriate Handling, Processing and Analysis of Blood Samples Is Essential to Avoid Oxidation of Vitamin C to Dehydroascorbic Acid. *Antioxidants* **2018**, *7*, 29. [CrossRef] [PubMed]

8

Influence of Vitamin C on Lymphocytes

Gwendolyn N. Y. van Gorkom [1,*], Roel G. J. Klein Wolterink [1], Catharina H. M. J. Van Elssen [1], Lotte Wieten [2], Wilfred T. V. Germeraad [1] and Gerard M. J. Bos [1]

1 Division of Hematology, Department of Internal Medicine, GROW-School for Oncology and Developmental Biology, Maastricht University Medical Center, 6202AZ Maastricht, The Netherlands; r.kleinwolterink@maastrichtuniversity.nl (R.G.J.K.W.); janine.van.elssen@mumc.nl (C.H.M.J.V.E.); w.germeraad@maastrichtuniversity.nl (W.T.V.G.); gerard.bos@mumc.nl (G.M.J.B.)

2 Department of Transplantation Immunology, Maastricht University Medical Center, 6202 AZ Maastricht, The Netherlands; Lotte.wieten@maastrichtuniversity.nl

* Correspondence: gwendolyn.van.gorkom@mumc.nl

Abstract: Vitamin C or ascorbic acid (AA) is implicated in many biological processes and has been proposed as a supplement for various conditions, including cancer. In this review, we discuss the effects of AA on the development and function of lymphocytes. This is important in the light of cancer treatment, as the immune system needs to regenerate following chemotherapy or stem cell transplantation, while cancer patients are often AA-deficient. We focus on lymphocytes, as these white blood cells are the slowest to restore, rendering patients susceptible to often lethal infections. T lymphocytes mediate cellular immunity and have been most extensively studied in the context of AA biology. In vitro studies demonstrate that T cell development requires AA, while AA also enhances T cell proliferation and may influence T cell function. There are limited and opposing data on the effects of AA on B lymphocytes that mediate humoral immunity. However, AA enhances the proliferation of NK cells, a group of cytotoxic innate lymphocytes. The influence of AA on natural killer (NK) cell function is less clear. In summary, an increasing body of evidence indicates that AA positively influences lymphocyte development and function. Since AA is a safe and cheap nutritional supplement, it is worthwhile to further explore its potential benefits for immune reconstitution of cancer patients treated with immunotoxic drugs.

Keywords: vitamin C; ascorbic acid; lymphocytes; natural killer cells; NK cells; B cells; T cells

---

1. Introduction

Vitamin C or ascorbic acid (AA) has often been linked to cancer treatment. Already in the 1970s, Cameron and Pauling reported that high doses of AA intravenously increased the survival time of terminal cancer patients more than four times [1] but this finding could not be repeated in other studies where AA supplementation was given orally [2,3]. However, subsequent studies show that AA has a wide variety of effects on cancer cells and the immune system. In this review, we discuss the effects of AA on lymphocytes in the light of cancer treatment.

AA is an essential micronutrient for humans with many functions in the human body. It is an antioxidant and a free radical scavenger and serves as an essential cofactor for many enzymatic reactions through iron-, copper- and 2-oxoglutarate-dependent dioxygenases. Among many other functions, these dioxygenases are important in epigenetic regulation by catalysing the hydroxylation of methylated nucleic acids (DNA and RNA) and histones [4]. While most mammals use the enzyme gulono-gamma-lactone oxidase to synthesize AA in the liver, many primates and humans carry a non-functional copy of the *GULO*-gene and consequently depend on dietary sources of AA. When studying the effects of AA and AA deficiency in vivo in animal models, this is a complicating factor. Guinea pigs, like humans, also have a defect in the GULO-gene and are thereby often chosen for AA deficiency studies. Alternatively, there are two knockout mouse models, a *Gulo* knockout ($Gulo^{-}/^{-}$) and a senescence marker protein-30 knockout (*SMP30KO*), in which biosynthesis of AA in the liver is blocked [5,6].

AA has an extensive role in the immune system. Its role in phagocytic cells like neutrophils, has been investigated thoroughly and was recently reviewed [7]. In summary, AA enhances chemotaxis and phagocytosis of phagocytes and thereby promotes microbial killing. In contrast, the role of AA in different subsets of lymphocytes is less clear. Since lymphocytes actively acquire AA via sodium-dependent vitamin C transporters (SVCT) and sodium independent glucose transporters (GLUT) (reviewed in [8] and have intracellular AA concentrations that are 10–100-fold higher than plasma levels [9,10], it is likely that AA has an essential function in these cells. There are three main subsets of lymphocytes, namely T cells, B cells and natural killer (NK cells). T cells are involved in cell-mediated, cytotoxic adaptive immunity, B cells are responsible for the adaptive, humoral immunity and NK cells are part of the innate, antigen-independent immunity.

In our laboratory, we are interested in lymphocytes in cancer treatment, because these cells are often destroyed by anticancer treatment and take time to recover. During this phase, patients are highly susceptible to possibly lethal infections. Depending on the intensity of the chemotherapy used, this period may be relatively short, for example in breast cancer, or long, for example in leukaemia. After so-called myeloablative chemotherapy, hematopoietic stem cells (HSC) that are located in the bone marrow have to be replaced in order to restore all types of blood cells, including leukocytes. In particular, the regeneration of T-lymphocytes, a subset of lymphocytes that are especially important to fight against viral infections, is slow as a consequence of age-dependent involution of the thymus, the organ that is required for their development [11,12]. Looking at ways to improve T cell recovery after cancer therapy, we investigated factors that influence human T-lymphocyte development and found that AA acts as a factor that promotes maturation of T cells. AA is also indispensable for T cell development in vitro [13]. Additionally, we showed that NK cells regenerate faster under the influence of AA [14].

We also found that haematological cancer patients often have severely decreased serum AA levels compared to healthy controls (20.5 $\pm$ 12 μM versus 65 $\pm$ 4 μM, respectively). Serum AA levels were even undetectable in 19% of patients with a haematological malignancy, irrespective of the choice of treatment [15]. Since AA is a cheap and readily available supplement with a safe profile, it is attractive to speculate that cancer patients who need to regenerate their immune system after chemotherapy with or without hematopoietic stem cell transplantation (HSCT) may benefit from the effects of AA on immune reconstitution. In this way, we hypothesize that mortality and morbidity resulting from opportunistic infections could be reduced. It could also be that NK cells regenerate faster and are able to kill cancer cells sooner. AA supplementation could also be used in cellular therapies, where in vitro proliferated and adapted subtypes of lymphocytes are used to eliminate tumour cells in vivo. However, before using AA in clinical applications, it is important to have a better understanding of the role of AA in these lymphocytes.

In this article, we highlight the effects of AA on different subsets of lymphocytes as far as they are known for this moment. We will focus on the effects on the physiology of these cells and on the role of AA on lymphocytes in health and disease and not on the potential mechanisms behind these effects, since this was extensively reviewed before [4].

2. AA and T Lymphocytes

T lymphocytes are a major component of the human immune system and are involved in cell-mediated, cytotoxic adaptive immunity. On their surface, T cells express the T cell receptor (TCR) that is responsible for recognizing and binding specific antigens bound to major histocompatibility complex (MHC) molecules. There are different types of T lymphocytes, including cytotoxic T cells, T helper cells, memory T cells and regulatory T cells. Cytotoxic T cells are characterized by a MHC class I binding CD8 protein on their cell surface. The TCR and CD8 receptor bind infected cells and tumour cells. After binding, the cytotoxic T cells mature and, upon activation by an infected cell, secrete perforin and granzymes, that kill the infected cells. T helper cells are CD4 positive cells that regulate immune responses. Their TCR binds to MHC class II on antigen presenting cells (APCs). After binding, T-helper cells secrete cytokines that activate other immune cells, including cytotoxic T cells. Memory T cells are long-living cells that recognize previously encountered pathogens and provide lifelong immunity. Regulatory T cells shut down T cell mediated immunity toward the end of an immune reaction and help to maintain tolerance to self-antigens.

Here we describe the effects on AA on general T cell development and summarize what is known about the influence of AA on these most important subsets of T cells. We will not discuss cytotoxic T cells since we found no studies examining the effects of AA on this specific subset.

2.1. T Cell Development and AA

T cell development is a tightly controlled process that takes place in the thymus, which can be simulated in vitro using foetal thymic organ cultures [16], stromal cells [17] or in feeder-free conditions [13]. While mature T lymphocytes express either CD4 or CD8 for helper and cytotoxic subsets respectively, immature T cells are called "double negative" (DN) because they lack CD4 and CD8 expression. Traveling through the highly-organized thymus, the developing T cells undergo numerous rounds of proliferation. The thymic stromal cells provide the structural support and cytokines necessary for selection of a functional TCR that does not recognize self-antigens. This process of "education" is required to generate a diverse repertoire of TCRs to ensure immunity against a wide variety of antigens. The various stages of human T cell development are characterized by sequential acquisition of CD7, CD5, intracellular CD3, CD1a, CD4 and CD8, TCR$\alpha\beta$ and surface CD3 [18].

In search for factors that enhance T cell differentiation after stem cell transplantation, we discovered that AA enhances human T cell proliferation in vitro [13]. Beside this effect on T cell proliferation, we also found multiple effects on early T cell development. Most importantly, we showed that AA is required in vitro for the transition of DN precursors to the next, so-called "double positive" (DP, CD4$^+$ CD8$^+$) stage in feeder-free cultures as well as in cultures with stromal cells when culturing T cells from cord blood or G-CSF stimulated hematopoietic stem cells. Furthermore, we found that in a feeder-free system, early maturation of T cells after 3 weeks was improved under the influence of AA in a dose dependent way with an optimum at 95 μM [13]. These results are in line with a murine study in which the investigators cultured adult bone marrow-derived hematopoietic progenitor cells on stromal cells and showed that these cells only differentiate to the DP stage in the presence of AA. To determine the effect of AA in vivo, foetal liver chimeric mice were generated by transfer of *Slc23a2*-deficient HCS into recipient mice. In the absence of *Slc23a2*, hematopoietic cells are unable to concentrate AA. Consequently, in animals with a *Slc23a2*-deficient hematopoietic system, T cell maturation was virtually absent compared to control mice [19].

Since AA functions as an antioxidant, we tested if other antioxidants could restore T cell development. As this was not the case, the effect of AA on developing human T cells cannot be attributed to its antioxidant properties [11]. This finding is supported by Manning et al. [19] who showed that induction and maintenance of *Cd8a* gene expression is dependent on AA-dependent removal of repressive histone modifications, rather than on its function as an antioxidant.

In summary, in humans and mice, AA is required in vitro for the early development of T cells as it overcomes a development block from DN to DP. Furthermore, AA speeds up the maturation process of T lymphocytes. In mice, at least part of this effect is due to AA-dependent epigenetic regulation.

2.2. *T Cell Proliferation and AA*

Multiple researchers studied the effect of vitamin C on the proliferation and survival of T cells, in vitro as well as in vivo.

One study describes the effect of AA on in vitro culture of in vivo activated mouse T cells. While more than 70% apoptotic cells were found in cultures without AA, the addition of AA (450 μM) decreased apoptosis by one-third and induced more proliferation was seen compared to cultures without AA [20]. In another study, evaluating the effects of AA on murine T cells during in vitro activation, it was found that that low concentrations (62.5 μM and 125 μM) of AA do not change proliferation or viability of T cells, while higher concentrations (250 μM and 500 μM) do decrease both [21]. In a third study, researchers examined how AA prevents oxidative damage using purified human T cells. They report similar effects: medium-high concentrations of AA (57–142 μM) decrease T cell proliferation, while at higher concentrations (284 μM), AA decreases cell viability and IL-2 secretion more than 90% [22]. In another study studying the expression of SVCT on T cells, the investigators show a similar effect. Peripheral blood T cells of healthy human volunteers were activated in vitro in the absence or presence of different doses AA, before and after activation. AA did not have any effect on proliferation or apoptosis in low doses (62.5–250 μM). At high doses (500–1000 μM), the proliferation was inhibited and there was an increase in apoptosis when AA was added before activation [23].

In a study on the effect of AA-deficiency on lymphocyte numbers in guinea pigs, the investigators found that in animals with an 4-week AA-free diet, the number of T-lymphocytes decreased continuously while T cell number slightly increased in AA-supplemented animals (25 and 250 mg intraperitoneally/day) [24]. Plasma and tissue concentrations of AA were significantly lower in animals without AA compared to AA-treated animals. In another in vivo study using AA-deficient *SMP30KO*$^{-/-}$ mice, the researchers determined the long-term effect of AA on immune cells using a diet with an increased AA level (200 mg/kg vs. 20 mg/kg). During the one-year study, T-lymphocytes in the peripheral blood increased in number. More specifically, the number of naive T cells, memory T cells in the spleen and mature T cells in the thymus [6] increased. Plasma concentrations of AA in mice with a low-dose AA diet were similar to wildtype mice, while plasma concentrations in the high-dose diet were significantly higher.

Badr et al., examined if the impaired T cell function in type I diabetes can be improved by AA supplementation using a streptozotocin-induced diabetes type I rat model. These animals have diminished T cell cytokine production, less proliferation and lower surface expression of CD28, a protein that is important for T cell activation and survival. AA supplementation (100 mg/kg/day for 2 months) restored the CD28 expression, cytokine secretion and proliferation [25].

Studies in humans are limited. Because elderly people often have lower serum levels of AA and are more prone to infections, a placebo-controlled trial was performed in which elderly people received either an intramuscular injection of AA (500 mg/day) or placebo for 1 month. Compared to the placebo group, an increase in T cell proliferation was seen in the AA-supplemented group [26]. The only other study in humans could not recapitulate this effect [27]. Healthy volunteers were kept on an AA-free diet during a 5-week period to induce AA deficiency. This did not lead to any changes in T cell numbers or function, while the induction of AA deficiency was confirmed in plasma and leukocytes.

In summary, both animal and human studies show that physiological AA concentrations have a beneficial effect on T cell proliferation, while supraphysiological concentrations are toxic for T cells. In vivo, restoration of AA in deficient patients positively influences T cell proliferation as well, while this observation could not be reproduced in induced AA-deficiency.

2.3. *T Helper Cells (Th) and AA*

There are several subsets of Th cells, the most important ones being Th1, Th2 and Th17. Th1 cells are part of the defence against intracellular bacteria and protozoa. Using their main effector cytokines IFN-γ and TNF-α, they activate cytotoxic T cells and macrophages. Th2 cells are effective against extracellular parasites and produce mainly IL-4, IL-5 and IL-13. They stimulate eosinophils, basophils, mast cells and B-cells. Th2 cells are important mediators of allergy and hypersensitivity. For this reason, Th2 cells are often investigated in animal models for asthma. Th17 cells have an important role in pathogen clearance of mucosal surfaces and produce IL-17, a cytokine that stimulates B-cells. The various Th subsets differentiate from naïve CD4$^+$ T cells in a process called "polarization". In vivo, dendritic cells (DC) are the most important antigen-presenting cells (APC) that steer Th polarization via the production of cytokines.

Several researchers report that AA induces a shift of immune responses from Th2 to Th1. In one of these studies, a mouse model was used to examine the effect of AA (5 mg/day) on delayed-type hypersensitivity response against 2,4,-dinitro-I-fluorobenzene (DNFB). In this study, mice were intraperitoneally injected with AA before, during or after sensitization with DNFB. If T cells of mice supplemented with AA during the sensitization were later stimulated ex vivo, higher levels of Th1 cytokines (TNF-α and IFN-γ) and lower levels of Th2 cytokines (IL-4) were observed. This effect was not observed when mice were supplemented with AA before or after sensitization [28]. This modulation of immune balance from Th2 to Th1 was also seen in another study, in which the effects of AA supplementation on asthma was studied. Here, AA supplementation (130 mg/kg/day for 5 weeks) of ovalbumin-sensitized mice significantly increased the IFN-γ/IL-5 secretion ratio in bronchoalveolar lavage fluid compared to control mice, confirming a shift from Th2 to Th1 [29]. The mechanism underpinning this effect has not been elucidated yet but it was suggested to be mediated by DCs. In an in vitro study, murine bone marrow-derived DCs were pre-treated with different doses of AA before being activated with lipopolysaccharide (LPS). The DCs that were treated with AA secreted more IL-12, a polarizing cytokine for Th1 cells. It also showed that naïve murine T cells, when co-cultured with these activated and AA treated murine DCs, produced more IFN-γ and less IL-5 verifying this effect [30].

While most studies focus on the Th1/Th2 balance, we found only one study that describes that Th17 polarization of sorted murine naïve CD4$^+$ cells is more effective in the presence of AA [31]. Interestingly, the investigators demonstrate that this effect is probably due to AA-mediated effects on histone demethylation that enhances the expression of the IL-17 locus.

In summary, multiple animal studies show that AA promotes Th1 differentiation at the expense of Th2 polarization. There is limited data showing that Th17 polarization is promoted by AA acting as an epigenetic regulator.

2.4. *Memory T Cells and AA*

Memory T cells constitute a small subset of lymphocytes but provide life-long immunity to previously encountered antigens. At this moment, the effects of AA on memory T cells is hardly investigated. Jeong et al. examined the effect of DCs pre-treated with AA on CD8$^+$ T cell differentiation. In vitro, murine bone marrow-derived DCs were pre-treated with AA before activation with LPS and, like in the earlier study from the same research group [30], secreted more IL12p70 but also more IL-15, a cytokine that is linked to memory T cell generation. These DCs in co-culture with murine T cells led to an enhanced CD8$^+$ memory T cell production. The effect was also seen in a mouse model for melanoma, in which the immune response and anti-melanoma effect of melanoma-primed DCs was enhanced if pre-treated with AA: the investigators observed increased generation of tumour-specific CD8$^+$ memory T cells and an increased protective effect for inoculated melanoma cells [32].

In summary, in vitro and in a mouse model AA increased the generation of CD8$^+$ memory T cells through increased production of stimulating cytokines by DCs.

2.5. *Regulatory T Cells (Tregs) and AA*

Tregs are important for the maintenance of immune-balance and self-tolerance. They are characterized by the expression of the transcription factor Foxp3, required for their immunosuppressive capacity. Stable expression of Foxp3 is dependent on DNA demethylation of a region in the first intron. Two recent in vivo and in vitro studies on murine Tregs found that AA stabilizes expression of

Foxp3 by promoting active Ten Eleven Translocation (TET) 2-mediated DNA methylation of this region. Thus, AA is required for the development and function of Tregs [33,34]. Concordantly, AA is a known co-factor for Ten Eleven Translocation (TET) family proteins that catalyse the first step of DNA demethylation: the conversion of 5-methyl-cytosine (5 mC) to 5-hydroxy-methyl-cytosine (5 hmC) [35,36]. For instance, in embryonic stem cells, AA was shown to be an important epigenetic regulator through this pathway [37]. The addition of AA to embryonic stem cell cultures induced demethylation of over 2000 genes within one hour [38].

In another study, the influence of AA on skin graft rejection in mice after treatment with ex vivo cultured and alloantigen-induced Tregs was investigated. The in vivo alloantigen-induced murine Tregs showed more DNA demethylation and stability of Foxp3 expression when cultured in the presence of AA. These Tregs also showed better suppressive capacity in vivo, thereby promoting skin allograft acceptance [39]. In a mouse model for graft-versus-host-disease (GVHD), the effects of AA on these ex vivo alloantigen-induced Tregs was determined [40]. GVHD is a serious and sometimes lethal complication following allogeneic hematopoietic stem cell transplantation caused by alloreactive donor T cells that induce tissue injury in the recipient. In this model, in vitro murine alloantigen-induced Tregs pre-treated with AA showed more stable Foxp3 expression when transferred into mice with acute GVHD and were clinically effective to diminish GVHD symptoms. Moreover, cultured human alloantigen-induced Tregs also had a higher Foxp3 expression if cultured with AA.

In contrast, in a mouse model for sepsis, AA was found to decrease the inhibition of Tregs [41]. Here, sepsis was induced in AA-deficient *Gulo*$^{-}/^{-}$ mice that were supplemented with AA (200 mg/kg twice) or not. AA administration improved survival in both wild type and *Gulo*$^{-}/^{-}$ mice and diminished the negative inhibition of Tregs by decreasing the expression of Foxp-3, CTLA-4, a protein that functions as an immune checkpoint and downregulates immune responses and the inhibitory cytokine TGF-β.

In summary, AA directly regulates Treg function via epigenetic regulation of the master transcription factor Foxp3. In most studies employing more chronic situations (transplantation, GVHD), Foxp3 expression is increased. In this way, AA can be useful in generating ex vivo allo-antigen-induced Tregs that can be used for clinical applications in transplantation and autoimmune disorders. In one model of acute sepsis in mice, AA administration decreased Foxp3 expression but was still beneficial for the outcome.

3. AA and B Lymphocytes

B lymphocytes are at the centre of the adaptive, humoral immune system. They are responsible for the production of antigen-specific immunoglobulin (Ig) directed against invasive pathogens (antibodies). Similar to other leukocytes, AA accumulated in B lymphocytes but there is only limited data on the function of AA in these cells.

3.1. B Lymphocyte Numbers and AA

In an early study investigating the effect of AA deficiency on numbers of lymphocytes in guinea pigs, animals on a 4-week AA-free diet showed a continuous increase in the percentage of B-lymphocytes while the percentage of T-lymphocytes decreased. The opposite effect was seen in animals on AA supplementation (25 and 250 mg intraperitoneally/day) [24]. In a more recent and extensive study, the effect of AA-2G, a stable vitamin C derivate, was investigated on mouse B cells in vitro. Mouse spleen B cells were cultured for 2 days with an anti-μ antibody in the presence of stimulating cytokines and then washed and recultured with and without AA-2G. In these cultures, the number of viable cells decreased much quicker without AA, resulting in about 70% more viable cells in cultures with AA than without AA. AA-2G also increased the production of IgM dose-dependently [42]. Another group that studied the effect of AA on mouse spleen B cells in vitro published contradictive results. They showed a slight dose-dependent increase of apoptosis (16% at a concentration of 1 mM) in murine IgM/CD40-activated B cells pre-treated with AA [43]. Tanaka et al. investigated the effect of AA on immune responses in human peripheral blood lymphocytes cultured for 7 days with and without AA-2G before stimulating them with pokeweed mitogen (PWM), a T cell dependent B cell stimulus. The cultures treated with AAS-2G showed an increased number of IgM and IgG-secreting cells after stimulation [44].

3.2. B Lymphocyte Function and AA

We only found limited and conflicting data on the effect of vitamin C on the production of antibodies by B lymphocytes. Two early studies in guinea pigs show that high-dose AA supplementation increases immunoglobulin levels after immunization with sheep red blood cells (SRBC) and bovine serum albumin (BSA) [45,46]. However, in two other animal models, AA supplementation did not have an effect on antigen-induced immunoglobulin levels after immunization [47,48]. One study determined the effect of high dose AA (2500 mg/day for 4 weeks) in mice sensitized by topical application of di-nitro-chlorobenzene (DNCB) and re-challenged 2 weeks later. They found no effect of AA on immunoglobulin levels [47]. In the other study, the effect of different low doses of AA (0, 30 and 60 mg) on the immune functions of dogs immunized with PWM was studied but no differences in PWM-specific IgG and IgA levels were observed [48]. However, the latter two studies were performed in animals that are able to synthetize AA, while guinea pigs cannot. In AA-synthetizing calves, AA supplementation (1.75 g/day) led to lower plasma IgG levels against keyhole limpet haemocyanin (KLH), a T cell dependent antigen that is often used in immunological studies in animals [49]. Two studies were performed in AA-sufficient chickens to investigate if AA supplementation is beneficial for vaccination against infectious bursal disease (IBD). Chickens with AA supplementation (1 g/mL) showed higher immunoglobulin levels compared to chickens without extra AA [50,51]. Furthermore, non-vaccinated chickens receiving AA supplementation did not show any symptoms or mortality after challenge with IBD while non-vaccinated chickens without AA all experienced clinical symptoms and only 70% survived [50].

In one study in healthy human volunteers, researchers found a correlation between serum IgG and plasma and leukocyte AA concentration and serum IgM and leukocyte AA concentration. After daily supplementation of 1 g AA during one week, serum IgG significantly rose in those healthy volunteers as did plasma and leukocyte AA concentration [52]. Likewise, another study in healthy human volunteers showed an increase in serum levels of IgM and IgA after 1 g/day supplementation of AA for 75 days [53]. These findings were contradicted in two other studies. In one study, the investigators examined the effect of 2–3 g AA supplementation per day on the production of all immunoglobins in healthy volunteers and did not find any change [54]. The other study is an earlier described placebo-controlled trial in elderly people where they received either an intramuscular injection of AA (500 mg/day) or a placebo for 1 month. Also in this trial, AA supplementation did not have any influence on serum IgA, IgM and IgG levels [26].

In conclusion, it is possible that vitamin C has an effect on the proliferation and function of B lymphocytes but the results until now are inconclusive. When conducting an intervention study of AA in cancer patients it would be interesting to also examine B cell levels and immunoglobulin changes.

4. AA and Natural Killer Cells

Next to B and T lymphocytes, NK cells are the most prominent lymphocyte subset as they make up to 20% of the blood lymphocyte population and are important for the immunity against pathogens (especially viruses) and for tumour surveillance. They are large granular lymphocytes arising from the same lymphoid progenitors as T and B lymphocytes and are primarily formed in the bone marrow. NK cells are innate lymphoid cells (ILCs) that provide fast, antigen-independent immunity. They exhibit direct cytotoxic effects, secrete cytokines and chemokines and regulate other immune cells. NK cell cytotoxicity is based on the absence of self MHC class I to discriminate between normal and diseased cells. Killing of these MHC class I missing target cells can only be initiated after simultaneous detection of activating signals, like stress signals, on the surface of tumour or infected cells.

Our knowledge about the effects of AA on NK cell development is limited. We previously described that AA (95 μM) enhances proliferation of mature NK cells from peripheral blood mononuclear cells (PBMCs) in vitro in a cytokine-stimulated culture [14]. AA also improved the generation and expansion of NK cell progenitors from hematopoietic stem cells and from T/NK cell progenitors in vitro in a cytokine-stimulated culture.

Other studies investigated the role of AA on the function of NK cells. In our previously described study, we tested functionality of the mature NK cells that were expanded in vitro in a cytotoxicity assay on K562 cells, a chronic myeloid leukaemia cell line that is often used to assess NK cell function in vitro. There was no difference in killing capacity between NK cells that were cultured with or without AA. [14]. In contrast, an earlier study on the cytotoxicity of fresh human NK cells isolated from peripheral blood that had different doses of AA (10 μM to 2.5 mM) present during the killing showed a dose-dependent decrease of NK cell mediated killing of K562 cells in vitro [55]. A similar experiment was repeated in another study but with different results. A presence of 3 mM AA increased the cytotoxicity of NK cells 105% in average, while no change was found using lower concentrations (10 μM, 0.1 mM and 1 mM) [56].

Another group also investigated the effect of AA on peripheral blood NK cell function using a cytotoxicity assay on K562 with NK cells from healthy volunteers that were supplemented with a single high dose of vitamin C. The study showed a biphasic effect on NK cell cytotoxicity: a slight decrease 1 to 2 h after supplementation followed by a significant enhancement at 8 h with a maximum effect after 24 h and return to normal after 48 h [57]. Plasma and leukocyte concentration of AA increased after 1 h and maximized after 2 to 4 h. After that, the levels declined but were still elevated up to 24 h after supplementation. Since NK cell function is often decreased after exposure to toxic chemicals, these researchers also performed a similar experiment in 55 patients that where accidently exposed to various toxic chemicals (for instance pesticides, metals and organic solvents). Almost half of these patients showed a very low baseline NK cell activity and in 78% of the patients there was significantly enhancement of cytotoxicity compared to baseline 24 h after ingestion of 60 mg/kg AA [58]. It is difficult to interpret these findings, since the patients were very diverse and there was no control group.

A comparable study was performed with NK cells isolated from peripheral blood of patients with β-thalassemia major. NK cells of these patients show a severe reduction in their cytotoxic function compared to healthy controls, possibly due to oxidative stress caused by iron overload after multiple blood transfusions [59]. AA (200 μg/mL) almost normalized the cytotoxic capacity of these NK cells, while the NK cell function of healthy controls did not change [60]. Remarkably, AA and iron are connected in many biological processes. For example, AA enhances the absorption of nonheme iron from the intestines [61] and AA is an essential cofactor in many enzymatic reaction by iron-dependent dioxygenases. The positive effect of AA on the NK cell function in this case is probably related to its antioxidant properties, since NK cells in patients with iron overload are known to have more intracellular reactive oxygen species (ROS) [62].

The effects of vitamin C on NK cell cytotoxicity against ovarian cancer cells was also studied in vivo in AA deficient mice. *Gulo*$^{-}$/$^{-}$ mice that are dependent on dietary AA were not supplemented for 2 weeks and sub sequentially inoculated with MOSECs (murine ovarian surface epithelial cells) and compared with *Gulo*$^{-}$/$^{-}$ mice that received normal AA supplementation. After the inoculation of tumour cells, all animals received normal AA supplementation. *Gulo*$^{-}$/$^{-}$ mice that were AA-depleted during this period survived shorter than supplemented mice. NK cells isolated from these AA-depleted mice showed a significant decrease in killing capacity in vitro compared to AA-supplemented mice and wildtype mice. In concordance, their NK cells showed reduced expression of the activating receptors CD69 and NKG2D. Furthermore, these NK cells produced less IFN-γ and displayed reduced production of the cytolytic proteins perforin and granzyme B [63].

In conclusion, AA might have different effects on NK cells during different stages. Early and late human NK cell development is enhanced by AA in vitro, however the effect in vivo remains to be shown. It is likely that the effect of AA at this time point is caused by its role as an epigenetic regulator, since this is also observed in T cells that share various developmental steps.

The influence of AA on NK cell function is not fully determined yet. In most in vitro studies in which NK cells of healthy volunteers (that probably have normal AA levels) were used, no effect of AA was observed. However, in AA-deficient mice, NK cell function was decreased compared to mice with normal levels of AA. Furthermore, in two human studies employing NK cells with an impaired function AA was able to restore NK cell function to almost normal. These results suggest that at least physiological levels of AA are necessary for normal NK cell function and AA is probably not able to increase the cytotoxicity of NK cells that function normally but can help to restore the function in NK cells that are impaired.

It is unknown whether next to NK cells, the development and function of recently identified other members of the ILC family are also enhanced by AA. This may be important, because other ILC subsets may also provide immunity while T cell immunity has not yet recovered. Furthermore, it has been shown that, in allogeneic HSCT higher ILC 3 numbers are associated with less GVHD [64].

5. Conclusions

AA has multiple effects on the development, proliferation and function of lymphocytes. An overview of these effects and the relationship between different cell types can be seen in Figure 1. T-lymphocytes have been most extensively studied in this context: AA positively influences T cell development and maturation, especially in case of AA deficiency. There is very limited and conflicting data on the effects of AA on B-lymphocyte biology. As for NK cells, AA positively influences NK cell proliferation but its role in NK cell function is less clear. A limited number of studies suggest that NK cell function required normal AA levels, while supraphysiological levels do not enhance NK cell function. Overall, most conclusions are based on in vitro studies, that are difficult to interpret and compare since there are many differences in experimental setups (multiple derivates of AA used in various concentrations and different incubation times). AA is also known to oxidate easily to dehydroascorbate in cell-cultures. The in vivo studies require careful interpretation as well: little data is available on local (intracellular) AA levels, while it is known that intracellular AA levels can be more than 1000-fold higher compared to plasma levels.

The studies discussed in the present review provide some insight in the mechanisms that underpin the effect on AA on lymphocytes. There are important indications that AA acts as an epigenetic regulator/cofactor in TET-mediated DNA and histone demethylation. Plausibly, AA's epigenetic functions are mostly seen in cells that undergo change (e.g., early T cell development, T helper cell differentiation). In situations of cells under stress (e.g., thalassemia, sepsis), the antioxidant properties of AA are probably more important.

Since AA is a cheap supplement with limited side-effects, it is worthwhile to speculate on its potential for cancer patients that are proven to have lower serum AA levels. Here, AA could enhance immune reconstitution after treatments that give long immunosuppression (for instance, patients receiving intensive chemotherapy for leukaemia or autologous HSCT) as most studies indicate a positive effect of AA supplementation on lymphocyte development. In this case, AA's effect on NK cells may be most significant, because NK cell reconstitution after myeloablative chemotherapy and HSCT is much faster than T cell reconstitution and could provide temporary immunity against infections [65]. Furthermore, NK cells are capable of recognizing and eliminating cancer cells. Currently, several clinical trials already study the anti-cancer potential of ex vivo generated NK cells. AA supplementation can be used to generate these NK cells in vitro but could also have an effect in vivo in the proliferation and survival of these cells. Furthermore, AA supplementation could may also positively influence T cell reconstitution after myeloablative therapy. It is possible that slow T cell regeneration is (partly) due to the AA-deficient state in these patients.

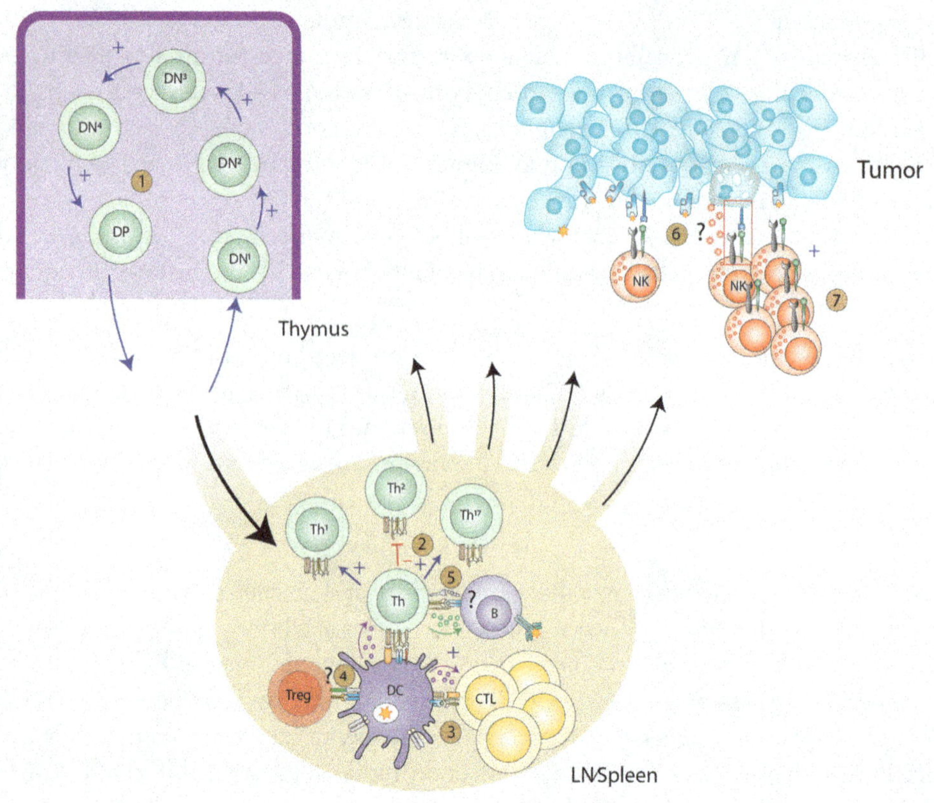

Figure 1. Effects of AA on Immune cells. **1**. T cell development: Enhanced T cell development due to fast transition from DN to DD stage. **2**. Th cell differentiation: skewing towards Th1 and Th17, with inhibition of Th2 polarization. **3**. CTL induction: Increased induction of CTLs due to production of IL-15 and IL-12 by DCs. **4**. Treg induction: Current data are conflicting. **5**. B cell: No conclusive data. **6**. NK cell function: No conclusive data. **7**. NK cell proliferation: increased NK cell proliferation.

On the other hand, AA supplementation in cancer patients may also have negative effects. Most of the curative effect of an allogeneic hematopoietic stem cell transplantation is attributed to the graft versus tumour effect mediated by the donor T cells that recognize cancer cells. This effect could potentially be diminished by increasing the amount and function of Tregs by vitamin C, as seen in some studies [33,34]. On the other hand, another study shows decreased Treg activity following AA administration [41]. In addition, stimulation of Tregs may also protect against GVHD.

Thus, AA plays a multitude of roles in lymphocyte development and function. However, its exact mechanism(s) of action and its effects in human health and disease are currently unknown. Given its safe profile and the fact that most animal studies have important limitations, we currently prepare a single arm phase II study to test the safety (GVHD) and efficacy of AA supplementation after allogeneic stem cell transplantation. This study is likely to provide important insights in how this vitamin functions in a complex, diseased organism and what groups of patients may benefit from this safe supplement.

Author Contributions: Gwendolyn N. Y. van Gorkom wrote the paper, Roel G. J. Klein Wolterink, Catharina H. M. J. Van Elssen, Lotte Wieten, Wilfred T. V. Germeraad and Gerard M. J. Bos were involved in the previous work on this topic in our group and/or substantively revised it.

Conflicts of Interest: The authors declare no conflict of interest.

References

1. Cameron, E.; Pauling, L. Supplemental ascorbate in the supportive treatment of cancer: Prolongation of survival times in terminal human cancer. *Proc. Natl. Acad. Sci. USA* **1976**, *73*, 3685–3689. [CrossRef] [PubMed]
2. Creagan, E.T.; Moertel, C.G.; O'Fallon, J.R.; Schutt, A.J.; O'Connell, M.J.; Rubin, J.; Frytak, S. Failure of high-dose vitamin C (ascorbic acid) therapy to benefit patients with advanced cancer. A controlled trial. *N. Engl. J. Med.* **1979**, *301*, 687–690. [CrossRef] [PubMed]
3. Moertel, C.G.; Fleming, T.R.; Creagan, E.T.; Rubin, J.; O'Connell, M.J.; Ames, M.M. High-dose vitamin C versus placebo in the treatment of patients with advanced cancer who have had no prior chemotherapy. A randomized double-blind comparison. *N. Engl. J. Med.* **1985**, *312*, 137–141. [CrossRef] [PubMed]
4. Young, J.I.; Zuchner, S.; Wang, G. Regulation of the Epigenome by Vitamin C. *Annu. Rev. Nutr.* **2015**, *35*, 545–564. [CrossRef] [PubMed]
5. Harrison, F.E.; Meredith, M.E.; Dawes, S.M.; Saskowski, J.L.; May, J.M. Low ascorbic acid and increased oxidative stress in gulo($^{-}/^{-}$) mice during development. *Brain Res.* **2010**, *1349*, 143–152. [CrossRef] [PubMed]
6. Uchio, R.; Hirose, Y.; Murosaki, S.; Yamamoto, Y.; Ishigami, A. High dietary intake of vitamin C suppresses age-related thymic atrophy and contributes to the maintenance of immune cells in vitamin C-deficient senescence marker protein-30 knockout mice. *Br. J. Nutr.* **2015**, *113*, 603–609. [CrossRef] [PubMed]
7. Carr, A.C.; Maggini, S. Vitamin C and Immune Function. *Nutrients* **2017**, *9*, 1211. [CrossRef] [PubMed]
8. Wilson, J.X. Regulation of vitamin C transport. *Annu. Rev. Nutr.* **2005**, *25*, 105–125. [CrossRef] [PubMed]
9. Omaye, S.T.; Schaus, E.E.; Kutnink, M.A.; Hawkes, W.C. Measurement of vitamin C in blood components by high-performance liquid chromatography. Implication in assessing vitamin C status. *Ann. N. Y. Acad. Sci.* **1987**, *498*, 389–401. [CrossRef] [PubMed]
10. Evans, R.M.; Currie, L.; Campbell, A. The distribution of ascorbic acid between various cellular components of blood, in normal individuals, and its relation to the plasma concentration. *Br. J. Nutr.* **1982**, *47*, 473–482. [CrossRef] [PubMed]
11. Roux, E.; Dumont-Girard, F.; Starobinski, M.; Siegrist, C.A.; Helg, C.; Chapuis, B.; Roosnek, E. Recovery of immune reactivity after T-cell-depleted bone marrow transplantation depends on thymic activity. *Blood* **2000**, *96*, 2299–2303. [PubMed]
12. Bosch, M.; Khan, F.M.; Storek, J. Immune reconstitution after hematopoietic cell transplantation. *Curr. Opin. Hematol.* **2012**, *19*, 324–335. [CrossRef] [PubMed]
13. Huijskens, M.J.; Walczak, M.; Koller, N.; Briede, J.J.; Senden-Gijsbers, B.L.; Schnijderberg, M.C.; Bos, G.M.; Germeraad, W.T. Technical advance: Ascorbic acid induces development of double-positive T cells from human hematopoietic stem cells in the absence of stromal cells. *J. Leukoc. Biol.* **2014**, *96*, 1165–1175. [CrossRef] [PubMed]
14. Huijskens, M.J.; Walczak, M.; Sarkar, S.; Atrafi, F.; Senden-Gijsbers, B.L.; Tilanus, M.G.; Bos, G.M.; Wieten, L.; Germeraad, W.T. Ascorbic acid promotes proliferation of natural killer cell populations in culture systems applicable for natural killer cell therapy. *Cytotherapy* **2015**, *17*, 613–620. [CrossRef] [PubMed]
15. Huijskens, M.J.; Wodzig, W.K.; Walczak, M.; Germeraad, W.T.; Bos, G.M. Ascorbic acid serum levels are reduced in patients with hematological malignancies. *Results Immunol.* **2016**, *6*, 8–10. [CrossRef] [PubMed]
16. Jenkinson, E.J.; Anderson, G.; Owen, J.J. Studies on T cell maturation on defined thymic stromal cell populations in vitro. *J. Exp. Med.* **1992**, *176*, 845–853. [CrossRef] [PubMed]
17. Schmitt, T.M.; Zuniga-Pflucker, J.C. Induction of T cell development from hematopoietic progenitor cells by delta-like-1 in vitro. *Immunity* **2002**, *17*, 749–756. [CrossRef]
18. Meek, B.; Cloosen, S.; Borsotti, C.; Van Elssen, C.H.; Vanderlocht, J.; Schnijderberg, M.C.; van der Poel, M.W.; Leewis, B.; Hesselink, R.; Manz, M.G.; et al. In vitro-differentiated T/natural killer-cell progenitors derived from human CD34^{+} cells mature in the thymus. *Blood* **2010**, *115*, 261–264. [CrossRef] [PubMed]
19. Manning, J.; Mitchell, B.; Appadurai, D.A.; Shakya, A.; Pierce, L.J.; Wang, H.; Nganga, V.; Swanson, P.C.; May, J.M.; Tantin, D.; et al. Vitamin C promotes maturation of T-cells. *Antioxid. Redox Signal.* **2013**, *19*, 2054–2067. [CrossRef] [PubMed]
20. Campbell, J.D.; Cole, M.; Bunditrutavorn, B.; Vella, A.T. Ascorbic acid is a potent inhibitor of various forms of T cell apoptosis. *Cell. Immunol.* **1999**, *194*, 1–5. [CrossRef] [PubMed]

21. Maeng, H.G.; Lim, H.; Jeong, Y.J.; Woo, A.; Kang, J.S.; Lee, W.J.; Hwang, Y.I. Vitamin C enters mouse T cells as dehydroascorbic acid in vitro and does not recapitulate in vivo vitamin C effects. *Immunobiology* **2009**, *214*, 311–320. [CrossRef] [PubMed]
22. Eylar, E.; Baez, I.; Navas, J.; Mercado, C. Sustained levels of ascorbic acid are toxic and immunosuppressive for human T cells. *P. R. Health Sci. J.* **1996**, *15*, 21–26. [PubMed]
23. Hong, J.M.; Kim, J.H.; Kang, J.S.; Lee, W.J.; Hwang, Y.I. Vitamin C is taken up by human T cells via sodium-dependent vitamin C transporter 2 (SVCT2) and exerts inhibitory effects on the activation of these cells in vitro. *Anat. Cell Biol.* **2016**, *49*, 88–98. [CrossRef] [PubMed]
24. Fraser, R.C.; Pavlovic, S.; Kurahara, C.G.; Murata, A.; Peterson, N.S.; Taylor, K.B.; Feigen, G.A. The effect of variations in vitamin C intake on the cellular immune response of guinea pigs. *Am. J. Clin. Nutr.* **1980**, *33*, 839–847. [CrossRef] [PubMed]
25. Badr, G.; Bashandy, S.; Ebaid, H.; Mohany, M.; Sayed, D. Vitamin C supplementation reconstitutes polyfunctional T cells in streptozotocin-induced diabetic rats. *Eur. J. Nutr.* **2012**, *51*, 623–633. [CrossRef] [PubMed]
26. Kennes, B.; Dumont, I.; Brohee, D.; Hubert, C.; Neve, P. Effect of vitamin C supplements on cell-mediated immunity in old people. *Gerontology* **1983**, *29*, 305–310. [CrossRef] [PubMed]
27. Kay, N.E.; Holloway, D.E.; Hutton, S.W.; Bone, N.D.; Duane, W.C. Human T-cell function in experimental ascorbic acid deficiency and spontaneous scurvy. *Am. J. Clin. Nutr.* **1982**, *36*, 127–130. [CrossRef] [PubMed]
28. Noh, K.; Lim, H.; Moon, S.K.; Kang, J.S.; Lee, W.J.; Lee, D.; Hwang, Y.I. Mega-dose Vitamin C modulates T cell functions in Balb/c mice only when administered during T cell activation. *Immunol. Lett.* **2005**, *98*, 63–72. [CrossRef] [PubMed]
29. Chang, H.-H.; Chen, C.; Lin, J.-Y. High dose vitamin C supplementation increases the Th1/Th2 cytokine secretion ratio, but decreases eosinophilic infiltration in bronchoalveolar lavage fluid of ovalbumin-sensitized and challenged mice. *J. Agric. Food Chem.* **2009**, *57*, 10471–10476. [CrossRef] [PubMed]
30. Jeong, Y.J.; Hong, S.W.; Kim, J.H.; Jin, D.H.; Kang, J.S.; Lee, W.J.; Hwang, Y.I. Vitamin C-treated murine bone marrow-derived dendritic cells preferentially drive naive T cells into Th1 cells by increased IL-12 secretions. *Cell. Immunol.* **2011**, *266*, 192–199. [CrossRef] [PubMed]
31. Song, M.H.; Nair, V.S.; Oh, K.I. Vitamin C enhances the expression of IL17 in a Jmjd2-dependent manner. *BMB Rep.* **2017**, *50*, 49–54. [CrossRef] [PubMed]
32. Jeong, Y.J.; Kim, J.H.; Hong, J.M.; Kang, J.S.; Kim, H.R.; Lee, W.J.; Hwang, Y.I. Vitamin C treatment of mouse bone marrow-derived dendritic cells enhanced CD8(+) memory T cell production capacity of these cells in vivo. *Immunobiology* **2014**, *219*, 554–564. [CrossRef] [PubMed]
33. Sasidharan Nair, V.; Song, M.H.; Oh, K.I. Vitamin C Facilitates Demethylation of the Foxp3 Enhancer in a Tet-Dependent Manner. *J. Immunol.* **2016**, *196*, 2119–2131. [CrossRef] [PubMed]
34. Yue, X.; Trifari, S.; Aijo, T.; Tsagaratou, A.; Pastor, W.A.; Zepeda-Martinez, J.A.; Lio, C.W.; Li, X.; Huang, Y.; Vijayanand, P.; et al. Control of Foxp3 stability through modulation of TET activity. *J. Exp. Med.* **2016**, *213*, 377–397. [CrossRef] [PubMed]
35. Tahiliani, M.; Koh, K.P.; Shen, Y.; Pastor, W.A.; Bandukwala, H.; Brudno, Y.; Agarwal, S.; Iyer, L.M.; Liu, D.R.; Aravind, L.; et al. Conversion of 5-methylcytosine to 5-hydroxymethylcytosine in mammalian DNA by MLL partner TET1. *Science* **2009**, *324*, 930–935. [CrossRef] [PubMed]
36. Ito, S.; D'Alessio, A.C.; Taranova, O.V.; Hong, K.; Sowers, L.C.; Zhang, Y. Role of Tet proteins in 5mC to 5hmC conversion, ES-cell self-renewal and inner cell mass specification. *Nature* **2010**, *466*, 1129–1133. [CrossRef] [PubMed]
37. Blaschke, K.; Ebata, K.T.; Karimi, M.M.; Zepeda-Martinez, J.A.; Goyal, P.; Mahapatra, S.; Tam, A.; Laird, D.J.; Hirst, M.; Rao, A.; et al. Vitamin C induces Tet-dependent DNA demethylation and a blastocyst-like state in ES cells. *Nature* **2013**, *500*, 222–226. [CrossRef] [PubMed]
38. Chung, T.L.; Brena, R.M.; Kolle, G.; Grimmond, S.M.; Berman, B.P.; Laird, P.W.; Pera, M.F.; Wolvetang, E.J. Vitamin C promotes widespread yet specific DNA demethylation of the epigenome in human embryonic stem cells. *Stem Cells* **2010**, *28*, 1848–1855. [CrossRef] [PubMed]
39. Nikolouli, E.; Hardtke-Wolenski, M.; Hapke, M.; Beckstette, M.; Geffers, R.; Floess, S.; Jaeckel, E.; Huehn, J. Alloantigen-Induced Regulatory T Cells Generated in Presence of Vitamin C Display Enhanced Stability of Foxp3 Expression and Promote Skin Allograft Acceptance. *Front. Immunol.* **2017**, *8*, 748. [CrossRef] [PubMed]

40. Kasahara, H.; Kondo, T.; Nakatsukasa, H.; Chikuma, S.; Ito, M.; Ando, M.; Kurebayashi, Y.; Sekiya, T.; Yamada, T.; Okamoto, S.; et al. Generation of allo-antigen-specific induced Treg stabilized by vitamin C treatment and its application for prevention of acute graft versus host disease model. *Int. Immunol.* **2017**, *29*, 457–469. [CrossRef] [PubMed]
41. Gao, Y.; Lu, B.; Zhai, J.; Liu, Y.; Qi, H.; Yao, Y.; Chai, Y.; Shou, S. The Parenteral Vitamin C Improves Sepsis and Sepsis-Induced Multiple Organ Dysfunction Syndrome via Preventing Cellular Immunosuppression. *Mediat. Inflamm.* **2017**, *2017*, 4024672. [CrossRef] [PubMed]
42. Ichiyama, K.; Mitsuzumi, H.; Zhong, M.; Tai, A.; Tsuchioka, A.; Kawai, S.; Yamamoto, I.; Gohda, E. Promotion of IL-4- and IL-5-dependent differentiation of anti-μ-primed B cells by ascorbic acid 2-glucoside. *Immunol. Lett.* **2009**, *122*, 219–226. [CrossRef] [PubMed]
43. Woo, A.; Kim, J.H.; Jeong, Y.J.; Maeng, H.G.; Lee, Y.T.; Kang, J.S.; Lee, W.J.; Hwang, Y.I. Vitamin C acts indirectly to modulate isotype switching in mouse B cells. *Anat. Cell Biol.* **2010**, *43*, 25–35. [CrossRef] [PubMed]
44. Tanaka, M.; Muto, N.; Gohda, E.; Yamamoto, I. Enhancement by ascorbic acid 2-glucoside or repeated additions of ascorbate of mitogen-induced IgM and IgG productions by human peripheral blood lymphocytes. *Jpn. J. Pharmacol.* **1994**, *66*, 451–456. [CrossRef] [PubMed]
45. Prinz, W.; Bloch, J.; Gilich, G.; Mitchell, G. A systematic study of the effect of vitamin C supplementation on the humoral immune response in ascorbate-dependent mammals. I. The antibody response to sheep red blood cells (a T-dependent antigen) in guinea pigs. *Int. J. Vitam. Nutr. Res.* **1980**, *50*, 294–300. [PubMed]
46. Feigen, G.A.; Smith, B.H.; Dix, C.E.; Flynn, C.J.; Peterson, N.S.; Rosenberg, L.T.; Pavlovic, S.; Leibovitz, B. Enhancement of antibody production and protection against systemic anaphylaxis by large doses of vitamin C. *Res. Commun. Chem. Pathol. Pharmacol.* **1982**, *38*, 313–333. [CrossRef]
47. Albers, R.; Bol, M.; Bleumink, R.; Willems, A.A.; Pieters, R.H. Effects of supplementation with vitamins A, C, and E, selenium, and zinc on immune function in a murine sensitization model. *Nutrition* **2003**, *19*, 940–946. [CrossRef]
48. Hesta, M.; Ottermans, C.; Krammer-Lukas, S.; Zentek, J.; Hellweg, P.; Buyse, J.; Janssens, G.P. The effect of vitamin C supplementation in healthy dogs on antioxidative capacity and immune parameters. *J. Anim. Physiol. Anim. Nutr.* **2009**, *93*, 26–34. [CrossRef] [PubMed]
49. Goodwin, J.S.; Garry, P.J. Relationship between megadose vitamin supplementation and immunological function in a healthy elderly population. *Clin. Exp. Immunol.* **1983**, *51*, 647–653. [PubMed]
50. Amakye-Anim, J.; Lin, T.L.; Hester, P.Y.; Thiagarajan, D.; Watkins, B.A.; Wu, C.C. Ascorbic acid supplementation improved antibody response to infectious bursal disease vaccination in chickens. *Poult. Sci.* **2000**, *79*, 680–688. [CrossRef] [PubMed]
51. Wu, C.C.; Dorairajan, T.; Lin, T.L. Effect of ascorbic acid supplementation on the immune response of chickens vaccinated and challenged with infectious bursal disease virus. *Vet. Immunol. Immunopathol.* **2000**, *74*, 145–152. [CrossRef]
52. Vallance, S. Relationships between ascorbic acid and serum proteins of the immune system. *Br. Med. J.* **1977**, *2*, 437–438. [CrossRef] [PubMed]
53. Prinz, W.; Bortz, R.; Bregin, B.; Hersch, M. The effect of ascorbic acid supplementation on some parameters of the human immunological defence system. *Int. J. Vitam. Nutr. Res.* **1977**, *47*, 248–257. [PubMed]
54. Anderson, R.; Oosthuizen, R.; Maritz, R.; Theron, A.; Van Rensburg, A.J. The effects of increasing weekly doses of ascorbate on certain cellular and humoral immune functions in normal volunteers. *Am. J. Clin. Nutr.* **1980**, *33*, 71–76. [CrossRef] [PubMed]
55. Huwyler, T.; Hirt, A.; Morell, A. Effect of ascorbic acid on human natural killer cells. *Immunol. Lett.* **1985**, *10*, 173–176. [CrossRef]
56. Toliopoulos, I.K.; Simos, Y.V.; Daskalou, T.A.; Verginadis, I.I.; Evangelou, A.M.; Karkabounas, S.C. Inhibition of platelet aggregation and immunomodulation of NK lymphocytes by administration of ascorbic acid. *Indian J. Exp. Biol.* **2011**, *49*, 904–908. [PubMed]
57. Vojdani, A.; Ghoneum, M. In vivo effect of ascorbic acid on enhancement of natural killer cell activity. *Nutr. Res.* **1993**, *13*, 753–764. [CrossRef]
58. Heuser, G.; Vojdani, A. Enhancement of natural killer cell activity and T and B cell function by buffered vitamin C in patients exposed to toxic chemicals: The role of protein kinase-C. *Immunopharmacol. Immunotoxicol.* **1997**, *19*, 291–312. [CrossRef] [PubMed]

59. Farmakis, D.; Giakoumis, A.; Polymeropoulos, E.; Aessopos, A. Pathogenetic aspects of immune deficiency associated with beta-thalassemia. *Med. Sci. Monit.* **2003**, *9*, Ra19–R22. [PubMed]
60. Atasever, B.; Ertan, N.Z.; Erdem-Kuruca, S.; Karakas, Z. In vitro effects of vitamin C and selenium on NK activity of patients with beta-thalassemia major. *Pediatr. Hematol. Oncol.* **2006**, *23*, 187–197. [CrossRef] [PubMed]
61. Lynch, S.R.; Cook, J.D. Interaction of vitamin C and iron. *Ann. N. Y. Acad. Sci.* **1980**, *355*, 32–44. [CrossRef] [PubMed]
62. Hua, Y.; Wang, C.; Jiang, H.; Wang, Y.; Liu, C.; Li, L.; Liu, H.; Shao, Z.; Fu, R. Iron overload may promote alteration of NK cells and hematopoietic stem/progenitor cells by JNK and P38 pathway in myelodysplastic syndromes. *Int. J. Hematol.* **2017**, *106*, 248–257. [CrossRef] [PubMed]
63. Kim, J.E.; Cho, H.S.; Yang, H.S.; Jung, D.J.; Hong, S.W.; Hung, C.F.; Lee, W.J.; Kim, D. Depletion of ascorbic acid impairs NK cell activity against ovarian cancer in a mouse model. *Immunobiology* **2012**, *217*, 873–881. [CrossRef] [PubMed]
64. Munneke, J.M.; Bjorklund, A.T.; Mjosberg, J.M.; Garming-Legert, K.; Bernink, J.H.; Blom, B.; Huisman, C.; van Oers, M.H.; Spits, H.; Malmberg, K.J.; et al. Activated innate lymphoid cells are associated with a reduced susceptibility to graft-versus-host disease. *Blood* **2014**, *124*, 812–821. [CrossRef] [PubMed]
65. Vacca, P.; Montaldo, E.; Croxatto, D.; Moretta, F.; Bertaina, A.; Vitale, C.; Locatelli, F.; Mingari, M.C.; Moretta, L. NK Cells and Other Innate Lymphoid Cells in Hematopoietic Stem Cell Transplantation. *Front. Immunol.* **2016**, *7*, 188. [CrossRef] [PubMed]

9

Profiling of Omega-Polyunsaturated Fatty Acids and their Oxidized Products in Salmon after Different Cooking Methods

Kin Sum Leung [1], Jean-Marie Galano [2], Thierry Durand [2] and Jetty Chung-Yung Lee [1,*]

1 School of Biological Sciences, The University of Hong Kong, Pokfulam Road, Hong Kong, China; sam612@connect.hku.hk

2 Institut des Biomolécules Max Mousseron (IBMM), UMR 5247, CNRS Université de Montpellier, ENSCM, F-34093 Montpellier, France; jgalano@univ-montp1.fr (J.-M.G.); thierry.durand@umontpellier.fr (T.D.)

* Correspondence: jettylee@hku.hk

Abstract: Consumption of food containing n-3 PUFAs, namely EPA and DHA, are known to benefit health and protect against chronic diseases. Both are richly found in marine-based food such as fatty fish and seafood that are commonly cooked prior to consumption. However, the elevated temperature during cooking potentially degrades the EPA and DHA through oxidation. To understand the changes during different cooking methods, lipid profiles of raw, boiled, pan-fried and baked salmon were determined by LC-MS/MS. Our results showed that pan-frying and baking elevated the concentration of peroxides in salmon, whereas only pan-frying increased the MDA concentration, indicating it to be the most severe procedure to cause oxidation among the cooking methods. Pan-frying augmented oxidized products of n-3 and n-6 PUFAs, while only those of n-3 PUFA were elevated in baked salmon. Notably, pan-frying and baking increased bioactive oxidized n-3 PUFA products, in particular F_{4t}-neuroprostanes derived from DHA. The results of this study provided a new insight into the application of heat and its effect on PUFAs and the release of its oxidized products in salmon.

Keywords: salmon; cooking; lipid peroxidation; polyunsaturated fatty acids; neuroprostanes

1. Introduction

Long chain n-3 polyunsaturated fatty acids (PUFA), including α-linolenic acid (ALA), eicosapentaenoic acid (EPA) and docosahexaenoic acid (DHA), are important to human health, as they have been reported to protect against cardiovascular disease and neurodegeneration and to reduce inflammation [1–6]. Consumption of dietary n-3 PUFAs is necessary, as ALA cannot be synthesized in the human body due to the absence of Δ^{12}- and Δ^{15}-desaturase enzymes and the low conversion efficiency of ALA to EPA and DHA in the metabolism. Both EPA and DHA are obtained through our diet, mainly from marine-based food such as fish oil, fatty fish and seafood [7]. However, due to hygiene reasons, it is rare to consume fish raw, and instead, it is commonly cooked by steaming, boiling, pan-frying, baking or roasting prior to consumption. The high temperature generated from these cooking methods could degrade EPA and DHA by breaking down the double bonds for oxidation. Some studies found that the levels of EPA and DHA in marine species were reduced after long-term storage and heat treatment [8–11], while others reported that the levels of EPA and DHA in certain fish species remained unchanged after cooking [12–14].

The high temperature generated during cooking increases the formation of free radicals and reactive oxygen species (ROS) and primarily releases products such as peroxides. On further oxidation, secondary products, namely the aldehydes or alcohol-derived compounds of the hydroperoxide primary metabolites, are released. For instance, F_2-isoprostanes derived from arachidonic (AA) is a well-known biomarker for oxidative stress in diseases [15], but little is known about its role or generation in food. Likewise, an increasing amount of studies has shown that oxidized products formed through peroxidation of EPA and DHA are beneficial to our health. For example, F_3-isoprostanes (F_3-IsoPs) derived from EPA are anti-inflammatory and anti-thrombotic, as they lower the production of pro-inflammatory prostaglandins and thromboxanes derived from arachidonic acid (AA) by competing for the cyclooxygenase enzyme activity [16]. In addition, some neuroprostanes derived from DHA such as 4-(*RS*)-4-F_4- neuroprostane (NeuroP) are cardio-protective by reducing the risk of ischemia injury in the heart. Furthermore, 4-(*RS*)-4-F_4-NeuroP was found to prevent post-translational modification of the type 2 ryanodine receptor (RyR2) in cardiac cells [17]. Such an effect restored calcium homeostasis in the heart and reduced arrhythmia. A_4-NeuroP and J_4-NeuroP are proposed to be have anti-inflammatory properties [17,18] that could bind and activate peroxisome proliferator-activated receptors (PPARs) to reduce the expression of cytokines IL-6 and TNF-α in response to the inflammation of macrophages [19].

Nevertheless, oxidation of DHA also releases other oxidized products such as 4-hydroxy-2-hexenal (4-HHE). It is the major secondary lipid peroxidation products of DHA that is claimed to be neurotoxic in neuronal cells by augmenting ROS activity and down-regulating antioxidant enzyme and glutathione (GSH) levels [20]. However, recently, there have been studies suggesting that low dose 4-HHE is cardioprotective through the activation of Nrf2 in the vascular cells [21,22].

In this study, the effect of cooking methods on the quality of the PUFA of fatty fish (salmon) was investigated by examining the level of lipid peroxidation and the quantification of PUFA and the oxidized product content of the raw and cooked salmons.

2. Materials and Methods

2.1. Fish Samples and Heat Treatment

Fresh, deskinned salmon filets were purchased from a local food market and stored in refrigerators (<4 °C) for 2 h before cooking and extraction for analysis. A total of 16 filets, each 100 g, was divided into four groups including raw as the control, boiling, pan-frying and oven-baking. Details of the cooking process are outlined below.

1. Boiling: Salmon filets were boiled individually on a heat plate in 800 mL of water initially at 99 ± 1 °C for 10 min.
2. Pan-frying: Salmon filets were fried on a medium-sized frying pan on a heat plate to a center temperature of 200 ± 10 °C for 10 min and were flipped over half way (5 min) through cooking.
3. Oven-baking: The oven was pre-heated to 200 °C. Salmon filets were individually placed on an aluminum foil-coated metal tray and baked at 200 °C for 15 min.

No cooking oil was added in any cooking method to ensure that the lipids of the samples were from the salmon only. Thereafter, the cooked salmons were cooled to room temperature and stored at −80 °C until analysis.

2.2. Extraction of Crude Oil

Raw and cooked salmon samples (50 g) were chopped finely by hand. The oil content was derived in a Soxhlet extractor with 500 mL of n-hexane/diethyl ether (80:20, *v*/*v*) for 8 h. The oil collected was cooled to room temperature and dried completely using nitrogen gas. The dried oil was purged with nitrogen and stored at −80 °C until further analysis.

2.3. Measurement of Lipid Peroxidation

A portion of the oil sample (1 g) collected was used for the peroxide value (PV) test to determine total lipid peroxides and the primary lipid peroxidation products, and another portion (1 g) of the oil sample extracted was used to estimate malondialdehyde (MDA) content using the thiobarbituric acid reactive substances (TBARS) test.

The peroxide levels, expressed as peroxide value of the oil, were measured by the conversion of potassium iodide to release iodine according to the Toru et al. method [23]. In brief, 1.0 g of the oil sample was weighed in an Erlenmeyer flask (125 mL) and dissolved with 30 mL acetic acid/chloroform (3:2, v/v) solution. A volume of 0.5 mL saturated potassium iodide solution was then added to the dissolved oil, and the mixture was diluted with 30 mL of distilled water. The sample mixture was first titrated with 0.01 M sodium thiosulfate until it turned pale yellow. Then, 1 mL of starch indicator was added, and titration was continued until the disappearance of the dark blue color in the solution.

TBARS test was measured based on the reaction between TBA with MDA and other confounding components according to the Papastergiadis et al. method [24]. In brief, 0.5 g of oil were dissolved in 10 mL toluene and reacted with 10 mL TBA reagent. The reaction mixture was swirled and vigorously shaken for 4 min, and the layers were separated by a separatory funnel. The lower phase was collected and heated in a boiling water bath for 10 min. After cooling down under running tap water, the absorbance of the samples was measured by spectrophotometer at 530 nm, and the concentration of MDA was calculated by using the equation generated by the MDA standard curve.

Corn oil (Lion & Globe, Hong Kong, China) purchased from a local market was stored at room temperature for 4 years to serve as the positive control for the PV and TBARS tests.

2.4. Extraction of Polyunsaturated Fatty Acids and Oxidized Products

PUFA and oxidized lipid products were extracted from salmon samples by Folch extraction as reported previously [25]. In brief, 0.05 g of finely-chopped salmon samples were homogenized in 10 mL of Folch solution (chloroform/methanol 2:1 v/v + 0.05% BHT) using a blade homogenizer (T25, ULTRA-TURRAX, IKA, Guangzhou, China). Afterwards, 2 mL of 0.9% NaCl were added to create a phase separation and extraction. After centrifugation at 800× g for 10 min at 4 °C, the lower organic phase was transferred to a glass vial, and the solvent was evaporated under a stream of nitrogen gas. The dried extract was re-suspended in 1 M potassium hydroxide in methanol (1:1). The samples were then hydrolyzed overnight, in the dark, at room temperature (25 °C). After hydrolysis, the samples were cooled and neutralized by hydrochloric acid. Finally, formic acid (pH 4.5) was added, mixed together with heavy isotope internal standards 4-(*RS*)-4-F_{4t}-NeuroP-d_4 and 10-F_{4t}-NeuroP-d_4 synthesized by Institut des Biomolécules Max Mousseron (IBMM, Montpellier, France) and isoprostanes (IsoP) including 5-F_{2t}-IsoP-d_{11}, 15-F_{2t}-IsoP-d_4, $PGF_{2\alpha}$-d_4, hydroxyeicosatetraenoic acid (HETE), namely 5(*S*)-HETE-d_8, 12(*S*)-HETE-d_8, 15(*S*)-HETE-d_8, 20-HETE-d_6, AA-d_8, EPA-d_5 and DHA-d_5 (Cayman Chemicals, Ann Arbor, MI, USA). Finally, the samples were cleaned and extracted using anionic exchange solid phase extraction columns (60 mg, Oasis MAX, Waters, Milford, MA, USA), as described in our previous study [26].

2.5. Quantification of Polyunsaturated Fatty Acids and Its Oxidized Products

The extracted PUFA and its oxidized products were analyzed according to previous studies with modifications [27,28]. A liquid chromatography tandem mass spectrometry (LC-MS/MS) system consisting of a 1290 Infinity LC system (Agilent, Santa Clara, CA, USA) with a C18 column (2.6 μm particle size, 150 × 2.1 mm, Phenomenex, Torrance, CA, USA) set to 30 °C was used. The mobile phase consisted of 0.1% formic acid in water (A) and 0.1% formic acid in acetonitrile (B). The flow rate was set to 200 μL/min, and the injection volume was 10 μL. The gradient was first maintained at 10% B from 0 to 1 min, then a linear gradient from 10% B to 98% B for 7 min, then 98% B held for 4 min and, finally, a linear gradient from 98% B to 10% B for 0.1 min. Thereafter, the column was re-equilibrated to the starting condition. A QTrap 3200 triple quadrupole mass spectrometer (Sciex Applied Biosystems, Framingham, MA, USA) coupled to the LC was operated at negative atmospheric pressure chemical ionization (APCI) mode. The spray voltage was set to −4000 V, and nitrogen gas was used as the curtain gas. The scan mode was multiple reaction monitoring (MRM), and the MS/MS transition (Figure 1) was monitored according to our previous reports [27,28]. Quantitation of each analyte was determined by relating the peak area with its corresponding deuterated internal standard peak including AA, EPA, DHA, 5(*S*)-, 12(*S*)-, 15(*S*)-, 20(*S*)-HETE, 15-F_{2t}-IsoP, 5-F_{2t}-IsoP, 4-(*RS*)-4-F_{4t}-NeuroP and 10-F_{4t}-NeuroP. For the analytes without the corresponding deuterated internal standards, i.e., adrenic acid (AdA), 8(*S*)-, 9(*S*)-, 11(*S*)-HETE, 7-F_{2t}-dihomo-IsoP, 17-F_{2t}-dihomo-IsoP, 7-F_{2t}-dihomo-isofuran, 17-F_{2t}-dihomo-isofuran, resolvin E1, 5-F_{3t}-IsoP, 8-F_{3t}-IsoP, 15-F_{3t}-IsoP, resolvin D1, 4(*RS*)-ST-Δ^5-8-neurofuran, 14(*RS*)-14-F_{3t}-IsoP and 4-F_{3t}-IsoP, quantitation was done by using deuterated internal standards with the relative response factor.

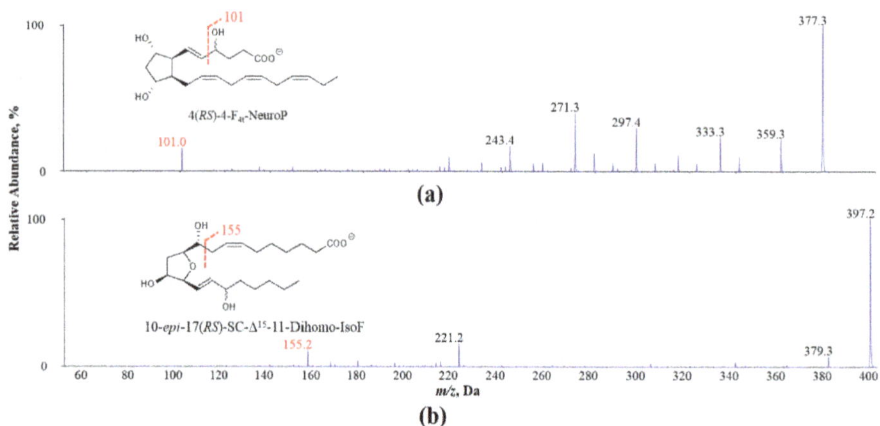

Figure 1. Exemplary MS/MS spectra of oxidized PUFA products (**a**) 4(*RS*)-4-F_{4t}-NeuroP derived from DHA and (**b**) 10-*epi*-17(*RS*)-SC-Δ^{15}-11-dihomo-IsoF derived from AdA: adrenic acid; NeuroP: neuroprostane; IsoF: isofuran.

2.6. Extraction of Reactive Aldehydes, 4-Hydroxy-2(E)-Hexenal and 4-Hydroxy-2-Nonenal

Reactive aldehydes including 4-HHE and 4-HNE were extracted and derivatized from salmon samples according to Douny et al., with modifications [29]. In brief, 1 g of salmon samples was homogenized with 200 µL of BHT solution (1 mg/mL in ethanol) and 2200 µL of ethanol-water (50:50 *v*/*v*) by using a blade homogenizer (T25, ULTRA-TURRAX, IKA). A volume of 100 µL of internal standard mix containing 4-HHE-d_3 and 4-HNE-d_3 (0.25 ng/µL in ethanol) was added to the homogenates and vortexed for 1 min. Afterwards, the samples were centrifuged at 2100× *g* for 10 min. A volume of 2 mL supernatant was collected, filtered with hydrophilic filter and transferred into a new glass tube. Then, 2 mL 0.05 M 2,4-dinitrophenylhydrazine (DNPH)solution in acetonitrile/acetic acid (9:1 *v*/*v*) were added to the extract, and the samples were incubated in a 60 °C water bath for 2 h to derivatize the reactive aldehydes and internal standards. Thereafter, 2 mL of Milli-Q water and 2 mL of hexane were added to the mixture. To increase the yield, the derivatized extract was collected again with 2 mL hexane. The hexane extracts were combined and dried under a stream of nitrogen. The dried extract was resuspended with 100 µL of 0.1% acetic acid/acetonitrile (60:40 *v*/*v*), and LC-MS/MS analysis was performed immediately.

2.7. Quantification of 4-HHE and 4-HNE

4-HHE and 4-HNE were measured in the samples by LC-MS/MS using ExionLC™ AC analytical HPLC with a C18 column (2.6 µm particle size, 150 × 2.1 mm, Phenomenex, Torrance, CA, USA) maintained at 30 °C. The mobile phase consisted of 0.1% acetic acid in water (A) and 0.1% acetic acid in acetonitrile (B). The flow rate was set to 300 µL/min, and the injection volume was 20 µl. The gradient was first increased from 40% B to 65% B for 8.5 min, then gradually increased to 100% B for 4 min and maintained for 7.5 min. Thereafter, the column was re-equilibrated to the starting condition. A Sciex X500R QTOF System mass spectrometer (Sciex Applied Biosystems, Framingham, MA, USA) coupled to the LC was operated at negative electrospray ionization, where the source temperature was set to 500 °C. The scan mode was multiple reaction monitoring (MRM), and the MS/MS transition was monitored as 293.09→167.01 for 4-HHE-DNPH, 335.14→167.01 for 4-HNE-DNPH, 296.09→167.01 for 4-HHE-d_3 and 338.14→167.01 for 4-HNE-d_3. Quantitation of 4-HHE and 4-HNE was determined by relating the peak area to its corresponding deuterated internal standard peak.

2.8. Statistical Analysis

Statistical analysis was performed using GraphPad Prism Version 6.0 (GraphPad Prism, La Jolla, CA, USA). All values were expressed as the mean ± standard deviation (SD). Differences between more than three groups were analyzed by 1-way analysis of variance (ANOVA), and $p < 0.05$ was noted as statistically significant.

3. Results

3.1. Different Cooking Methods Did Not Reduce PUFAs' Levels in Salmon

The content of PUFAs determined in the prepared salmon samples is shown in Figure 2. Surprisingly, different cooking methods did not significantly reduce the concentration of AA, AdA, EPA and DHA of the salmons. Although there was a tendency for a significant change in some PUFA levels by the heat treatments, the large standard deviation of the mean (~50%) hampered the statistical relevance. Notably, the large deviation was more prominent when the salmon was fried or baked.

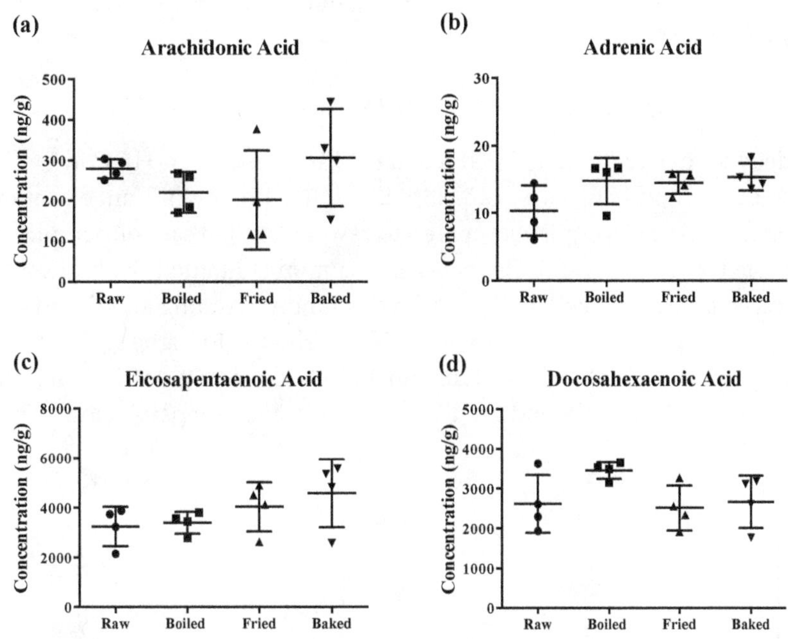

Figure 2. Concentration of polyunsaturated fatty acids measured in salmon samples. Graphs represent (**a**) arachidonic acid, (**b**) adrenic acid, (**c**) eicosapentaenoic acid and (**d**) docosahexaenoic acid measured in salmon samples. Data are presented as the mean ± S.D. ($n = 4$). Raw: control salmons without any cooking; boiled: salmons cooked by boiling; fried: salmons cooked by pan-frying; baked: salmons cooked by oven-baking.

3.2. Elevated Lipid Peroxidation Was Found in Pan-Fried and Oven-Baked Salmons

Lipid peroxidation was assessed in the cooked salmon and in old corn oil by the PV and TBARS tests (Figure 3). The corn oil (expired for four years) was used as a positive control and had approximately a 60-fold higher level for the PV value and a five-fold higher MDA level compared to raw salmon. Boiling did not increase PV and MDA significantly compared to raw salmon. However, a significant increase in PV was found in pan-fried and oven-baked salmon, and increased MDA was found in pan-fried salmon only, compared to other salmon samples. The elevation of peroxides showed that pan-frying and oven-baking indeed increased the extent of primary oxidation in the salmon. In addition, the higher level of MDA observed in pan-fried salmon suggested it to be more detrimental compared to other cooking methods.

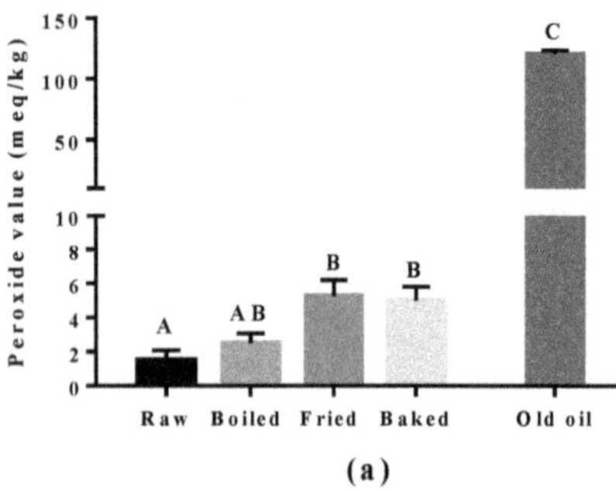

(a)

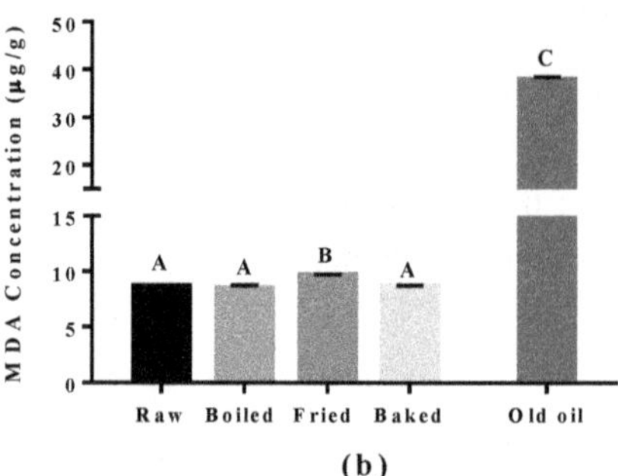

(b)

Figure 3. Level of lipid peroxidation in salmon samples measured by the peroxide value (PV) test and the thiobarbituric acid (TBARS) test. Graphs showing (**a**) PV and (**b**) malondialdehyde (MDA) measured in the oil extracted from salmon samples. Data are presented as the mean ± S.D. ($n = 4$). Raw: control salmons without any cooking; boiled: salmons cooked by boiling; fried: salmons cooked by pan-frying; baked: salmons cooked by oven-baking; old oil: corn oil expired for four years as the positive control. A similar letter denotes no statistical differences between samples, otherwise it is statistically significant at $p < 0.05$.

3.3. Elevated 4-HHE and 4-HNE Were Found in Cooked Salmons

Reactive aldehydes derived from n-3 PUFA and n-6 PUFA, namely 4-HHE and 4-HNE respectively, were measured in the salmon samples by LC-MS/MS (Figure 4). A significant elevation of 4-HHE and 4-HNE was found in pan-fried samples compared to raw and boiled salmon samples. Similar to what was observed in the PV and TBARS tests, pan-fried salmon contained the highest levels of 4-HHE and 4-HNE, followed by oven-baked, boiled and raw salmons. Among all salmon samples, the level of 4-HHE was higher compared to the level of 4-HNE likely due to higher n-3 PUFA than n-6 PUFA content in the salmons. The elevation of 4-HHE and 4-HNE found in pan-fried salmons indicated that lipid peroxidation of both n-3 PUFA and n-6 PUFA was escalated by pan-frying.

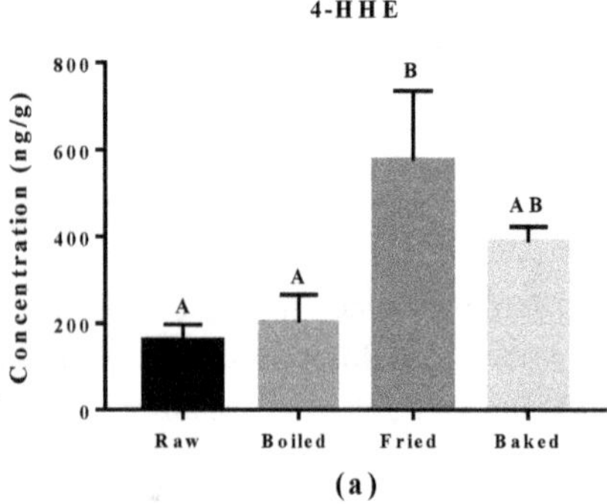

(a)

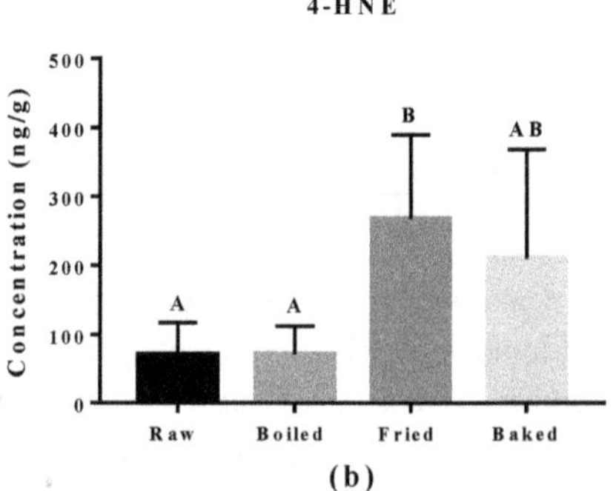

(b)

Figure 4. Levels of 4-hydroxy-2(E)-hexenal (4-HHE) and 4-hydroxy-2-nonenal (4-HNE) in salmon samples measured by LC-MS/MS. Graphs showing (**a**) 4-HHE and (**b**) 4-HNE in salmon samples. Data are presented as the mean ± S.D. ($n = 6$). Raw: control salmons without any cooking; boiled: salmons cooked by boiling; fried: salmons cooked by pan-frying; baked: salmons cooked by oven-baking. Similar letters denote no statistical differences between samples, otherwise it is statistically significant at $p < 0.05$.

3.4. Elevated Oxidized PUFA Products Were Found in Cooked Salmons

Oxidized PUFA products released by enzymatic and non-enzymatic oxidation of the salmon samples were measured by using LC-MS/MS. A total of 25 out of 42 were successfully detected. No cooking methods showed much effect on the level of enzymatic-oxidized PUFA products of the salmon. Only two types of analytes, RvE1 enzymatically derived from EPA, after pan-frying, and 14-hydroxy-DHA (HDHA) derived from DHA by both enzymatic and non-enzymatic oxidation, after oven-baking, were elevated significantly (Table 1).

The effect of cooking methods on the level of non-enzymatic-oxidized lipid products was more obvious (Figures 5 and 6). The cooking method that led to the strongest lipid peroxidation in salmon was pan-frying, where a significant increase in the amount of 15-F_{2t}-IsoP derived from AA, 15-F_{3t}-IsoP and 8-F_{3t}-IsoP derived from EPA, and 10-HDHA and 16-HDHA derived from DHA were detected. On the other hand, oven-baking also increased the levels of certain oxidized lipid products including 15-F_{3t}-IsoP derived from EPA and 4-(*RS*)-4-F_{4t}-NeuroPs, 10-HDHA and 16-HDHA derived from DHA. However, boiling the salmon only increased the concentration of 15-F_{3t}-IsoP.

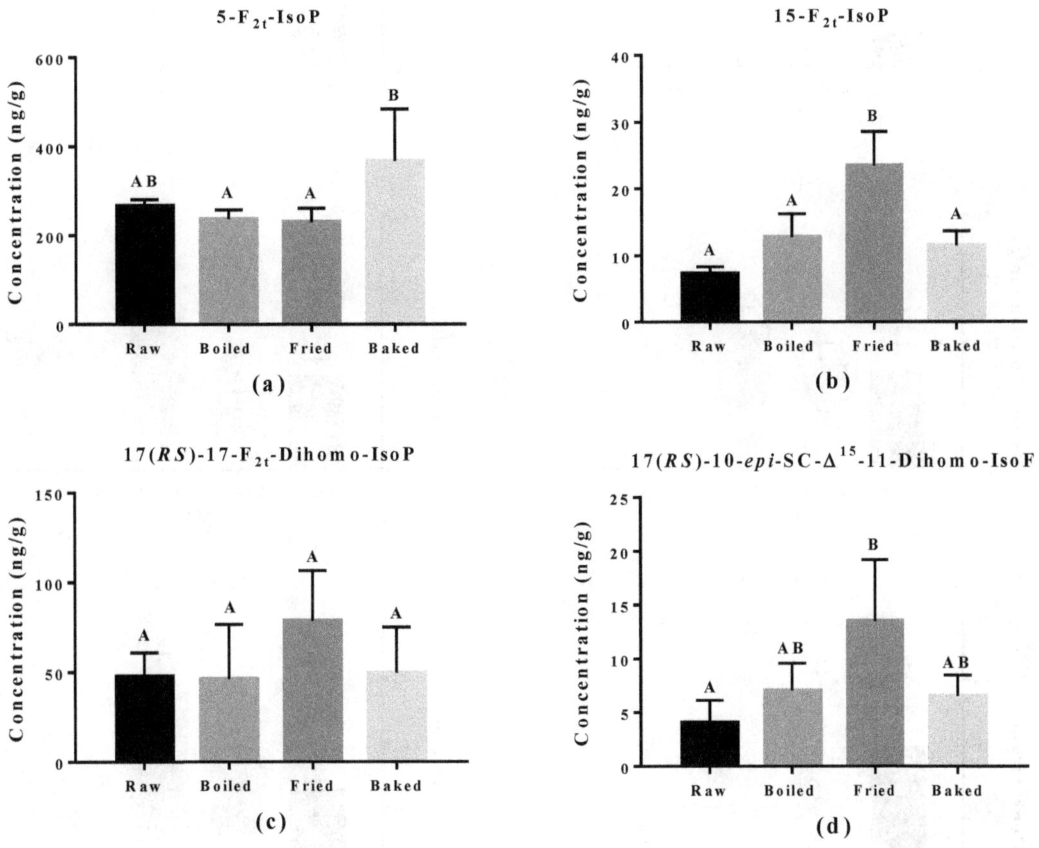

Figure 5. Concentration of non-enzymatically oxidized n-6 PUFA products measured in salmon samples. Graphs represent (**a**,**b**) F_2-IsoPs derived from arachidonic acid and (**c**,**d**) dihomo-IsoP and dihomo-isofuran derived from adrenic acid. Data are presented as the mean ± S.D. (n = 4). Raw: control salmons without any cooking; boiled: salmons cooked by boiling; fried: salmons cooked by pan-frying; baked: salmons cooked by oven-baking. Similar letters denote no statistical differences between samples, otherwise it is statistically significant at $p < 0.05$.

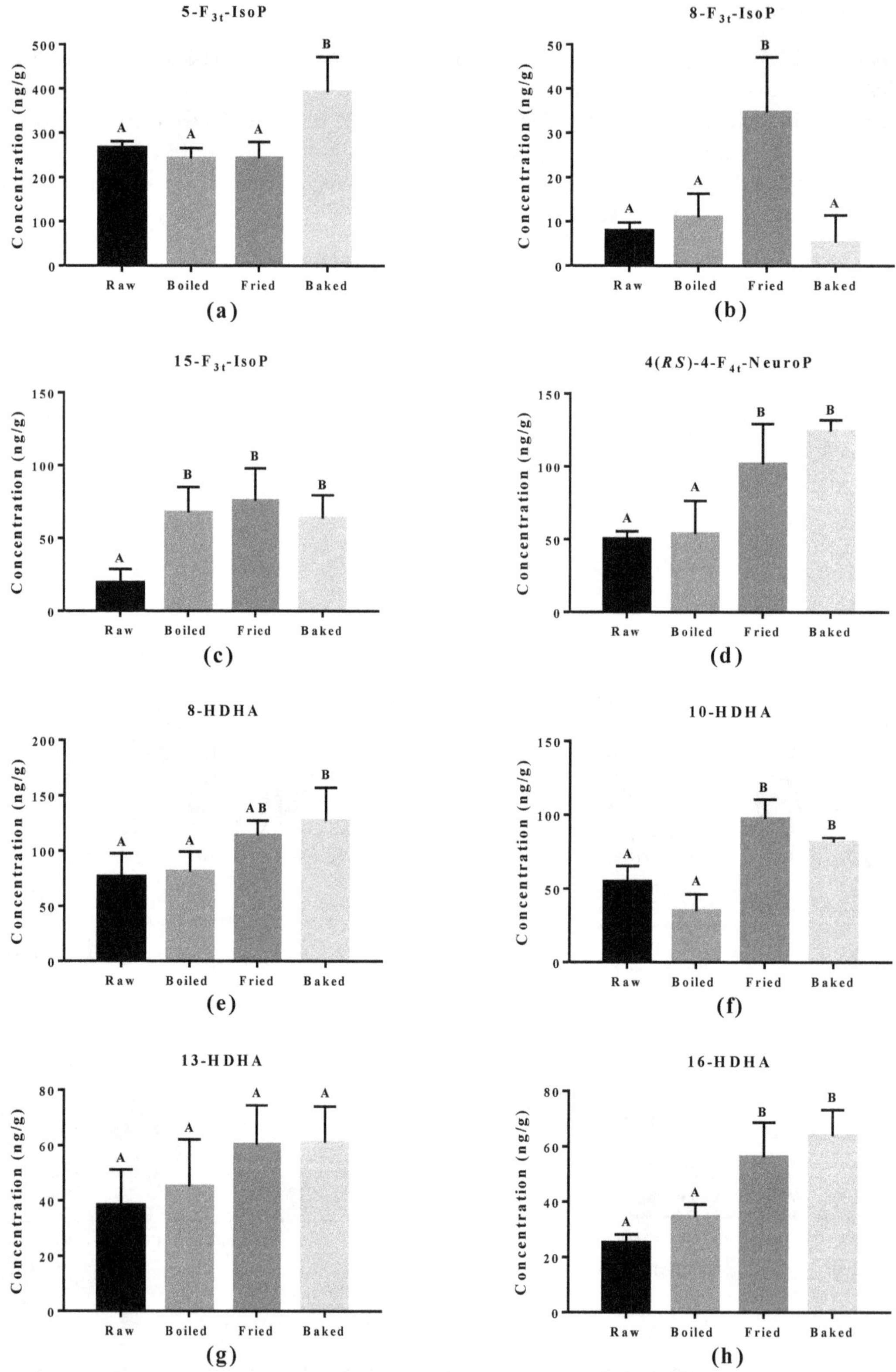

Figure 6. Concentration of non-enzymatically oxidized n-3 PUFA products measured in salmon samples. Graphs represent (**a**–**c**) F_3-IsoPs derived from eicosapentaenoic acid and (**d**–**h**) NeuroPs and hydroxy-DHA (HDHA) derived from docosahexaenoic acid. Data are presented as the mean ± S.D. ($n = 4$). Raw: control salmons without any cooking; boiled: salmons cooked by boiling; fried: salmons cooked by pan-frying; baked: salmons cooked by oven-baking. Similar letters denote no statistical differences between samples, otherwise it is statistically significant at $p < 0.05$.

Table 1. Concentration of enzymatically-oxidized products derived from n-3 and n-6 PUFAs measured in salmon samples.

	Raw	Boiled	Fried	Baked
Enzymatic oxidized lipid products derived from AA				
5(*S*)-HETE	134.12 ± 29.53 ^{a}	150.46 ± 33.12 ^{a}	265.91 ± 92.79 ^{a}	201.24 ± 7.79 ^{a}
8(*S*)-HETE	19.98 ± 8.02 ^{a}	21.30 ± 2.45 ^{a}	56.83 ± 35.47 ^{a}	29.80 ± 4.81 ^{a}
11(*S*)-HETE	32.15 ± 9.16 ^{a}	30.73 ± 7.76 ^{a}	81.76 ± 43.66 ^{a}	55.31 ± 27.44 ^{a}
12(*S*)-HETE	138.95 ± 50.97 ^{a}	235.53 ± 198 ^{a}	142.66 ± 86.35 ^{a}	98.54 ± 42.05 ^{a}
15(*S*)-HETE	8.71 ± 4.42 ^{a}	9.62 ± 4.32 ^{a}	6.71 ± 2.77 ^{a}	7.90 ± 2.69 ^{a}
Enzymatic oxidized lipid products derived from EPA				
RvE1	8.97 ± 2.94 ^{a}	14.31 ± 2.84 ^{a}	25.55 ± 3.86 ^{b}	11.80 ± 3.41 ^{a}
Enzymatic oxidized lipid products derived from DHA				
4-HDHA	63.36 ± 17.08 ^{a}	51.03 ± 10.09 ^{a}	78.24 ± 15.16 ^{a}	88.54 ± 17.42 ^{a}
7-HDHA	36.45 ± 6.32 ^{a}	35.28 ± 7.88 ^{a}	47.03 ± 11.73 ^{a}	54.47 ± 16.39 ^{a}
11-HDHA	38.21 ± 4.84 ^{a}	33.86 ± 8.98 ^{a}	55.02 ± 7.74 ^{a}	48.91 ± 13.09 ^{a}
14-HDHA	40.43 ± 3.42 ^{a}	35.62 ± 10.38 ^{a}	84.71 ± 22.08^b	89.26 ± 13.17 ^{b}
17-HDHA	391.58 ± 43.80 ^{a}	539.14 ± 149.46 ^{a}	489.99 ± 36.43 ^{a}	790.34 ± 273.12 ^{a}
RvD1	19.46 ± 8.50 ^{a}	19.11 ± 2.90 ^{a}	23.82 ± 3.81 ^{a}	37.43 ± 12.13 ^{a}
NPD1	11.41 ± 3.01 ^{a}	15.44 ± 2.70 ^{a}	24.68 ± 6.20 ^{s}	11.93 ± 2.33 ^{a}

Data are presented as the mean ± S.D. (n = 4), ng/g of tissue. Raw: control salmons without any cooking; boiled: salmons cooked by boiling; fried: salmons cooked by pan-frying; baked: salmons cooked by oven-baking. HETE: hydroxyeicosatetraenoic acid; HDHA: hydroxy-DHA; RvD1: resolving D1; NPD1: neuroprotection D1. Similar letters in superscript denote no statistical differences between samples, otherwise it is statistically significant at $p < 0.05$.

4. Discussion

Regular consumption of long chain n-3 PUFAs, namely EPA and DHA, has been proposed to have health benefits such as improving blood flow and blood pressure, cardiovascular disease prevention and neurodegenerative disease protection [2,4,30]. In general, fatty fish is a rich source of EPA and DHA. American Heart Association recommended to the public to consume regular fatty fish at least twice a week to obtain the health benefits of EPA and DHA [31]. However, fish in most countries is consumed cooked and not raw; therefore, concerns about the method of cooking may lead to the reduction of n-3 PUFAs and the generation of potentially toxic oxidized lipid products due to the high heat.

In this study, the content of PUFAs, oxidized PUFA products and level of lipid peroxidation in raw, boiled, pan-fried and oven-baked salmon were examined. None of the cooking methods was able to significantly reduce either n-3 or n-6 PUFAs in the salmon samples, which indicates that the quality of n-3 PUFAs in benefitting health was not altered after cooking. This matched the findings in the study of Bastias et al., where the fatty acid profile in salmon remained unchanged after cooking by four different methods [32]. In a similar study, cooking methods including boiling, frying and roasting of humpback salmon showed that only frying significantly reduced EPA and DHA [13]. The group suggested that the decreased PUFAs in the salmon may be caused by the longer frying time. The frying time used was 15-20 min, but in this study, it took 10 min; in comparison, the longer frying time may have raised the oxidation of PUFAs in the salmon and subsequent loss of PUFAs. Although in this study, cooking oil was not used in the frying process, the reduction of PUFAs in pan-fried salmon may occur if cooking oil is added during frying. Flaskerud et al. found that pan-frying trout in corn oil and canola oil had no effect on the level of PUFAs in the fish, but pan-frying with peanut oil and high oleic sunflower oil induced the reduction of EPA and of EPA and DHA, respectively [33]. This matched the findings from Gladyshev et al., who used sunflower oil to fry the salmon [13]. The decline of EPA and DHA is the result of the fat of fish filets transferring to the cooking oil when pan-frying in sunflower oil. Sioen et al. proposed that the fat of the fish is leached out during the frying process to the cooking oil, and the free radicals generated in the hot cooking oil in return oxidize the fat of the fish [34]. Thereafter, another similar study was conducted by Gladyshev et al. with four different fish species including sea trout, herring, rock sole and cod [35]. They concluded that the difference of EPA and DHA content in fish depends on the fish type and the use of cooking oil, and not the cooking methods. In their report, only the fried Norwegian trout showed a significant reduction of EPA and DHA compared to raw trout. Again, the loss of EPA and DHA in fried Norwegian trout was mainly due to the sunflower oil during frying.

Heating PUFA will generate numerous types of oxidized products that may be advantageous and disadvantageous to human health. Unexpectedly, PUFA levels were not significantly reduced by the cooking methods, but the results of the PV test, TBARS test, quantification of 4-HHE and 4-HNE and the oxidized products showed alteration. The large standard deviation of the mean PUFAs particularly after frying or baking signified that cooking methods perhaps had an impact on the PUFA concentration. Of the salmon samples, frying and baking induced lipid peroxidation in the salmon where frying had the strongest effect among the three cooking methods. The difference observed in the level of lipid peroxidation in salmon cooked by the different methods is attributed to the heat temperature. Boiling is a mild cooking method, and the temperature generated through boiling was the lowest compared to other cooking methods where the maximum is 100 °C, i.e., the boiling point of water. Moreover, the cooking time was not long compared to baking since the heat transfer by boiling is very effective as the salmon is immersed into the hot water, allowing energy transfer to the food by constant collision of the food molecules through water convection [36]. The short cooking time and low temperature may explain the low level of peroxides and reactive aldehydes in boiled fish compared to raw fish.

On the other hand, pan-frying transfers heat through conduction at a temperature between 190 °C and 210 °C. Even though the temperature used in pan-frying is twice that of boiling, the cooking time is similar to boiling, as the temperature can only transfer to the surface of the food through conduction, which then rapidly dehydrates the food surface and causes Maillard browning and flavor development [35]. The interior of the food can remain moist, and the temperature usually does not exceed 100 °C, as it is insulated by the outer surface and the fat of the food. However, the temperature of the salmon surface is highly exposed to free radicals of the oil released by thermal oxidation in the presence of oxygen, i.e., air and water. As a consequence, the lipid peroxidation caused by frying is strong compared to other methods, and as a result, the levels of peroxides and reactive aldehydes are high.

As for baking, the temperature used was 200 °C and the cooking time was the longest (15 min) since the heat transfer in baking is air convection and radiation, which is not as efficient as boiling and frying. The air in the oven is a thousand-times less dense than water, so the energy transfer by collisions of hot air molecules and food are low [36]. Therefore, it takes more time to heat up the food in the oven, and the inner temperature of the food is much lower than the surrounding temperature. Subsequently, the rate of lipid peroxidation by baking is less strong compared to pan-frying, although the temperature used is similar and the cooking time longer.

The elevation of lipid peroxidation in salmon fillet after frying was further supported by the oxidized PUFA products measured. One product, 15-F_{2t}-IsoP derived from AA, is formed via ROS/free radicals non-enzymatically and is a renowned in vivo oxidative stress biomarker in vivo. It was also significantly induced in the fried salmon sample compared to boiling or baking. This observation indicates frying does increase the free radical production through thermal oxidation of the salmon fillet. Similar products from n-3 PUFA, namely 15-F_{3t}-IsoP and 8-F_{3t}-IsoP from EPA and 4(*RS*)-4-F_{4t}-NeuroP from DHA, are also formed through ROS/free radicals in non-enzymatic oxidation. Elevation of 15-F_{3t}-IsoP was also found in boiled and baked salmon and no change in 8-F_{3t}-IsoP, which matched the PV and TBARS findings that the level of lipid peroxidation produced from boiling and baking is less strong compared to frying. It was surprising to discover that the baking and frying methods increased several DHA-derived oxidized products, but most notably 4(*RS*)-4-F_{4t}-NeuroP. Recent studies found that 4(*RS*)-4-F_{4t}-NeuroP is cardio-protective, containing an anti-arrhythmic factor that can repair the RyR2 ryanodine receptor in the heart and maintain calcium homeostasis [17,18,37]. Furthermore, 4(*RS*)-4-F_{4t}-NeuroP improved heart variability, reduced pro-inflammatory cytokines and reduced thrombosis with improved blood flow [17].

In this study, pan-frying the salmon generated high levels of DHA-derived oxidized products. This is probably due to the strong heat contact in pan frying and potentially promoted secondary lipid peroxidation to generate aldehydes such as 4-HHE and 4-HNE that can cross-link with the protein [38] in the salmon. The elevation of 4-HHE in pan-fried salmon may not be disadvantageous to human health. Although 4-HHE is known to be neurotoxic, to increase during digestion of fatty fish and even to induce gut inflammation [39,40], a low concentration of 4-HHE was found to be cardioprotective by activating Nrf2 [21,22]. Furthermore, the results of the TBARS assay also showed pan-frying to be the only cooking method strong enough to increase the level of MDA in salmon. Both results support that the high temperature contact and heat conduction of the frying led to further degradation of the oxidized products of DHA.

5. Conclusions

The results of this study provided a new insight into how cooking methods affect the composition of PUFAs and oxidized PUFA products in salmon. Prior to the study, we hypothesized that it was possible to reduce the amount of PUFAs and increase their oxidized products in salmon through common cooking methods since the high temperature used could oxidize PUFAs due to the numerous double bonds in the structure. However, the results were unexpected. While the quantified inherent margin of error of the PUFAs showed no reduction after cooking, oxidized products of PUFAs were clearly increased, suggesting that indeed a proportion of the n-3 PUFA, namely EPA and DHA, was modified and generated bioactive compounds such as 4(*RS*)-4-F_{4t}-NeuroP.

Author Contributions: K.S.L. and J.C.-Y.L. designed the study. Analytical measurements were performed by K.S.L. and J.-M.G. T.D. synthesized the IBMM compounds. Data interpretation was made by K.S.L. and J.C.-Y.L. K.S.L., J.-M.G., T.D. and J.C.-Y.L. contributed in the writing of the manuscript.

Funding: This research was funded by The University of Hong Kong, Small Project Funding (No. 201409176019).

Conflicts of Interest: The authors declare no conflict of interest.

References

1. Rajaram, S. Health benefits of plant-derived α-linolenic acid. *Am. J. Clin. Nutr.* **2014**, *100* (Suppl. 1), 443S–448S. [CrossRef] [PubMed]
2. Tapiero, H.; Ba, G.N.; Couvreur, P.; Tew, K.D. Polyunsaturated fatty acids (PUFA) and eicosanoids in human health and pathologies. *Biomed. Pharmacother.* **2002**, *56*, 215–222. [CrossRef]
3. Calder, P.C. N-3 polyunsaturated fatty acids, inflammation, and inflammatory diseases. *Am. J. Clin. Nutr.* **2006**, *83*, 1505S–1519S. [CrossRef] [PubMed]
4. Zhang, W.; Li, P.; Hu, X.; Zhang, F.; Chen, J.; Gao, Y. Omega-3 polyunsaturated fatty acids in the brain: Metabolism and neuroprotection. *Front. Biosci.* **2011**, *16*, 2653–2670. [CrossRef]
5. Thomas, J.; Thomas, C.J.; Radcliffe, J.; Itsiopoulos, C. Omega-3 fatty acids in early prevention of inflammatory neurodegenerative disease: A focus on Alzheimer's disease. *Biomed. Res. Int.* **2015**, *2015*, 172801. [CrossRef] [PubMed]
6. Eser, P.O.; Vanden Heuvel, J.P.; Araujo, J.; Thompson, J.T. Marine- and plant-derived omega-3 fatty acids differentially regulate prostate cancer cell proliferation. *Mol. Clin. Oncol.* **2013**, *1*, 444–452. [CrossRef] [PubMed]
7. Burdge, G.C.; Calder, P.C. Conversion of α-linolenic acid to longer-chain polyunsaturated fatty acids in human adults. *Reprod. Nutr. Dev.* **2005**, *45*, 581–597. [CrossRef] [PubMed]
8. Ohshima, T.; Shozen, K.; Ushio, H.; Koizumi, C. Effects of grilling on formation of cholesterol oxides in seafood products rich in polyunsaturated fatty acids. *Food Sci. Technol.* **1996**, *29*, 94–99. [CrossRef]

9. Sampaio, G.R.; Bastos, D.H.M.; Soares, R.A.M.; Queiroz, Y.S.; Torres, E.A.F.S. Fatty acids and cholesterol oxidation in salted and dried shrimp. *Food Chem.* **2006**, *95*, 344–351. [CrossRef]
10. Sant'Ana, L.S.; Mancini, J. Influence of the addition of antioxidants in vivo on the fatty acid composition of fish fillets. *Food Chem.* **2000**, *68*, 175–178. [CrossRef]
11. Tarley, C.R.T.; Visentainer, J.V.; Matsushita, M.; de Souza, N.E. Proximate composition, cholesterol and fatty acids profile of canned sardines (*Sardinella brasiliensis*) in soybean oil and tomato sauce. *Food Chem.* **2004**, *88*, 1–6. [CrossRef]
12. Echarte, M.; Zulet, M.A.; Astiasaran, I. Oxidation process affecting fatty acids and cholesterol in fried and roasted salmon. *J. Agric. Food Chem.* **2001**, *49*, 5662–5667. [CrossRef] [PubMed]
13. Gladyshev, M.I.; Sushchik, N.N.; Gubanenko, G.A.; Demirchieva, S.M.; Kalachova, G.S. Effect of way of cooking on content of essential polyunsaturated fatty acids in muscle tissue of humpback salmon (*Oncorhynchus gorbuscha*). *Food Chem.* **2006**, *96*, 446–451. [CrossRef]
14. Stolyhwo, A.; Kolodziejska, I.; Sikorski, Z.E. Long chain polyunsaturated fatty acids in smoked atlantic mackerel and baltic sprats. *Food Chem.* **2006**, *94*, 589–595. [CrossRef]
15. Milne, G.L.; Dai, Q.; Roberts, L.J., 2nd. *The isoprostanes—25 years later. Biochim. Biophys. Acta* **2015**, *1851*, 433–445. [PubMed]
16. Alkazemi, D.; Jackson, R.L., 2nd; Chan, H.M.; Kubow, S. Increased F3-isoprostanes in the canadian inuit population could be cardioprotective by limiting F2-isoprostane production. *J. Clin. Endocrinol. Metab.* **2016**, *101*, 3264–3271. [CrossRef] [PubMed]
17. Roy, J.; Oger, C.; Thireau, J.; Roussel, J.; Mercier-Touzet, O.; Faure, D.; Pinot, E.; Farah, C.; Taber, D.F.; Cristol, J.P.; et al. Nonenzymatic lipid mediators, neuroprostanes, exert the antiarrhythmic properties of docosahexaenoic acid. *Free Radic. Biol. Med.* **2015**, *86*, 269–278. [CrossRef] [PubMed]
18. Roy, J.; Fauconnier, J.; Oger, C.; Farah, C.; Angebault-Prouteau, C.; Thireau, J.; Bideaux, P.; Scheuermann, V.; Bultel-Ponce, V.; Demion, M.; et al. Non-enzymatic oxidized metabolite of DHA, 4(RS)-4-F4T-neuroprostane protects the heart against reperfusion injury. *Free Radic. Biol. Med.* **2017**, *102*, 229–239. [CrossRef] [PubMed]
19. Gladine, C.; Newman, J.W.; Durand, T.; Pedersen, T.L.; Galano, J.M.; Demougeot, C.; Berdeaux, O.; Pujos-Guillot, E.; Mazur, A.; Comte, B. Lipid profiling following intake of the omega 3 fatty acid DHA identifies the peroxidized metabolites F4-neuroprostanes as the best predictors of atherosclerosis prevention. *PLoS ONE* **2014**, *9*, e89393. [CrossRef] [PubMed]
20. Long, E.K.; Murphy, T.C.; Leiphon, L.J.; Watt, J.; Morrow, J.D.; Milne, G.L.; Howard, J.R.H.; Picklo, M.J. *Trans*-4-hydroxy-2-hexenal is a neurotoxic product of docosahexaenoic (22:6; n-3) acid oxidation. *J. Neurochem.* **2008**, *105*, 714–724. [CrossRef] [PubMed]
21. Ishikado, A.; Morino, K.; Nishio, Y.; Nakagawa, F.; Mukose, A.; Sono, Y.; Yoshioka, N.; Kondo, K.; Sekine, O.; Yoshizaki, T.; et al. 4-hydroxy hexenal derived from docosahexaenoic acid protects endothelial cells via NRF2 activation. *PLoS ONE* **2013**, *8*, e69415. [CrossRef] [PubMed]
22. Ishikado, A.; Nishio, Y.; Morino, K.; Ugi, S.; Kondo, H.; Makino, T.; Kashiwagi, A.; Maegawa, H. Low concentration of 4-hydroxy hexenal increases heme oxygenase-1 expression through activation of NRF2 and antioxidative activity in vascular endothelial cells. *Biochem. Biophys. Res. Commun.* **2010**, *402*, 99–104. [CrossRef] [PubMed]
23. Toru, T.; Yuichiro, M.; Mayumi, M. Determination of peroxide value by the colorimetric iodine method with protection of iodide as cadmium complex. *Lipids* **1978**, *13*, 147–151.
24. Papastergiadis, A.; Mubiru, E.; Van Langenhove, H.; De Meulenaer, B. Malondialdehyde measurement in oxidized foods: Evaluation of the spectrophotometric thiobarbituric acid reactive substances (TBARS) test in various foods. *J. Agric. Food Chem.* **2012**, *60*, 9589–9594. [CrossRef] [PubMed]
25. Dupuy, A.; Le Faouder, P.; Vigor, C.; Oger, C.; Galano, J.M.; Dray, C.; Lee, J.C.; Valet, P.; Gladine, C.; Durand, T.; et al. Simultaneous quantitative profiling of 20 isoprostanoids from omega-3 and omega-6 polyunsaturated fatty acids by LC-MS/MS in various biological samples. *Anal. Chim. Acta* **2016**, *921*, 46–58. [CrossRef] [PubMed]
26. Lee, C.Y.; Jenner, A.M.; Halliwell, B. Rapid preparation of human urine and plasma samples for analysis of F2-isoprostanes by gas chromatography-mass spectrometry. *Biochem. Biophys. Res. Commun.* **2004**, *320*, 696–702. [CrossRef] [PubMed]

27. Lee, Y.Y.; Wong, C.K.; Oger, C.; Durand, T.; Galano, J.M.; Lee, J.C. Prenatal exposure to the contaminant perfluorooctane sulfonate elevates lipid peroxidation during mouse fetal development but not in the pregnant dam. *Free Radic. Res.* **2015**, *49*, 1015–1025. [CrossRef] [PubMed]
28. Lee, Y.Y.; Crauste, C.; Wang, H.; Leung, H.H.; Vercauteren, J.; Galano, J.M.; Oger, C.; Durand, T.; Wan, J.M.; Lee, J.C. Extra virgin olive oil reduced polyunsaturated fatty acid and cholesterol oxidation in rodent liver: Is this accounted for hydroxytyrosol-fatty acid conjugation? *Chem. Res. Toxicol.* **2016**, *29*, 1689–1698. [CrossRef] [PubMed]
29. Douny, C.; Bayram, P.; Brose, F.; Degand, G.; Scippo, M.L. Development of an LC-MS/MS analytical method for the simultaneous measurement of aldehydes from polyunsaturated fatty acids degradation in animal feed. *Drug Test. Anal.* **2016**, *8*, 458–464. [CrossRef] [PubMed]
30. Gluck, T.; Alter, P. Marine omega-3 highly unsaturated fatty acids: From mechanisms to clinical implications in heart failure and arrhythmias. *Vasc. Pharmacol.* **2016**, *82*, 11–19. [CrossRef] [PubMed]
31. Kris-Etherton, P.M.; Harris, W.S.; Appel, L.J.; American Heart Association. Nutrition, C. Fish consumption, fish oil, omega-3 fatty acids, and cardiovascular disease. *Circulation* **2002**, *106*, 2747–2757. [CrossRef] [PubMed]
32. Bastias, J.M.; Balladares, P.; Acuna, S.; Quevedo, R.; Munoz, O. Determining the effect of different cooking methods on the nutritional composition of salmon (*Salmo salar*) and chilean jack mackerel (*Trachurus murphyi*) fillets. *PLoS ONE* **2017**, *12*, e0180993. [CrossRef] [PubMed]
33. Flaskerud, K.; Bukowski, M.; Golovko, M.; Johnson, L.; Brose, S.; Ali, A.; Cleveland, B.; Picklo, M.; Raatz, S. Effects of cooking techniques on fatty acid and oxylipin content of farmed rainbow trout (*Oncorhynchus mykiss*). *Food Sci. Nutr.* **2017**, *5*, 1195–1204. [CrossRef] [PubMed]
34. Sioen, I.; Haak, L.; Raes, K.; Hermans, C.; De Henauw, S.; De Smet, S.; Van Camp, J. Effects of pan-frying in margarine and olive oil on the fatty acid composition of cod and salmon. *Food Chem.* **2006**, *98*, 609–617. [CrossRef]
35. Gladyshev, M.I.; Sushchik, N.N.; Gubanenko, G.A.; Demirchieva, S.M.; Kalachova, G.S. Effect of boiling and frying on the content of essential polyunsaturated fatty acids in muscle tissue of four fish species. *Food Chem.* **2007**, *101*, 1694–1700. [CrossRef]
36. McGee, H. *On Food and Cooking: The Science and Lore of the Kitchen*; Scribner: New York, NY, USA, 2004.
37. Roy, J.; Le Guennec, J.Y.; Galano, J.M.; Thireau, J.; Bultel-Ponce, V.; Demion, M.; Oger, C.; Lee, J.C.; Durand, T. Non-enzymatic cyclic oxygenated metabolites of omega-3 polyunsaturated fatty acid: Bioactive drugs? *Biochimie* **2016**, *120*, 56–61. [CrossRef] [PubMed]
38. Long, E.K.; Picklo, M.J. *Trans*-4-hydroxy-2-hexenal, a product of n-3 fatty acid peroxidation: Make some room HNE. *Free Radic. Biol. Med.* **2010**, *49*, 1–8. [CrossRef] [PubMed]
39. Larsson, K.; Harrysson, H.; Havenaar, R.; Alminger, M.; Undeland, I. Formation of malondialdehyde (MDA), 4-hydroxy-2-hexenal (HHE) and 4-hydroxy-2-nonenal (HNE) in fish and fish oil during dynamic gastrointestinal in vitro digestion. *Food Funct.* **2016**, *7*, 1176–1187. [CrossRef] [PubMed]
40. Awada, M.; Soulage, C.O.; Meynier, A.; Debard, C.; Plaisancié, P.; Bérengère, B.; Picard, G.; Loizon, E.; Chauvin, M.A.; Estienne, M.; et al. Dietary oxidized n-3 PUFA induce oxidative stress and inflammation: Role of intestinal absorption of 4-HHE and reactivity in intestinal cells. *J. Lipid Res.* **2012**, *53*, 3069–3080. [CrossRef] [PubMed]

10

A Naturally Occurring Antioxidant Complex from Unripe Grapes: The Case of Sangiovese (v. *Vitis vinifera*)

Giovanna Fia [1,*], Claudio Gori [2], Ginevra Bucalossi [1], Francesca Borghini [3] and Bruno Zanoni [1]

1 Dipartimento di Gestione dei Sistemi Agrari, Alimentari e Forestali, University of Florence, Via Donizetti, 6, 50144 Firenze, Italy; ginevra.bucalossi@unifi.it (G.B.); bruno.zanoni@unifi.it (B.Z.)

2 Vino Vigna, Via Claudio Monteverdi, 9, 50053 Empoli, Italy; c.gori@vinovigna.com

3 ISVEA Srl, Servizi Analitici di Eccellenza per i Settori Enologico, Viticolo e il Comparto Alimentare, Via Basilicata 1/3, Poggibonsi, 53036 Siena, Italy; f.borghini@isvea.it

* Correspondence: giovanna.fia@unifi.it

Abstract: The wine industry is well known for its production of a large amount of wastes and by-products. Among them, unripe grapes from thinning operations are an undervalued by-product. Grapes are an interesting source of natural antioxidants such as flavonoids, non-flavonoids and stilbenes. A potential strategy to exploit unripe grapes was investigated in this study. Juice from unripe grapes, v. Sangiovese, was obtained by an innovative technique of solid-liquid extraction without the use of solvents. The juice was dried by a spray-drying technique with the addition of arabic gum as support to obtain powder; juice and powder were characterized for antioxidant activity, phenolic concentration and profile. Phenolic acids, flavonols, flava-3-ols, procyanidins and resveratrol were detected in the juice and powder. The powder was used as anti-browning additive in white wine to test the potential re-use of the unripe grapes in the wine industry. The results indicated that the antioxidant complex from unripe grapes contributed to increasing the anti-browning capacity of white wine. Other applications, such as food and nutraceutical products development, can be considered for the antioxidant complex extracted from unripe grapes. In conclusion, the method proposed in this study may contribute to the exploitation of unripe grapes as a by-product of the winemaking process.

Keywords: unripe grapes; Sangiovese; phenolic compounds; antioxidant activity; solid-liquid extraction

---

1. Introduction

Grapes are rich in bio-active compounds such as vitamins and polyphenols, which act as powerful antioxidants able to scavenge diverse reactive oxygen species (ROS) or inhibit their formation, and hence the oxidation of biomolecules [1]. Polyphenols are involved in the transfer of electrons to free radicals, chalation metal catalyst (Fe^{2+} and Cu^{+}), reduction of alpha-tocopherol radicals, and inhibition of oxidase [2]. Beyond the usual antioxidant activities, the protective effects of polyphenols could be due to their ability to act as modulators of cell signaling [3–5]. The antioxidant properties of grapes have been associated with their phenolic composition and, in particular, with the high content in anthocyanins, flavonols, flava-3-ols, procyanidins and phenolic acids [6,7]. Other polyphenols, such as resveratrol, unique to red grapes, can contribute to the health properties of matrices derived from this fruit. Polyphenols in grapes exist in a free form but the majority of these compounds are glycosides of different sugar units and acylated at different positions of the polyphenol skeleton. Each class of grape phenol compounds showed different antioxidant capacity in vitro and in vivo, with often inconsistent data [6,8]. The differences observed among in vitro and in vitro tests could be ascribed to the bioavailability of polyphenols that contribute to the effectiveness of these compounds in a biological system [9].

Winemaking is well-known for its generation of large amounts of organic wastes and by-products, such as marcs, pomace and lees. The industrial wine sector is exploring solutions to develop marketable products resulting from the exploitation of the industry's wastes, by converting waste materials into food ingredients and other bio-products with high added value [10]. One undervalued by-product of the wine sector is unripe grapes derived from thinning operations carried out to increase the quality of production. The aim of thinning is to remove bunches that do not have the ability to achieve a suitable maturation, thus promoting the maturation of those that remain on the plant. Unripe grapes of low quality, such as table grapes, are traditionally processed into various food products [11]. A potential use of unripe grapes in winemaking to reduce the alcohol concentration and pH of wine was investigated by other authors, who observed a partial reduction of alcohol content and simultaneous decrease of pH of both Cabernet Sauvignon and Merlot experimental wines [12]. Although the bioactive compounds and antioxidant activities of grapes at maturity and by-products of the wine production chain have been the subject of many investigations, unripe grapes and their potential application in the food industry have been scarcely studied [13,14]. Unripe grapes are a source of natural antioxidants such as polyphenols and resveratrol. Indeed, the biosynthesis of these compounds can start before veraison (change of color), when berries are still green, and continue over the course of ripening. It is known that the phenolic composition of grapes depends on many factors, such as variety, maturation stage and environmental conditions [15]. Antioxidant compounds from unripe grapes are potentially exploitable in the food industry as functional ingredients and protective agents against oxidation. Sangiovese is one of the most cultivated varieties of grapes in Italy, and has considerable economic importance. The phenolic composition of Sangiovese has been well studied [15], while information about the antioxidant properties of unripe grapes, v. Sangiovese, and their potential applications are lacking.

The aim of the present study was to obtain an antioxidant complex from unripe grapes, v. Sangiovese, and to evaluate its composition and antioxidant capacity. In addition, the potential protective effect toward white wine oxidation was investigated.

2. Materials and Methods

2.1. Chemicals

Standards, solvents and reagents were purchased from Sigma-Aldrich (Milan, Italy), except for quercetin-3-Oglucoside, quercetin-3-*O*-glucuronide and rutin, which were supplied by HWI Analytik GmbH (Rülzheim, Germany). Methanol and ethanol were supplied by Carlo Erba (Milan, Italy). Ultrapure water was obtained from a Milli-Q Gradient water purification system (Thermo Scientific, Waltham, MA, USA).

2.2. Sangiovese Grapes

Sangiovese grapes were obtained from thinning operations during "green harvesting" on a vineyard located in Lucca, Tuscany, Italy. The grapes were manually harvested on 18 August 2015 during berry ripening at growth stage 36 according to the modified Eichhorn-Lorenz (E-L) system [16]. Only the healthy grapes were transported to the winery in small cases for further operations.

2.3. Wines

Three unfinished wines, Viognier, Chardonnay and Bellone (sparkling base wine), vintage 2015, were provided by the La Torre farm, Velletri, Italy. These commercial wines were used in this study to evaluate the anti-browning capacity of the anti-oxidant complex from unripe grapes.

2.4. Preparation of Juice and Powder

The grapes were crushed and destemmed at the winery, using a Delta E2 destemmer (Bucher Vaslin, Zurich, Switzerland), then transferred to an industrial system [17] for the solid-liquid extraction phase, also performed at the winery (Figure 1).

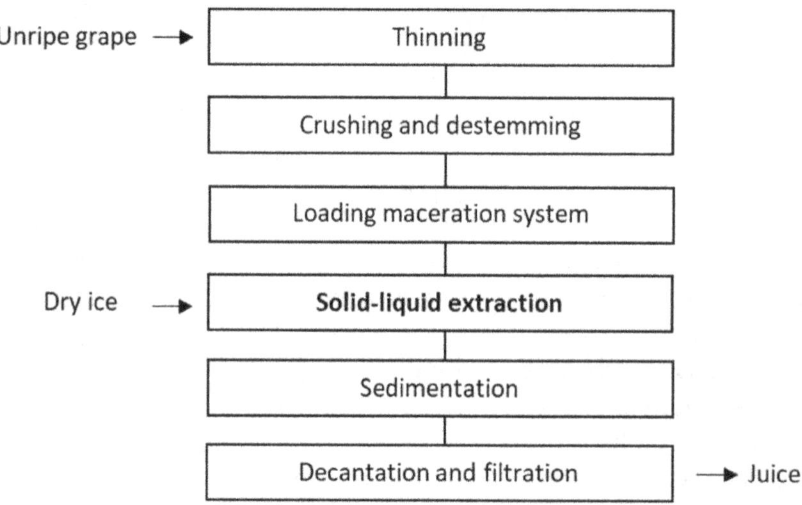

Figure 1. Scheme of process for juice production from unripe grapes.

The system is a stainless-steel tank, of 12,500 L capacity, covered for 75% of its surface by a low-temperature thermostated jacket. Inside the system, there are four whorls to stir up the crushed grapes. A device automatically controls temperature and remixing. The system is also equipped with accessories for loading the grapes, draining the juice, and the discharge of semi-solid residue (pomace). A total of 650 kg of grapes were processed with the addition of 1 kg of dry ice to every 10 kg of grapes. The grapes were remixed every 6 h for 30 min, for a total period of 3 days, at a temperature of 6 °C. During the process, samples of juice (500 mL) were taken immediately after mixing, at the start (2 h), and after 6, 18, 24, 30, 42, 48, 54, 66 and 72 h. Furthermore, after 2 and 72 h, three samples of juice (500 mL) were taken for phenolic composition evaluation. All samples were stored at −20 °C for further analysis. After 72 h, the product was maintained still inside the system at 6 °C for 48 h for sedimentation. After this period, the juice was decanted and large-particle (Ø 1 mm) filtered before freezing. The juice (250 L) was stored at −20 °C until the moment of spray-drying. After thawing, the juice was combined with arabic gum (16% w/v) (Nexira Food, Rouen, France) as support for spray-drying, mixed well and spray-dried to obtain powder. It was necessary to use a support because of the sugar content (153 g/L) of the juice. Arabic gum was chosen from among different types of support because its use is allowed in winemaking. Spray-drying was performed using an industrial turbine spry-dryer (Gea Niro, Milan, Italy). The rotational speed of the turbine was 18,000 revolutions per minute, and the flow rate of the peristaltic pump automatically controlled the drying air temperature, which was 180 °C (input) and 80 °C (outlet). The powder, placed in polyethylene pouches, was stored in a desiccator containing silica, in the dark, for further analysis.

2.5. General Analyses

Alcohol, reducing sugar, total acidity, pH, total and free sulphur dioxide were evaluated in duplicate according to the official or usual methods recommended by the International Organisation of the Vine and Wine, (OIV) [18].

2.6. Total Polyphenols (TP) Determination

Total polyphenols were quantified according to the Folin-Ciocalteau (FC) method [19] with some modifications. Undiluted juice and powder solutions (10%, *w/v*) prepared in distilled water were filtered on a membrane (Ø 0.45 μm). Phenolic compounds were purified from 1 mL of undiluted juice or powder solution on C18 Sep-pak cartridge (Waters, Milan, Italy) following the method described by Di Stefano et al. [20]. 4 mL of sodium carbonate (10%, *w/v*) was added to 1 mL of each sample, mixed well, and left to stand for 5 min. A volume of 1 mL of diluted FC reagent was added to the mixture, and it was then well shaken. Samples were left in the dark for 90 min at room temperature, and then the absorbance was measured spectrophotometrically at 700 nm with a Perkin Elmer Lambda 10 spectrophotometer (Waltham, MA, USA). TP was expressed as (+)-catechin equivalents (CATeq)/L of juice or (CATeq)/g powder. A standard curve was obtained with (+)-catechin solutions at concentrations ranging from 5 to 500 mg/L.

2.7. Total Anthocyanins Determination

Wine sample was diluted with a solution consisting of $C_2H_5OH/H_2O/HCl$ = 69/30/1 (*v/v/v*) and the absorbance was measured at 540 nm [20], using a Perkin Elmer Lambda 10 spectrophotometer. The total anthocyanin (TA) content was expressed as malvidin-3-glucoside equivalents and calculated using the following formula:

$$TA_{540\ nm}\ (mg/L) = A_{540nm} \times 16.7 \times d$$

where A_{540nm}, absorbance at the wavelength of 540 nm; d, dilution; 16.7, molar extinction coefficient of malvidin-3-glucoside.

2.8. 2,2-Diphenyl-1-Picryhydrazil (DPPH) Antioxidant Test

Free-radical-scavenging activity was evaluated by the 2,2-diphenyl-1-picryhydrazil (DPPH) test [21], with some modifications. Briefly, a solution of DPPH (6×10^{-5} M) was prepared by dissolving 0.236 mg of DPPH in 100 mL of methanol. Undiluted juice or powder solution (10%, *w/v*) prepared in distilled water were filtered on a membrane (Ø 0.45 μm). For the reaction, 0.1 mL of either undiluted juice or powder solution was mixed with 3.9 mL of DPPH stock solution. For the reference sample, 0.1 mL of solvent was added to 3.9 mL of DPPH solution to measure the maximum DPPH absorbance. Samples were left in the dark for 30 min at 30 °C for the reaction and immediately afterwards the decrease of absorbance was measured at 515 nm with a Perkin Elmer Lambda 10 spectrophotometer (Waltham, MA, USA). Antioxidant activity was expressed as μmoL of Trolox equivalents antioxidant capacity (TEAC)/L of juice and (TEAC)/g of powder. Trolox standard solutions were prepared in ethanol at concentrations ranging from 10 to 600 μmoL/L. Each assay was performed in triplicate.

2.9. Liquid Chromatography-High-Resolution Mass Spectrometry (LC-HRMS) Analysis

Phenolic compounds and glutathione analysis was performed via liquid chromatography-high-resolution mass spectrometry (LC-HRMS), coupled with a diode array detector (DAD) (Ultimate 3000, Dionex, Thermo Fisher Scientific (Waltham, MA, USA)). All samples and standards were handled to minimize light exposure. The samples were filtrated to 0.45 μm and then analyzed, without any other preparation step. The liquid chromatograph was an Accela (Accela 1250, Thermo Fisher Scientific, (Waltham, MA, USA) equipped with a quaternary pump and a thermostated autosampler. A kinetex F5 column (2.1 × 100 mm 1.7 μm; Phenomenex (Torrance, CA, USA)) was used. Autosampler tray temperature was set at 10 °C, and the column at 40 °C. Gradient elution was performed with water/0.05% formic acid/5 mM ammonium formate (solvent A) and methanol/0.05% formic acid/5 mM ammonium formate (solvent B) at a constant flow rate of 400 μL/min; and injection volume was 3 μL. An increasing linear gradient of solvent B was used. Separation was carried out in 45 min under the following conditions: 0 min, 5% B; 13 min, 5% B; 22 min, 35% B; 24 min, 35% B; 27 min,

90%; 32 min 90% B and from 33 min to 45 min, 5% B. An LTQ Orbitrap Exactive mass spectrometer (Thermo Fisher Scientific, (Waltham, MA, USA)) equipped with an electrospray ionization (ESI) source in negative mode was used to acquire mass spectra in a full mass spectrometry (MS) data dependent MS^2 experiment. Operation parameters were as follows: source voltage, 4 kV; sheath gas, 35 (arbitrary units); auxiliary gas, 10 (arbitrary units); sweep gas, 0 (arbitrary units); capillary temperature, 300 °C, S-lens radio frequency (RF) level, 60 and automatic gain control (AGC) target, 1×10^6 for MS mode and 2×10^5 for MS^2 mode. Samples were first analyzed in full MS mode with the resolution set at 70,000, whereas the subsequent analyses were performed in dd-MS^2 mode with the resolution set at 17,500. An isolation width of 2 amu was used, and precursors were fragmented by stepped normalized collision energy of 25, 30 and 35. The maximum injection time was set to 200 ms with one microscan both for MS mode and for MS^n mode. The mass range was from m/z 150 to 1000. Data analyses were performed using TraceFinder™ 4.1 software (Thermo Fisher Scientific (Waltham, MA, USA)). Peak assignment was carried out on the basis of the exact mass of the molecular ions and the cis and trans forms were recognized by comparison of the retention times with the standard sample. Quantitative analysis was performed by TraceFinder™ 4.1 software (Thermo Fisher Scientific (Waltham, MA, USA)) with external standard method, using a linear regression of five standard solutions of a mix of the above reported substances from 0.05 to 1 g L^{-1}. For coutaric and fertaric acids, due to the lack of reference materials, corresponding free acids (coumaric and ferulic acids) were used as standard. The samples out of calibration range were conveniently diluted in 12% water/ethanol solution. The recovery and matrix effects were checked for all the samples by standard additions and consecutive dilutions as well. The analysis was carried out in triplicate. All chromatographic runs were collected in the same work session and the resulting relative standard deviation (RSD) was less than 10%.

2.10. HPLC-Determination of Anthocyanins

The relative composition of anthocyanins was determined by high-performance liquid chromatography (HPLC) analysis performed with an HPLC 1290 (AGILENT, Santa Clara, CA, USA), using a reverse phase column and ultraviolet-visible (UV-VIS) detection [17].

2.11. Polyphenols Oxidative Medium (POM) Test

The wine's predisposition towards browning was determined by the so-called POM-test [22,23]. A volume of 15 mL of wine was heated at 60 °C for 1 h, then 60 μL of a 3% hydrogen peroxide solution was added to accelerate the oxidation of color. The browning produced was estimated on the basis of the percent increase (% Oxidation $(OX)_{H2O2}$) of the absorbance at 420 nm and calculated by the following formula:

$$\%\ OX_{H2O2} = [(A_{OX} - A_{BOX})/A_{BOX}] \times 100$$

The absorbance was measured using a Perkin Elmer Lambda 10 spectrophotometer before oxidation (A_{BOX}) and after oxidation (A_{OX}), after cooling the solution at room temperature. The POM-test was performed in triplicate with and without the addition of the antioxidant complex (powder) at a concentration of 2 g/L.

2.12. Statistics Analysis

Chemical analyses were performed in duplicate or triplicate and the data are presented as mean ± standard deviation. Analysis of variance (ANOVA) (Least Significant Differences (LSD), 5% level) was performed using Statgraphics plus 3.1 by Statgraphics (The Plains, VA, USA).

3. Results and Discussion

3.1. Solid-Liquid Extraction and Juice Composition

The antioxidant complex of unripe grapes was obtained according to the process scheme shown in Figure 1. At the end of processing, juice yield was about 40% of the grapes used. The analytical parameters of the juice were compatible with unripe grapes: total acidity (11.09 g/L as tartaric acid), pH 2.97, L-malic acid 3.43 (g/L), sugar content (153 g/L), non-detectable alcohol. Low temperature (6 °C) prevented unwanted fermentation.

Solid-state carbon dioxide (dry ice) is the most-used cryogen to lower temperature in winemaking. The sublimation of dry ice induces a thermal shock that is responsible for immediate cooling of grapes and must. The rapid lowering of the temperature and reduction of the environment due to the CO_2 gaseous state can contribute to protecting phenolics from the activity of oxidase enzymes and oxygen. Moreover, the addition of dry ice to the grapes causes freezing, leading to a breakdown of cells which can then more easily release pigment and other phenolic compounds [24].

The evolution of total polyphenols (TP) and anthocyanins was evaluated during processing (Figure 2). Both TP and anthocyanins were rapidly extracted from the grapes. The evolution of phenolic compounds extracted from the grapes reflected a typical solid-liquid extraction phenomenon: an almost instantaneous dissolution of "free" solutes at grape surface (i.e., leaching) was followed by diffusion of solutes from the interior of the grapes [25]. Comparing the polyphenol and anthocyanin content after 24 h with those obtained at the end of processing, about 92% of polyphenols and 78% of anthocyaninswere extracted after only 24 h. At 72 h, when the process was stopped, the concentration of anthocyanins (197 mg/L) in the juice showed a slight increase while that of TP (822 mg/L) was stable.

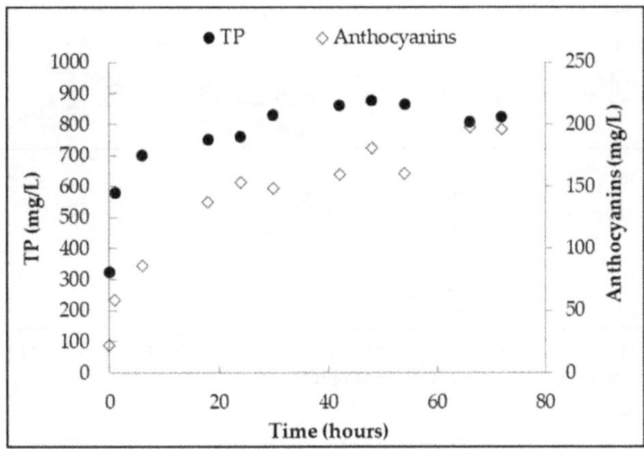

Figure 2. Evolution of total polyphenols (TP) and anthocyanins during processing.

Phenolic composition of the juice was assayed by LC–HRMS both at the beginning (2 h) and at the end of the process (Table 1).

Phenolic acids, flavonols, flava-3-ols, procyanidins and resveratrol were detected in the juice. At the beginning, the concentrations of free hydroxycinnamic acids were lower than those of their tartaric esters (caftaric, coutaric and fertaric acid), which are the most abundant forms contained in cells of grape pulp (Table 1). During processing, the concentration of the esters of hydroxycinnamic acids decreased to a significantly lower level after 72 h. The esters of hydroxycinnamic acids are rapidly oxidized via enzymatic reaction during crushing and juice extraction performed by pressing [26]. Gallic acid and flavonols were extracted in the juice during processing, reaching significantly higher concentrations by the end (72 h) with respect to those observed after 2 h. At the same time, cathechin, epichatechin, procyanidins B1 and B2, and resveratrol were efficiently extracted from the grapes. The five different anthocyanins were found in the juice in the proportions typical of Sangiovese grapes and, at lower concentration, their acetate and cumarate forms (Figure 3) [15]. The phenolic composition of powder obtained by spray-drying (S-D) with the addition of arabic gum (AG) reflected that of the juice (Table 1). Gluthatione was not detected while its oxidized form was, at a concentration of 6.6 μg/g of powder.

Table 1. Phenolic composition of the juice at the beginning (2 h) and at the end (72 h) of the process, and powder obtained by spray-drying (S-D) with the addition of arabic gum (AG).

Phenolic Compounds	Concentration (mg/L) of Juice *		Concentration (μg/g of Powder) *
	Time		S-D + AG
	2 h	72 h	
Phenolic Acids			
Caffeic acid	0.06 ± 0.01 [a]	0.43 ± 0.16 [b]	0.8 ± 0.0
Coumaric acid	0.03 ± 0.00	nd	0.5 ± 0.1
Ferulic acid	1.7 ± 0.4 [b]	0.14 ± 0.00 [a]	29.4 ± 4.7
Caftaric acid	50.0 ± 6.6 [b]	27.5 ± 1.7 [a]	191 ± 5
Coutaric acid	15.9 ± 1.8 [b]	9.4 ± 0.1 [a]	27.6 ± 4.4
Fertaric acid	16.8 ± 3.1 [a]	30.1 ± 3.3 [b]	291 ± 73
Gallic acid	0.05 ± 0.00 [a]	9.4 ± 2.1 [b]	9.5 ± 0.3
Flavonols			
Quercetin	0.07 ± 0.00 [a]	0.29 ± 0.01 [b]	1.3 ± 0.0
Quercetin 3-*O*-glucoside	0.13 ± 0.02 [a]	19.8 ± 0.8 [b]	11.8 ± 0.8
Quercetin 3-*O*-glucuronide	0.38 ± 0.07 [a]	27.0 ± 1.2 [b]	56.6 ± 3.1
Rutin	0.02 ± 0.00 [a]	0.40 ± 0.03 [b]	0.4 ± 0.0
Isorhamnetin	0.04 ± 0.00	nd	0.7 ± 0.0
Kaempferol	0.02 ± 0.00	nd	0.5 ± 0.0
Myricetin	nd	0.03 ± 0.00 [b]	nd
Flava-3-Ols			
(−)-Epicatechin	0.24 ± 0.02 [a]	39.5 ± 1.6 [b]	64 ± 12
(+) Catechin	6.3 ± 0.2 [a]	38.4 ± 1.3 [b]	327 ± 19
Procyanidins			
Procyanidin B1	0.82 ± 0.11 [a]	23.9 ± 0.9 [b]	19.0 ± 1.5
Procyanidin B2	0.15 ± 0.00 [a]	2.0 ± 0.1 [b]	10.1 ± 1.0
Stilbenes			
Resveratrol	0.01 ± 0.00 [a]	± 0.00 [b]	0.2 ± 0.0

* Data are presented as mean ± Standard Deviation (SD). Data are the mean of three replications. Significant differences ($p < 0.05$) are shown by [a,b] letters in the same line; nd, not detected.

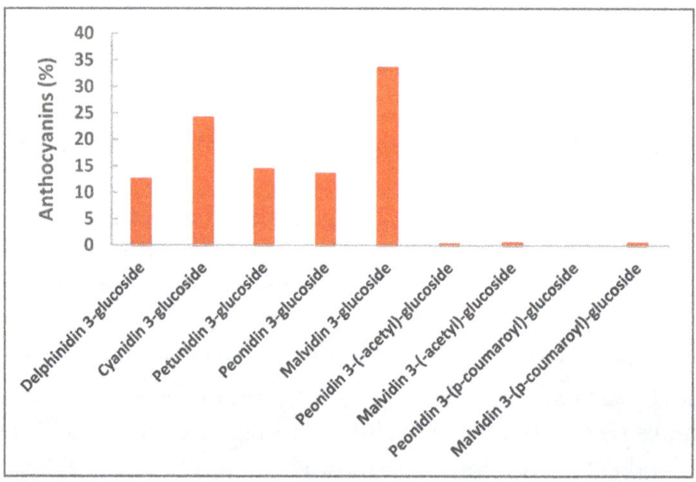

Figure 3. Composition (%) of anthocyanins in the juice at the end of processing.

3.2. *Antioxidat Activity and Effect on White Wine*

The juice and powder (spray-drying (S-D) + arabic gum (AG)) were assayed for total polyphenols by Folin–Ciocalteu method and antioxidant activity (DPPH-test) (Table 2).

Table 2. Total polyphenols content (TP) and antioxidant capacity of the juice and powder obtained by spray-drying (S-D) with the addition of arabic gum (AG).

Sample	Total Polyphenols * (mg CATeq/L of Juice or g of Powder)	Antioxidant Capacity * (μmoL TEAC/L of Juice or g of Powder)
Juice	1214.6 ± 37.8	5345.8 ± 119.3
S-D + AG	2.3 ± 0.01	24.4 ± 0.00

* Data are presented as means ± SD. Data are the mean of three replications. TEAC: Trolox equivalents antioxidant capacity. CATeq: (+)-catechin equivalents.

A phenolic concentration of 1214.6 mg CATeq/L was detected in the juice. Similar results were obtained by other authors [13], who assayed the phenolic content of juice extracted from unripe Merlot and Barbera grapes. Antioxidant activity (5345.8 μmoL TEAC/L) of the juice was almost five-fold more concentrated with respect to that observed by other authors [13]. Other compounds such as glutathione, an important constituent of grapes, can play a role in the anti-oxidant capacity of the juice [27].

About 2.6 g of juice (16.87 Brix) was required to produce 1 g of powder; 1 g of powder was composed of dry residue from juice (44.5%) and gum arabic (55.5%). Spray-dried sample had a total phenolic concentration of 2.3 mg CATeq/g of powder and antioxidant activity of 24.4 TEAC/g of powder. Regarding the total phenolic content, retention percentage for the spray-dried sample was about 70%, when compared with the juice.

The powder (S-D + AG) was used to enhance the antioxidant capacity of white wine. For this purpose, three white wines (Viognier, Chardonnay and Bellone) were combined with the powder, and their predisposition to browning was evaluated by POM-test, based on the absorbance increase at a wavelength of 420 nm after strong oxidation of the samples. The Viognier, Chardonnay and Bellone were unfinished wines with low sulfur dioxide concentrations and different chemical characteristics (Table 3).

Table 3. General analysis of three white wines.

Sample	PH	Total Acidity (g/L as Tartaric Acid Equivalents)	Free SO_2 (mg/L)	Total SO_2 (mg/L)
Viognier	3.35	5.5	5.0	11.0
Chardonnay	3.06	5.6	15.5	42.3
Bellone	2.90	7.1	12.8	16.6

The wines had a pH ranging from 2.90 (Bellone) to 3.35 (Viognier). Bellone was the wine with the highest acid concentration (7.1 g/L Tartaric Acid Equivalents, while Viognier showed the lowest total acidity of 5.5 g/L H_2T.

The results of the POM-test on white wines are presented in Table 4 Each sample was tested in triplicate without and with the addition of the powders at a concentration of 2 g/L.

All the wines showed an increase of absorbance ranging from 9% (Bellone) to 34% (Chardonnay) after the addition of hydrogen peroxide. The predisposition to browning with addition of the powder was lower than that observed without any addition (Table 4). Indeed, with the addition of powder, the Chardonnay, Bellone and Viognier wines showed an increase of absorbance of 5%, 0% and −15%, respectively, after the addition of hydrogen peroxide. Several factors can contribute to the oxidizability of wine, such as phenolic composition, pH and sulphur dioxide content [28]. From our data, the anti-browning capacity of the wines does not seem related to the SO_2 content, both free and total, while this important trait of white wine could mainly be due to the phenolic concentration and composition [28]. The obtained results show that the addition of unripe grape powder to a white wine may increase its antioxidant capacity and potentially replace the protective effect of sulphur dioxide.

Table 4. POM-test performed without and with the addition of powder (2 g/L). Percent increase (% OX_{H2O2}) of the absorbance at 420 nm.

Wine	Wine	Wine + Powder
	% OX_{H2O2}	**% OX_{H2O2}**
Viognier	12	−15
Chardonnay	34	5
Bellone	9	0

4. Conclusions

Results from this research demonstrated that it is possible to obtain a natural occurring antioxidant complex from unripe grapes. The extract had good polyphenol content and was composed by many bioactive compounds. For the first time, an extract from unripe grapes was used to prevent oxidation of white wine with promising results. Moreover, the extract from unripe grapes could find applications in food industry as functional ingredient. The processing technique used in this study can be easily implemented in larger scale for the effective production of the extract. In conclusion, this study confirm that it is possible to exploit an undervalued by-product, such as unripe grapes, as source of natural antioxidants through a simply technique.

Acknowledgments: This research did not receive any specific grant from funding agencies in the public, commercial, or not-for-profit sectors.

Author Contributions: Giovanna Fia and Claudio Gori conceived and designed the experiments; Ginevra Bucalossi performed the antioxidant tests and POM-tests; Francesca Borghini performed the LC-HRMS analysis; Giovanna Fia, Ginevra Bucalossi and Bruno Zanoni analyzed the data; Giovanna Fia wrote the paper.

Conflicts of Interest: The authors declare no conflict of interest.

References

1. Dani, C.; Bonatto, D.; Salvador, M.; Pereira, M.D.; Henriques, J.A.P.; Eleutherio, E. Antioxidant protection of resveratrol and catechin in Saccharomyces cerevisiae. *J. Agric. Food Chem.* **2008**, *56*, 4268–4272. [CrossRef] [PubMed]
2. Heim, K.E.; Tagliaferro, A.R.; Bobilya, D.J. Flavonoid antioxidants: Chemistry, metabolism and structure-activity relationships. *J. Nutr. Biochem.* **2002**, *13*, 572–584. [CrossRef]
3. Williams, R.J.; Spencer, J.P.E.; Rice-Evans, C. Flavonoids: Antioxidants or signalling molecules? *Free Radic. Biol. Med.* **2004**, *36*, 838–849. [CrossRef] [PubMed]
4. Tsao, R. Chemistry and biochemistry of dietary polyphenols. *Nutrients* **2010**, *2*, 1231–1246. [CrossRef] [PubMed]
5. Xia, E.; He, X.; Li, H.; Wu, S.; Li, S.; Deng, G. Biological Activities of Polyphenols from Grapes. *Int. J. Mol. Sci.* **2010**, *11*, 622–646. [CrossRef] [PubMed]
6. Dumitriu, D.; Peinado, R.A.; Peinado, J.; de Lerma, N.L. Grape pomace extract improves the in vitro and in vivo antioxidant properties of wines from sun light dried Pedro Ximnez grapes. *J. Funct. Foods* **2015**, *17*, 380–387. [CrossRef]
7. Hogan, S.; Zhang, L.; Li, J.; Zoecklein, B.; Zhou, K. Antioxidant properties and bioactive components of Norton (*Vitis aestivalis*) and Cabernet Franc (*Vitis vinifera*) wine grapes. *LWT Food Sci. Technol.* **2009**, *42*, 1269–1274. [CrossRef]
8. Muñoz, A.; Ramos, F. Componentes fenólicos de la dieta y sus propiedades biomedicinales. *Horiz. Med.* **2007**, *7*, 23–31.

9. Hollman, P.C.H.; Bijsman, M.N.C.P.; Van Gameren, Y.; Cnossen, E.P.J.; De Vries, J.H.M.; Katan, M.B. The sugar moiety is a major determinant of the absorption of dietary flavonoid glycosides in man. *Free Radic. Res.* **1999**, *31*, 569–573. [CrossRef] [PubMed]
10. Makris, D.P.; Boskou, G.; Andrikopoulos, N.K. Polyphenolic content and in vitro antioxidant characteristics of wine industry and other Agri-food solid waste extracts. *J. Food Compos. Anal.* **2007**, *20*, 125–132. [CrossRef]
11. Öncül, N.; Karabiyikli, Ş. Factors affecting the quality attributes of unripe grape functional food products. *J. Food Biochem.* **2015**, *39*, 689–695. [CrossRef]
12. Kontoudakis, N.; Esteruelas, M.; Fort, F.; Canals, J.M.; Zamora, F. Use of unripe grapes harvested during cluster thinning as a method for reducing alcohol content and pH of wine. *Aust. J. Grape Wine Res.* **2011**, *17*, 230–238. [CrossRef]
13. Tinello, F.; Lante, A. Evaluation of antibrowning and antioxidant activities in unripe grapes recovered during bunch thinning. *Aust. J. Grape Wine Res.* **2017**, *23*, 33–41. [CrossRef]
14. Shojaee-Aliabadi, S.; Hosseini, S.M.; Tiwari, B.; Hashemi, M.; Fadavi, G.; Khaksar, R. Polyphenols content and antioxidant activity of Ghure (unripe grape) marc extract: Influence of extraction time, temperature and solvent type. *Int. J. Food Sci. Technol.* **2013**, *48*, 412–418. [CrossRef]
15. Mattivi, F.; Guzzon, R.; Vrhovsek, U.; Stefanini, M.; Velasco, R. Metabolite profiling of grapes: Flavonols and anthocyanins. *J. Agric. Food Chem.* **2006**, *54*, 7692–7702. [CrossRef] [PubMed]
16. Coombe, B.G. Adoption of a system for identifying grapevine growth stages. *Aust. J. Grape Wine Res.* **1995**, *1*, 104–110. [CrossRef]
17. Gori, C.; Menichetti, S.; Fia, G. Multi-Functional Oenological Machine and Use in the Oenological Production Chain. European Patent 2,957,627, 22 June 2014.
18. International Organisation of the Vine and Wine (OIV). International Organisation of the Vine and Wine Website. 2014. Available online: http://www.oiv.int/oiv/info/frmethodesanalyses (accessed on 15 June 2015).
19. Singleton, V.L.; Rossi, J.A. Colorimetry of total phenolics with phosphomolybdic-phosphotungstic acid reagents. *Am. J. Enol. Vitic.* **1965**, *16*, 144–158.
20. Di Stefano, R.; Cravero, M.C.; Gentilini, N. Metodi per lo studio dei polifenoli dei vini. *Enotecnico* **1989**, *25*, 83–89.
21. Brand-Williams, W.; Cuvelier, M.E.; Berset, C. Use of a free radical method to evaluate antioxidant activity. *LWT Food Sci. Technol.* **1995**, *28*, 25–30. [CrossRef]
22. Muller-Spath, H. Der POM-test. *Deutsche Weinbau* **1992**, *23*, 1099–1100.
23. Camuzzo, P.; Battistutta, F.; Vendrane, M.; Páez, M.S.; Luisi, G.; Zironi, R. Antioxidant properties of different products and additives in white wine. *Food Chem.* **2015**, *168*, 107–114. [CrossRef] [PubMed]
24. Gambacorta, G.; Antonacci, D.; Pati, S.; La Gatta, M.; Faccia, M.; Coletta, A.; La Notte, E. Influence of winemaking technologies on phenolic composition of Italian red wines. *Eur. Food Res. Technol.* **2011**, *233*, 1057–1066. [CrossRef]
25. Zanoni, B.; Siliani, S.; Canuti, V.; Rosi, I.; Bertuccioli, M. A kinetic study on extraction and transformation phenomena of phenolic compounds during red wine fermentation. *Int. J. Food Sci. Technol.* **2010**, *45*, 2080–2088. [CrossRef]
26. Singleton, V.L.; Salgues, M.; Zaya, J.; Trousdale, E. Caftaric acid disappearance and conversion to products of enzymic oxidation in grape must and wine. *Am. J. Enol. Vitic.* **1985**, *36*, 50–56.
27. Kritzinger, E.C.; Bauer, F.F.; Du Toit, W.J. Role of glutathione in winemaking: A review. *J. Agric. Food Chem.* **2013**, *61*, 269–277. [CrossRef] [PubMed]
28. Fernández-Zurbano, P.; Ferreira, V.; Peña, C.; Escudero, A.; Serrano, F.; Cacho, J. Prediction of oxidative browning in white wines as a function of their chemical composition. *J. Agric. Food Chem.* **1995**, *43*, 2813–2817. [CrossRef]

11

Biological Implications of Differential Expression of Mitochondrial-Shaping Proteins in Parkinson's Disease

Sara Rocha [1,2,†], Ana Freitas [1,3,4,†], Sofia C. Guimaraes [1,3], Rui Vitorino [5,6], Miguel Aroso [1,3] and Maria Gomez-Lazaro [1,3,*]

1 i3S—Instituto de Investigação e Inovação em Saúde, Universidade do Porto, 4200-135 Porto, Portugal; sara.rocha@i3s.up.pt (S.R.); anafreitas@ineb.up.pt (A.F.); sofia.guimaraes@i3s.up.pt (S.C.G.); miguel.aroso@i3s.up.pt (M.A.)
2 IBMC—Instituto de Biologia Molecular e Celular, Universidade do Porto, 4200-135 Porto, Portugal
3 INEB—Instituto de Engenharia Biomédica, Universidade do Porto, 4200-135 Porto, Portugal
4 FMUP—Faculdade de Medicina da Universidade do Porto, 4200-319 Porto, Portugal
5 iBiMED, Department of Medical Sciences, University of Aveiro, 3810-193 Aveiro, Portugal; rvitorino@ua.pt
6 Unidade de Investigação Cardiovascular, Departamento de Cirurgia e Fisiologia, Universidade do Porto, 4200-319 Porto, Portugal
* Correspondence: maria.glazaro@ineb.up.pt
† These authors contributed equally to this work.

Abstract: It has long been accepted that mitochondrial function and morphology is affected in Parkinson's disease, and that mitochondrial function can be directly related to its morphology. So far, mitochondrial morphological alterations studies, in the context of this neurodegenerative disease, have been performed through microscopic methodologies. The goal of the present work is to address if the modifications in the mitochondrial-shaping proteins occurring in this disorder have implications in other cellular pathways, which might constitute important pathways for the disease progression. To do so, we conducted a novel approach through a thorough exploration of the available proteomics-based studies in the context of Parkinson's disease. The analysis provided insight into the altered biological pathways affected by changes in the expression of mitochondrial-shaping proteins via different bioinformatic tools. Unexpectedly, we observed that the mitochondrial-shaping proteins altered in the context of Parkinson's disease are, in the vast majority, related to the organization of the mitochondrial cristae. Conversely, in the studies that have resorted to microscopy-based techniques, the most widely reported alteration in the context of this disorder is mitochondria fragmentation. Cristae membrane organization is pivotal for mitochondrial ATP production, and changes in their morphology have a direct impact on the organization and function of the oxidative phosphorylation (OXPHOS) complexes. To understand which biological processes are affected by the alteration of these proteins we analyzed the binding partners of the mitochondrial-shaping proteins that were found altered in Parkinson's disease. We showed that the binding partners fall into seven different cellular components, which include mitochondria, proteasome, and endoplasmic reticulum (ER), amongst others. It is noteworthy that, by evaluating the biological process in which these modified proteins are involved, we showed that they are related to the production and metabolism of ATP, immune response, cytoskeleton alteration, and oxidative stress, amongst others. In summary, with our bioinformatics approach using the data on the modified proteins in Parkinson's disease patients, we were able to relate the alteration of mitochondrial-shaping proteins to modifications of crucial cellular pathways affected in this disease.

Keywords: Parkinson's disease; proteomics; bioinformatics; biological processes; mitochondria

1. Introduction

Mitochondria are pivotal organelles for several cellular functions, namely, the production of ATP through oxidative phosphorylation, the regulation of the Krebs cycle, fatty acid metabolism, gluconeogenesis, heme-synthesis, calcium and redox homeostasis, cell signaling, and the amplification of apoptosis [1]. They are highly dynamic organelles, as they can change their shape in response to cellular stimuli by fusion and fission processes and by their movement along the cellular cytoskeleton [2]. Alterations of mitochondria morphology can significantly influence several functions of the cellular metabolism, not only related to energy production but also in communication with the cytosol and the import and export of proteins, lipids, solutes, and metabolites or even the cytosol protection from possible harmful effects of certain mitochondrial components [3]. Mitochondria dynamic processes are of utmost importance for the mitochondrial growth rate, their redistribution within the cell, and for the maintenance of healthy mitochondria and proper functioning hence their alterations are frequently associated with different pathological conditions [4].

Parkinson's disease is a highly debilitating condition, being a common neurodegenerative disease, and more than 10 million people worldwide are affected by this disease [5]. Currently, its etiology is not fully unraveled; however, evidences point to the importance of mitochondria in its pathobiology. Clinical features include mainly motor-based dysfunctions such as bradykinesia, resting tremor, or cogwheel rigidity [6]. Those features are a consequence of the loss of dopaminergic (DA) neurons in the substantia nigra (SN). The association between mitochondrial dysfunction and the pathobiology of Parkinson's disease was first described in 1989. By using post mortem tissue from human patients, a functional deficiency was found on the mitochondrial Complex I from the respiratory chain [7,8]. Accumulating evidence shows the occurrence of mitochondria fragmentation in the context of different models of the pathology. Furthermore, alteration of the expression levels of different proteins linked to Parkinson´s disease (e.g., PINK1, Parkin, or DJ-1) are known to induce mitochondria fragmentation in DA neurons [9,10]. Recently, it was observed that alterations of the mitochondrial morphology can be related to their functional state and new tools were consequently designed to analyze mitochondrial shape and predict mitochondrial function [11].

Interestingly, several hypotheses for the specific loss of the DA neurons from the SN are also related to the vulnerability associated with the mitochondria of these neurons [12]. It has been suggested that DA neurons from the SN are more susceptible to oxidative stress due to the production of reactive oxygen species (ROS) during dopamine degradation, and these neurons present fewer amounts of antioxidants than other DA neurons within the brain [12]. They have very long axons in which mitochondria travel and also fragment to be able to accommodate within the synaptic terminals. Besides, it is known that DA neurons from the SN present lower mitochondria mass in the soma than in the dendrites, indicating that alterations of either fragmentation or movement along the cytoskeleton might have a bigger impact on these neurons [12]. Additionally, most of the substances that are used to model the disease directly target the mitochondria and induce the specific degeneration of the DA neurons.

In this study we made a thorough literature search to identify the mitochondrial proteins involved in controlling mitochondrial morphology that are differentially expressed in Parkinson's disease. The altered biological pathways that might be affected by changes in the expression of these mitochondrial-shaping proteins in Parkinson's disease were identified and analyzed. Considerations were made to better understand the biological mechanisms involved in this debilitating disease.

2. Methods

Literature Search

For the compilation of the mitochondrial proteins involved in controlling mitochondrial morphology (Table 1), two independent users performed a search on PubMed, Science Direct, and Google up to 7 July 2017 using the following keywords in separate queries: "mitochondrial morphology", "mitochondrial shape", "mitochondrial organization", "mitochondrial fusion", "mitochondrial fission", and "mitochondrial dynamics". Only *Homo sapiens* proteins were gathered. The corresponding gene name and synonyms were collected in Table 1 by searching at the Universal Protein Resource (UniProt) databases [13].

Table 1. List of mitochondrial-shaping proteins.

Gene Name (with Synonyms)	Protein Name	Function	Localization	Shaping Function	References
APOO, FAM121B, MIC23, MIC26, My025, UNQ1866/PRO4302	MICOS Complex subunit MIC26 (Apolipoprotein O) (MICOS Complex subunit MIC23) (Protein FAM121B)	Component of the MICOS Complex, a large protein Complex of the inner mitochondrial membrane that plays crucial roles in the maintenance of crista junctions, inner membrane architecture, and formation of contact sites to the outer membrane	IMM	Cristae shape	[14–16]
APOOL, CXorf33, FAM121A, MIC27, UNQ8193/PRO23204	MICOS Complex subunit MIC27 (Apolipoprotein O-like) (Protein FAM121A)	Component of the MICOS Complex, a large protein Complex of the inner mitochondrial membrane that plays crucial roles in the maintenance of crista junctions, inner membrane architecture, and formation of contact sites to the outer membrane	IMM	Cristae shape	[14,15,17,18]
ATP5A1, ATP5B, ATP5C1, ATP5D, ATP5E, ATP5F1, ATP5G1, ATP5G2, ATP5G3, ATP5H, ATP5I, ATP5J, ATP5J2, ATP5L, ATP5O, MT-ATP6, MT-ATP8	ATP synthase	ATP production	IMM	Cristae shape	[3,15,19]
ATPIF1, ATPI	ATPase inhibitor, mitochondrial (Inhibitor of F(1)F(o)-ATPase) (IF(1)) (IF1)	ATP production regulation	Matrix	Cristae shape	[3,20]
BAK1, BAK, BCL2L7, CDN1	Bcl-2 homologous antagonist/killer (Apoptosis regulator BAK)	Promotes apoptosis	OMM	OMM permeabilization	[3,21]
BAX, BCL2L4	Apoptosis regulator BAX	Accelerates apoptosis	OMM	OMM permeabilization	[3,19,21,22]
BCL2	Apoptosis regulator Bcl-2	Promotes cell survival	OMM	OMM permeabilization	[3,22]
BCL2A1, BCL2L5, BFL1, GRS, HBPA1	Bcl-2-related protein A1 (A1-A) (Hemopoietic-specific early response protein) (Protein BFL-1)	Promotes cell survival	OMM	Not clear function	[23,24]
BCL2L11, BIM	Bcl-2-like protein 11 (Bcl2-L-11) (Bcl2-interacting mediator of cell death)	Induces apoptosis and anoikis	IMM	Cristae remodeling	[25,26]
BID	BH3-interacting domain death agonist	The major proteolytic product p15 BID allows the release of cytochrome c	IMM	Cristae remodeling	[25,27]
BIK, NBK	Bcl-2-interacting killer (Apoptosis inducer NBK) (BIP1) (BP4)	Promotes apoptosis	IMM	Cristae remodeling	[25,28]
CHCHD3, MIC19, MINOS3	MICOS Complex subunit MIC19 (Coiled-coil-helix-coiled-coil-helix domain-containing protein 3)	Component of the MICOS Complex, a large protein Complex of the inner mitochondrial membrane that plays crucial roles in the maintenance of crista junctions, inner membrane architecture, and formation of contact sites to the outer membrane	IMM	Cristae shape	[14,16,18]

Table 1. *Cont.*

Gene Name (with Synonyms)	Protein Name	Function	Localization	Shaping Function	References
COA3, CCDC56, MITRAC12, HSPC009	Cytochrome c oxidase assembly factor 3 homolog, mitochondrial (Coiled-coil domain-containing protein 56) (Mitochondrial translation regulation assembly intermediate of cytochrome c oxidase protein of 12 kDa)	Core component of the MITRAC (mitochondrial translation regulation assembly intermediate of cytochrome c oxidase) Complex, which regulates cytochrome c oxidase assembly.	IMM	Cytochrome c oxidase	[29,30]
COX4I1, COX4I2, COX5A, COX5B, COX6A1, COX6A2, COX6B1, COX6B2, COX6C, COX7A1, COX7A2, COX7B, COX7B2, COX7C, COX8A, COX8C, MT-CO1, MT-CO2, MT-CO3	Mitochondrial Complex IV: cytochrome c oxidase subunits	ATP production	IMM	Cristae shape	[18]
CYC1, MT-CYB, UQCR10, UQCR11, UQCRB, UQCRC1, UQCRC2, UQCRFS1, UQCRH, UQCRQ	Mitochondrial Complex III: ubiquinol-cytochrome c reductase Complex subunits (UQCR)	ATP production	IMM	Cristae shape	[18]
DNAJC19, TIM14, TIMM14	Mitochondrial import inner membrane translocase subunit TIM14 (DnaJ homolog subfamily C member 19)	Probable component of the PAM Complex, a Complex required for the translocation of transit peptide-containing proteins from the inner membrane into the mitochondrial matrix in an ATP-dependent manner	IMM	Crista shape	[15,31,32]
DNM1L, DLP1, DRP1	Dynamin-1-like protein (EC 3.6.5.5) (Dnm1p/Vps1p-like protein) (DVLP) (Dynamin family member proline-rich carboxyl-terminal domain less) (Dymple) (Dynamin-like protein) (Dynamin-like protein 4) (Dynamin-like protein IV) (HdynIV) (Dynamin-related protein 1)	Mitochondrial and peroxisome division	OMM and cytosol	Fission	[3,18,22]
DNM2, DYN2	Dynamin-2 (EC 3.6.5.5)	Microtubule-associated force-producing protein involved in producing microtubule bundles and able to bind and hydrolyze GTP	Cytosol	Fission	[4,33]
FIS1, TTC11, CGI-135	Mitochondrial fission 1 protein (FIS1 homolog) (hFis1) (Tetratricopeptide repeat protein 11) (TPR repeat protein 11)	Mitochondrial fragmentation	OMM	Fission	[3,19,22]
FUNDC1	FUN14 domain-containing protein 1FUN14 domain-containing protein 1	Mitophagy	OMM	Fission	[29,34–36]
GDAP1	Ganglioside-induced differentiation-associated protein 1	Mitochondrial fission	OMM	Fission	[1,19,22]
hfzo1	Mitochondrial transmembrane GTPase Fzo-1	FUNDC1 mediates highly selective mitochondrial clearance under hypoxic conditions without impacting general autophagy	OMM	Fusion	[19]

Table 1. *Cont.*

Gene Name (with Synonyms)	Protein Name	Function	Localization	Shaping Function	References
IMMT, HMP, MIC60, MINOS2, PIG4, PIG52	MICOS Complex subunit MIC60(Cell proliferation-inducing gene 4/52 protein) (Inner mitochondrial membrane protein) (Mitofilin) (p87/89)	Component of the MICOS Complex, a large protein Complex of the inner mitochondrial membrane that plays crucial roles in the maintenance of crista junctions, inner membrane architecture, and formation of contact sites to the outer membrane	IMM	Cristae shape	[15,16,18,19,37]
INF2, C14orf151, C14orf173	Inverted formin-2 (HBEBP2-binding protein C)	Severs actin filaments and accelerates their polymerization and depolymerization	Cytosol	Mitochondrial constriction	[29,38]
LETM1	Mitochondrial proton/calcium exchanger protein (Leucine zipper-EF-hand-containing transmembrane protein 1)	Mitochondrial proton/calcium antiporter that mediates proton-dependent calcium efflux from mitochondria	IMM	Fission	[1,22,39]
MARCH5, RNF153	E3 ubiquitin-protein ligase MARCH5 (EC 2.3.2.27) (Membrane-associated RING finger protein 5) (Membrane-associated RING-CH protein V) (MARCH-V) (Mitochondrial ubiquitin ligase) (MITOL) (RING finger protein 153) (RING-type E3 ubiquitin transferase MARCH5)	Membrane-bound E3 ligase for mitochondrial morphology control	OMM	Fission	[1,19]
MAVS, IPS1, KIAA1271, VISA	Mitochondrial antiviral-signaling protein (MAVS) (CARD adapter inducing interferon beta) (Cardif) (Interferon beta promoter stimulator protein 1) (IPS-1) (Putative NF-kappa-B-activating protein 031N) (Virus-induced-signaling adapter) (VISA)	Required for innate immune response against viruses	OMM	Fusion	[22,40]
MCL1, BCL2L3	Induced myeloid leukemia cell differentiation protein Mcl-1 (Bcl-2-like protein 3) (Bcl2-L-3) (Bcl-2-related protein EAT/mcl1) (mcl1/EAT)	Regulation of apoptosis	IMM and OMM	Cristae shape (IMM isoform)	[18,29,41,42]
MFF, C2orf33, AD030, AD033, GL004	Mitochondrial Fission Factor	Mitochondrial and peroxisome division	OMM	Fission	[3,19]
MFN1	Mitofusin-1 (EC 3.6.5.-) (Fzo homolog) (Transmembrane GTPase MFN1)	Mitochondrial fusion	OMM	Fusion	[18,22,43]
MFN2, CPRP1, KIAA0214	Mitofusin-2 (EC 3.6.5.-) (Transmembrane GTPase MFN2)	Regulates mitochondrial clustering and fusion	OMM	Fusion	[18,22,43]
MIC13, C19orf70, QIL1	MICOS Complex subunit MIC13 (Protein P117)	Component of the MICOS Complex, a large protein Complex of the inner mitochondrial membrane that plays crucial roles in the maintenance of crista junctions, inner membrane architecture, and formation of contact sites to the outer membrane	IMM	Cristae shape	[15,18]
MIEF1, MID51, SMCR7L	Mid51/Mief, mitochondrial dynamics proteins of 51	Component of the MICOS Complex, a large protein Complex of the inner mitochondrial membrane that plays crucial roles in the maintenance of crista junctions, inner membrane architecture, and formation of contact sites to the outer membrane	OMM	Fission	[3,19]

Table 1. *Cont.*

Gene Name (with Synonyms)	Protein Name	Function	Localization	Shaping Function	References
MIEF2, MID49, SMCR7	Mitochondrial dynamics protein MID49 (Mitochondrial dynamics protein of 49 kDa) (Mitochondrial elongation factor 2) (Smith-Magenis syndrome chromosomal region candidate gene 7 protein)	Component of the MICOS Complex, a large protein Complex of the inner mitochondrial membrane that plays crucial roles in the maintenance of crista junctions, inner membrane architecture, and formation of contact sites to the outer membrane	OMM	Fission	[3,19]
MIGA1, FAM73A	Mitoguardin 1 (Protein FAM73A)	Regulator of mitochondrial fusion	OMM	Fusion	[4,44]
MIGA2, C9orf54, FAM73B, PSEC0112	Mitoguardin 2 (Protein FAM73B)	Regulator of mitochondrial fusion	OMM	Fusion	[4,44]
MINOS1, C1orf151, MIC10	MICOS Complex subunit MIC10 (Inner mitochondrial membrane organizing system protein 1)	Maintenance of cristae junctions, inner membrane architecture, and formation of contact sites to the outer membrane	IMM	Cristae shape	[15,18]
MTFP1, MTP18, HSPC242, My022	Mitochondrial fission process protein 1(Mitochondrial 18 kDa protein) (MTP18)	Involved in the mitochondrial division probably by regulating membrane fission	IMM	Fission	[1,22,45]
MUL1, C1orf166, GIDE, MAPL, MULAN, RNF218	Mitochondrial ubiquitin ligase activator of NFKB 1 (EC 2.3.2.27) (E3 SUMO-protein ligase MUL1) (E3 ubiquitin-protein ligase MUL1) (Growth inhibition and death E3 ligase) (Mitochondrial-anchored protein ligase) (MAPL) (Putative NF-kappa-B-activating protein 266) (RING finger protein 218) (RING-type E3 ubiquitin transferase NFKB 1)	Ubiquitin ligase activity	OMM	Fusion	[19,29]
NFE2L2, NRF2	Nuclear factor erythroid 2-related factor 2 (NF-E2-related factor 2) (NFE2-related factor 2) (HEBP1) (Nuclear factor, erythroid derived 2, like 2)	Transcription activator that binds to antioxidant response (ARE) elements in the promoter regions of target genes	Cytosol	Fusion	[29,46,47]
NRF1	Nuclear respiratory factor 1 (NRF-1) (Alpha palindromic-binding protein) (Alpha-pal)	Transcription factor implicated in the control of nuclear genes required for respiration, heme biosynthesis, and mitochondrial DNA transcription and replication	Cytosol	Fission	[29,46,48,49]
OMA1, MPRP1	Metalloendopeptidase OMA1, mitochondrial (EC 3.4.24.-) (Metalloprotease-related protein 1) (MPRP-1) (Overlapping with the m-AAA protease 1 homolog)	Metalloprotease that is part of the quality control system in the inner membrane of mitochondria	IMM	Fusion	[1,19]
OPA1, KIAA0567	Dynamin-like 120 kDa protein, mitochondrial (EC 3.6.5.5) (Optic atrophy protein 1) (Cleaved into: Dynamin-like 120 kDa protein, form S1)	Opa1 mediates dynamics changes in cristae morphology that correlate with the metabolic state of the organelle	IMM	Cristae shape, fusion	[1,3,15,18,22,50]
PARL, PSARL, PRO2207	Presenilins-associated rhomboid-like protein, mitochondrial (EC 3.4.21.105) (Mitochondrial intramembrane cleaving protease PARL) (Cleaved into: P-beta (Pbeta))	Required for the control of apoptosis	IMM	Mitochondrial morphology	[1,51]

Table 1. *Cont.*

Gene Name (with Synonyms)	Protein Name	Function	Localization	Shaping Function	References
PGAM5	Serine/threonine-protein phosphatase PGAM5, mitochondrial (EC 3.1.3.16) (Bcl-XL-binding protein v68) (Phosphoglycerate mutase family member 5)	Displays phosphatase activity for serine/threonine residues, as well as dephosphorylates and activates MAP3K5 kinase	OMM	Fission	[1,29,52]
PHB	Prohibitin	Prohibitin inhibits DNA synthesis; it has a role in regulating proliferation	IMM	Cristae shape	[1,15,18,31,53]
PHB2, BAP, REA	Prohibitin-2 (B-cell receptor-associated protein BAP37) (D-prohibitin) (Repressor of estrogen receptor activity)	Acts as a mediator of transcriptional repression by nuclear hormone receptors via the recruitment of histone deacetylases (by similarity); functions as an estrogen receptor (ER)-selective coregulator that potentiates the inhibitory activities of antiestrogens and represses the activity of estrogens	IMM	Cristae shape	[1,15,18]
PINK1	Serine/threonine-protein kinase PINK1, mitochondrial (EC 2.7.11.1) (BRPK) (PTEN-induced putative kinase protein 1)	Protects against mitochondrial dysfunction during cellular stress by phosphorylating mitochondrial proteins	OMM	Fission	[1,54]
PLD6	Mitochondrial cardiolipin hydrolase (EC 3.1.-.-) (Choline phosphatase 6) (Mitochondrial phospholipase) (MitoPLD) (Phosphatidylcholine-hydrolyzing phospholipase D6) (Phospholipase D6) (PLD 6) (Protein zucchini homolog)	Proposed to act as a cardiolipin hydrolase to generate phosphatidic acid at the mitochondrial surface	OMM	Fusion	[4,19,22,45]
PPARGC1A, LEM6, PGC1, PGC1A, PPARGC1	Peroxisome proliferator-activated receptor gamma coactivator 1-alpha (PGC-1-alpha) (PPAR-gamma coactivator 1-alpha) (PPARGC-1-alpha) (Ligand effect modulator 6)	Transcriptional coactivator for steroid receptors and nuclear receptors	Cytoplasm and nucleus	Fusion	[29,49,55]
PPARGC1B, PERC, PGC1, PGC1B, PPARGC1	Peroxisome proliferator-activated receptor gamma coactivator 1-beta (PGC-1-beta) (PPAR-gamma coactivator 1-beta) (PPARGC-1-beta) (PGC-1-related estrogen receptor alpha coactivator)	Plays the role of stimulator of transcription factors and nuclear receptors activities	Nucleus	Fusion	[29,55,56]
PRELID1, PRELI, CGI-106, SBBI12	PRELI domain-containing protein 1, mitochondrial (25 kDa protein of relevant evolutionary and lymphoid interest) (Px19-like protein)	Involved in the modulation of the mitochondrial apoptotic pathway by ensuring the accumulation of cardiolipin (CL) in mitochondrial membranes	Intermembrane space	Fission	[57,58]
PRKN, PARK2	E3 ubiquitin-protein ligase parkin (Parkin) (EC 2.3.2.-) (Parkin RBR E3 ubiquitin-protein ligase) (Parkinson juvenile disease protein 2) (Parkinson disease protein 2)	Functions within a multiprotein E3 ubiquitin ligase Complex, catalyzing the covalent attachment of ubiquitin moieties onto substrate proteins	Cytosol and mitochondria	Fission	[1,54,59,60]
ROMO1, C20orf52	Reactive oxygen species modulator 1(ROS modulator 1) (Epididymis tissue protein Li 175) (Glyrichin) (Mitochondrial targeting GxxxG motif protein) (MTGM) (Protein MGR2 homolog)	Induces the production of reactive oxygen species (ROS), which are necessary for cell proliferation	IMM	Fusion	[29,61]

Table 1. *Cont.*

Gene Name (with Synonyms)	Protein Name	Function	Localization	Shaping Function	References
SAMM50, SAM50, CGI-51, TRG3	Sorting and assembly machinery component 50 homolog (Transformation-related gen 3 protein) (TRG-3)	Plays a crucial role in the maintenance of the structure of mitochondrial cristae and the proper assembly of the mitochondrial respiratory chain Complexes	OMM	Cristae shape	[18]
SH3GLB1, KIAA0491, CGI-61	Endophilin-B1 (Bax-interacting factor 1) (Bif-1) (SH3 domain-containing GRB2-like protein B1)	Outer mitochondrial dynamics	OMM	OMM permeability	[1,22,62]
SH3GLB2, KIAA1848, PP578	Endophilin-B2 (SH3 domain-containing GRB2-like protein B2)	Mitophagy	Cytosol	Fission	[63]
SLC25A10, DIC	Mitochondrial dicarboxylate carrier (Solute carrier family 25 member 10)	Involved in the translocation of malonate, malate, and succinate in exchange for phosphate, sulfate, sulfite, or thiosulfate across the inner mitochondrial membrane	IMM	Cristae shape	[18,50]
SLC25A11, SLC20A4	Mitochondrial 2-oxoglutarate/malate carrier protein (OGCP) (Solute carrier family 25 member 11)	Catalyzes the transport of 2-oxoglutarate across the inner mitochondrial membrane in an electroneutral exchange for malate or other dicarboxylic acids, and plays an important role in several metabolic processes, including the malate-aspartate shuttle, the oxoglutarate/isocitrate shuttle, in gluconeogenesis from lactate, and in nitrogen metabolism	IMM	Cristae shape	[18,50]
SLC25A12, ARALAR1	Calcium-binding mitochondrial carrier protein Aralar1 (Mitochondrial aspartate glutamate carrier 1) (Solute carrier family 25 member 12)	Catalyzes the calcium-dependent exchange of cytoplasmic glutamate with mitochondrial aspartate across the inner mitochondrial membrane; may have a function in the urea cycle	IMM	Cristae shape	[18,50]
SLC25A13, ARALAR2	Calcium-binding mitochondrial carrier protein Aralar2 (Citrin) (Mitochondrial aspartate glutamate carrier 2) (Solute carrier family 25 member 13)	Catalyzes the calcium-dependent exchange of cytoplasmic glutamate with mitochondrial aspartate across the inner mitochondrial membrane; may have a function in the urea cycle	IMM	Cristae shape	[18,50]
SLC25A38	Solute carrier family 25 member 38, Appoptosin	Mitochondrial import machinery	IMM	Fusion	[29,64]
SMAD2, MADH2, MADR2	Mothers against decapentaplegic homolog 2 (MAD homolog 2) (Mothers against DPP homolog 2) (JV18-1) (Mad-related protein 2) (hMAD-2) (SMAD family member 2) (SMAD 2) (Smad2) (hSMAD2)	Receptor-regulated SMAD (R-SMAD) that is an intracellular signal transducer and transcriptional modulator activated by TGF-beta (transforming growth factor) and activin type 1 receptor kinases	Cytosol	Fusion	[29,65]
SPG7, CAR, CMAR, PGN	Paraplegin (EC 3.4.24.-) (Cell matrix adhesion regulator) (Spastic paraplegia 7 protein)	ATP-dependent zinc metalloprotease	IMM	Cristae shape	[18]
SPG7, CAR, CMAR, PGN	Paraplegin (EC 3.4.24.-) (Cell matrix adhesion regulator) (Spastic paraplegia 7 protein)	ATP-dependent zinc metalloprotease	IMM	Fusion	[1,22,51]

Table 1. *Cont.*

Gene Name (with Synonyms)	Protein Name	Function	Localization	Shaping Function	References
STOML2, SLP2, HSPC108	Stomatin-like protein 2, mitochondrial(SLP-2) (EPB72-like protein 2) (Paraprotein target 7) (Paratarg-7)	Mitochondrial protein that probably regulates the biogenesis and the activity of mitochondria; stimulates cardiolipin biosynthesis, binds cardiolipin-enriched membranes where it recruits and stabilizes some proteins including prohibitin, and may therefore act in the organization of functional microdomains in mitochondrial membranes	IMM	Cristae shape/Stabilize IM structure	[15,18]
SYNJ2, KIAA0348	Synaptojanin-2(EC 3.1.3.36) (Synaptic inositol 1,4,5-trisphosphate 5-phosphatase 2)	Membrane trafficking and signaling transduction	Cytosol	Mitochondrial aggregation	[66]
TAZ, EFE2, G4.5	Tafazzin (Protein G4.5)	Some isoforms may be involved in cardiolipin (CL) metabolism	OMM	Cristae shape	[15,16,67,68]
TFAM, TCF6, TCF6L2	Transcription factor A, mitochondrial (mtTFA) (Mitochondrial transcription factor 1) (MtTF1) (Transcription factor 6) (TCF-6) (Transcription factor 6-like 2)	Binds to the mitochondrial light strand promoter and functions in mitochondrial transcription regulation	Matrix	Mitochondrial biogenesis	[29,46]
TRAK1, KIAA1042, OIP106	Trafficking kinesin-binding protein 1 (106 kDa O-GlcNAc transferase-interacting protein)	Organelle trafficking	OMM and cytosol	Fusion	[1,4,19]
TRAK2, ALS2CR3, KIAA0549	Trafficking kinesin-binding protein 2 (Amyotrophic lateral sclerosis 2 chromosomal region candidate gene 3 protein)	Organelle trafficking	OMM and cytosol	Fusion	[1,4,19]
UQCC3, C11orf83, UNQ655/PRO1286	Ubiquinol-cytochrome-c reductase Complex assembly factor 3	Required for the assembly of the ubiquinol-cytochrome c reductase Complex (mitochondrial respiratory chain Complex III or cytochrome b-c1 Complex), mediating cytochrome b recruitment and probably stabilization within the Complex	IMM	Cristae shape	[18,69]
VAT1	Synaptic vesicle membrane protein VAT-1 homolog (EC 1.-.-.-) (Mitofusin-binding protein) (Protein MIB)	Negatively regulates mitochondrial fusion	OMM	Fusion	[1,19,22,70]
YME1L1, FTSH1, YME1L, UNQ1868/PRO4304	ATP-dependent zinc metalloprotease YME1L1 (EC 3.4.24.-) (ATP-dependent metalloprotease FtsH1) (Meg-4) (Presenilin-associated metalloprotease) (PAMP) (YME1-like protein 1)	Putative ATP-dependent protease; plays a role in mitochondrial organization and mitochondrial protein metabolism, including the degradation of PRELID1 and OPA1	IMM	Cristae shape	[19,58]

To collect the information from proteomic-based studies of the differentially expressed proteins in the context of Parkinson's disease, a search on PubMed and Web of Science (version v5.24) (up to 28 July 2017) was performed using the following keywords: "Parkinson's disease mass spectrometry", "Parkinson's disease proteomics". Studies working with samples from human patients and cellular models (from cell lines of human origin) were used to build the Supplementary Table S1. Three experienced reviewers selected the list of articles relevant for data extraction, taking into consideration only the studies that match the following criteria: proteomics studies, with information on differentially expressed proteins related to control conditions, employing samples either from human patients or cellular models (using cell lines of human origin).

Mitochondrial-shaping proteins were crossed with the proteins that have been found to be altered in Parkinson's disease using the respective gene names in Venny web tool (v.2.1.0) [71]. The gene name of the common proteins (proteins that are involved in mitochondrial shape and are modified in Parkinson's disease) were further used to determine the binding partners in HIPPIE web tool [72].

Network analysis was performed using the Cytoscape software (version v3.5.1) (Cytoscape Consortium, San Diego, CA, US)) with the plugins ClueGo (version v2.3.2) and Cluepedia (version v1.3.2). We used ClueGO's default settings: merge redundant groups with >50.0% overlap; the minimum GO level used was 3 and the maximum GO level was 8; statistical test used was "Enrichment/Depletion (Two-sided hypergeometric test)"; Kappa Score Threshold was 0.4; and number of genes was set at 2 with a minimum percentage at 4.0.

3. Results

3.1. *Differentially Expressed Mitochondrial Proteins Associated with Parkinson's Disease*

The interplay between mitochondria function and Parkinson's disease was first described as a deficiency of the mitochondrial respiratory chain Complex I [7,8]. Alterations of the mitochondrial shape have been related to their functional state [11] and, in the past few years, an increasing number of reports have shown alterations of mitochondrial morphology in the context of Parkinson's disease [73–76]. Mitochondrial morphology is tightly regulated by the combined action of proteins involved in fusion, fission, and movement along the cytoskeleton [3]. In this study we aimed to integrate the proteins related to mitochondria morphology with Parkinson's disease pathology. The flowchart followed in the present work is represented in Figure 1. The complete list of mitochondrial proteins that have been described to play a role in the control and regulation of mitochondrial morphology is depicted in Table 1. To integrate the alterations of the mitochondrial dynamics in the context of the pathobiology of Parkinson's disease, a literature search for proteomics-based studies in this disorder, that used samples from patients or cellular models (cell lines of human origin) (Supplementary Table S1), was performed. These proteins were then cross-referenced with the mitochondrial-shaping proteins listed in Table 1 (Figure 1).

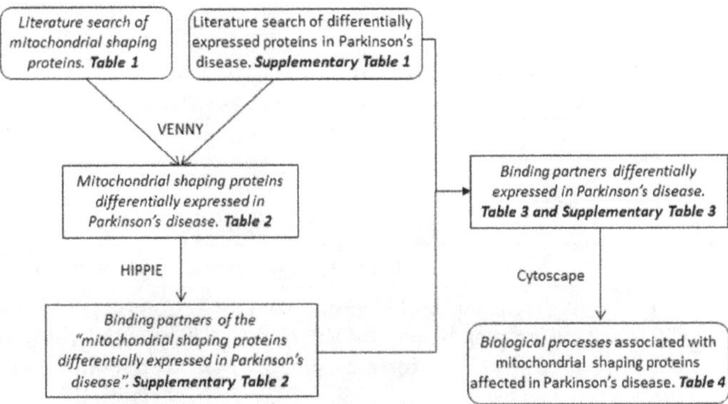

Figure 1. Flowchart showing the main steps used to identify the biological processes related to the mitochondrial-shaping proteins affected in Parkinson's disease.

From this analysis, 32 different gene names (Figure 2), related to mitochondrial morphology, were found to be modified in the context of Parkinson's disease, which correspond to 22 different proteins (Table 2). The vast majority of these mitochondrial proteins are related to the cristae morphology (82%), whereas only 9% are reported to be involved in the fusion and fission processes.

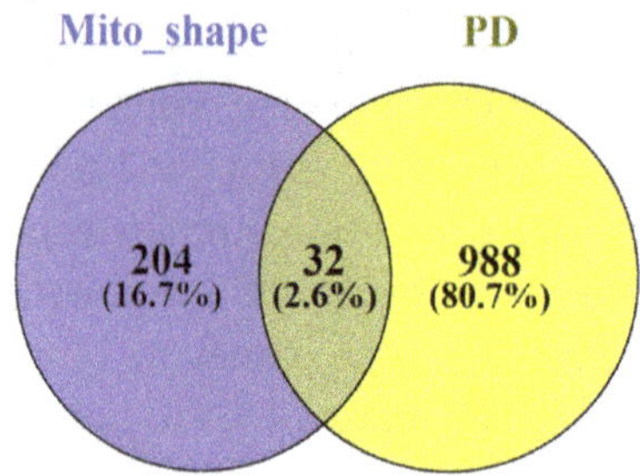

Figure 2. Venn diagram displaying the comparison of the number of the proteins found differentially expressed in the context of Parkinson's disease (Supplementary Table S1) and the mitochondrial-shaping proteins described in the literature (Table 1). The Venn diagram was constructed using the Venny 2.1 software [71]. PD—Parkinson's disease.

Table 2. List of mitochondrial-shaping proteins found to be modified in Parkinson's disease.

Gene Symbol (bioDBnet)	Name	Mito_Shaping
APOO, FAM121B, MIC23, MIC26, My025, UNQ1866/PRO4302	MICOS Complex subunit MIC26 (Apolipoprotein O) (MICOS Complex subunit MIC23) (Protein FAM121B)	Cristae shape
ATP5A1, ATP5A, ATP5AL2, ATPM	ATP synthase subunit alpha, mitochondrial	Cristae shape
ATP5B, ATPMB, ATPSB	ATP synthase subunit beta, mitochondrial	Cristae shape
ATP5H	ATP synthase subunit d	Cristae shape
ATP5I	ATP synthase subunit e, mitochondrial	Cristae shape
SAMM50, SAM50, CGI-51, TRG3	Sorting and assembly machinery component 50 homolog (Transformation-related gene 3 protein) (TRG-3)	Cristae shape
COX4I1, COX4	Cytochrome c oxidase subunit 4 isoform 1, mitochondrial (Cytochrome c oxidase polypeptide IV) (Cytochrome c oxidase subunit IV isoform 1) (COX IV-1)	Cristae shape
COX5A	Cytochrome c oxidase subunit 5A, mitochondrial (Cytochrome c oxidase polypeptide Va)	Cristae shape
COX6C	Cytochrome c oxidase subunit 6C (Cytochrome c oxidase polypeptide VIc)	Cristae shape
COX7C	Cytochrome c oxidase subunit 7C, mitochondrial (Cytochrome c oxidase polypeptide VIIc)	Cristae shape
MFN2, CPRP1, KIAA0214	Mitofusin-2 (EC 3.6.5.-) (Transmembrane GTPase MFN2)	Fusion
DNM1L	Dynamin-like protein	Fission
IMMT	Mitofilin	Cristae shape
MT-CO1	Cytochrome c oxidase polypeptide I	Cristae shape
PHB	Prohibitin	Cristae shape
PHB2	Prohibitin-2	Cristae shape
SH3GLB2	SH3-containing protein SH3GLB2	Fission
SLC25A13	Calcium-binding mitochondrial carrier protein Aralar2	Cristae shape
UQCRB, UQBP	Cytochrome b-c1 Complex subunit 7 (Complex III subunit 7) (Complex III subunit VII) (QP-C) (Ubiquinol-cytochrome c reductase Complex 14 kDa protein)	Cristae shape
UQCRFS1	Ubiquinol cytochrome c reductase iron–sulfur subunit	Cristae shape
UQCRH	Cytochrome b-c1 Complex subunit 6, mitochondrial	Cristae shape
VAT1	Synaptic vesicle membrane protein VAT-1 homolog	Fusion

Curiously, in Parkinson's disease the most reported mitochondrial morphology alterations are associated with mitochondrial fragmentation and movement impairment [74,77]. Mechanisms proposed for these alterations include: the alteration of the interaction between mitochondria and the motor complexes, and mitophagy impairment [78–83].

In our analysis, the fusion- and fission-related proteins found to be altered were Mitofusin-2 and the synaptic vesicle membrane protein VAT-1 homolog, as well as the dynamin-like protein (Drp1) and the SH3-containing protein SH3GLB2, respectively.

Although commonly accepted as a protein involved in mitochondrial fusion, the Mitofusin-2 protein also plays a key role in Ca^{2+} signaling. This function is facilitated by the physical interaction between the ER and the mitochondria for the delivery of Ca^{2+} to the mitochondrial matrix, enabling mitochondrial signaling. Hence, Mitofusin-2 is involved in both mitochondrial morphology and crosstalk between the ER and the mitochondria [84]. In the process of mitochondrial fusion both Mitofusin-1 and -2 have been reported to contribute, and although they share a common function in this process; deficiency in Mitofusion-2, but not Mitofusin-1, has been linked to neurodegenerative diseases [85]. Interestingly, the synaptic vesicle membrane protein VAT-1 homolog was found to be negatively regulate mitochondrial fusion in cooperation with Mitofusin-2 [70].

Regarding the mitochondrial fission process, in the context of Parkinson's disease, the role of Drp1 has been extensively recognized in mitochondrial fragmentation in different animal and cellular models preceding neuronal death [73,86,87]. This large GTPase is a cytosolic protein that, following mitochondrial fragmentation stimuli, translocates to the outer mitochondrial membrane where it assembles into large complexes in a spiral form, enabling the constriction of the mitochondria [19]. Endophilins might be involved in membrane shaping, e.g., Endophilin B2, although they have also been described to play a role in mitophagy by promoting the degradation of the inner mitochondrial membrane [63].

Nevertheless, as reported above, most of the proteins related to mitochondrial morphology that we found to be altered in the context of Parkinson's disease are associated with the regulation of the mitochondrial cristae morphology. Interestingly, accumulating evidence shows an association between the morphology of the mitochondrial cristae and the OXPHOS complexes. This fact brings forward the idea that the formation of the supercomplexes of the respiratory chain is related to the organization of the inner mitochondrial membrane [18]. The involvement of the mitochondria in Parkinson's disease is clear, and several indications also reveal that alterations in the balance of fission and fusion processes increase the occurrence of fragmented mitochondria. However, the data collected in the present work points to a major contribution of the modification of the mitochondrial cristae. The major drawback when studying mitochondrial morphology is the fact that many studies have employed immunofluorescence using antibodies against mitochondrial membrane proteins and subsequent observation in optical microscopes. This methodology exhibits a lack of resolution needed to visualize the morphological subtleties in the mitochondrial cristae [88]. Therefore, for the study of mitochondrial dynamics, super-resolution and immunoelectron microscopy are better options since it is then possible to visualize the inner mitochondrial compartment [88,89].

The mitochondrial contact site and the cristae-organizing system (MICOS) have been described as a multiprotein complex relevant to inner membrane architecture [1,90]. In fact, it was described that some of the MICOS subunits control the morphology of the cristae in coordination with the mitochondrial Complexes III and IV from the respiratory chain [18]. In the absence of MICOS, cristae morphology is aberrant and these respiratory chain complexes are not functional [14]. Interestingly, in our study we found that two of the MICOS core subunits were altered in the context of Parkinson's disease (Table 2): Mitofilin [18] and Mic26 [14]. The MICOS Complex interacts with proteins of the outer mitochondrial membrane, specifically with the sorting and assembly machinery component 50 (SAM50). Its depletion has been found to affect the mitochondria ultrastructure and the loss of cristae, thus affecting the assembly of the complexes of the mitochondrial respiratory chain [91]. Curiously, the SAM50 protein expression was also found to be altered in our analysis (Table 2).

Other modified proteins retrieved in our study included proteins from the mitochondrial respiratory chain such as members of the Complex III (the cytochrome b-c1 Complex subunit, the ubiquinol cytochrome c reductase iron–sulphur subunit, and the cytochrome b-c1 Complex subunit 6) and Complex IV (the cytochrome c oxidase subunit 4, the cytochrome c oxidase subunit 5A, the cytochrome c oxidase subunit 6C, the cytochrome c oxidase subunit 7C, and the cytochrome c oxidase polypeptide I).

Pivotal for the proper architecture of the mitochondrial cristae is the protein OPA1 [3]. Alterations were found to occur in the expression of the calcium-binding mitochondrial carrier protein Aralar2 (Slc25A), which acts in conjunction with OPA1 to sense modifications of the substrate levels for energy production. Following this interaction, the cristae are narrowed and the dimerization of the ATP synthase is stimulated [18].

The mitochondrial cristae structure is not solely maintained by proteins, but also by cardiolipin lipids [18], and several cardiolipin binding proteins have been described to be present at the mitochondrial membrane, amongst them the Prohibitin protein family. Prohibitin and Prohibitin-2 appeared to be altered in the context of Parkinson's disease in our analysis (Table 2). These proteins are known to be organized in complexes within the inner mitochondrial membrane and are important for the proper organization of the cristae morphology and mitochondrial respiration [53,92]. Moreover, these proteins are involved in the turnover of the subunits of the mitochondrial respiratory chain and participate in the assembly of the Complex IV from the respiratory chain [93,94].

There is evidence that aberrant cristae morphology affects the proper assembly of the OXPHOS complexes, but also that the lack of ATP synthase subunits impacts the morphology of the cristae [95,96]. The latter has been supported by studies showing that ATP synthase dimerization forces membrane curvature [97]. Interestingly, mitochondrial morphology also relies on the cellular energetic state since, by compromising mitochondrial membrane potential, mitochondrial fragmentation is induced [98]. In addition, dimer formation of the F1F0-ATP synthase affects mitochondrial cristae structure [95].

3.2. Binding Partners of Mitochondrial Proteins Differentially Expressed in Parkinson's Disease

Mitochondria are organelles with important roles in many cellular processes, hence we next explored the binding partners described for the mitochondrial proteins differentially expressed in Parkinson's disease (Table 2). Using the HIPPIE tool [72,99–101], we determined the complete list of binding partners, which is depicted in Supplementary Table S2 (Figure 1). This software provides information on human protein-protein interactions with high confidence scores that are due to the amount of supporting data available as well as derived from annotated information [72,99]. In total, for the 22 mitochondrial-shaping proteins altered in Parkinson's disease, we found 1683 hints of interacting proteins. Since some of the mitochondrial-shaping proteins have interacting proteins in common, these hints correspond to 1008 different proteins. When we cross-referenced these binding partners with the list of proteins found to be modified in the context of Parkinson's disease (Supplementary Table S1), 108 common hints were identified (Figure 3, Table 3, and Supplementary Table S3). In Supplementary Table S3, the different hints of the proteins listed in Table 3 within the different proteomics-based studies used in the present work are described.

As a first approach we assessed the cellular components, which are represented by these proteins using the plugin ClueGO in Cytoscape software (Figure 1). In Figure 4 it is possible to see the network built from the different cellular components and their upregulation (green nodes) or downregulation (red nodes) in Parkinson's disease. The cluster of proteins that were found to be upregulated fall into diverse cellular components: mitochondrial respiratory chain Complex III, proteasome complex, muscle thin filament tropomyosin, and melanosome. On the other hand, the downregulated are represented by: inner mitochondrial membrane, integral component of the lumenal side of the endoplasmic reticulum membrane, and mitochondrial proton-transporting ATP synthase complex.

Table 3. List of binding partners of the mitochondrial-shaping proteins altered in Parkinson's disease (Table 2) that are found in the list of proteins modified in the context of Parkinson's disease (Supplementary Table S1).

Gene Names	Protein Names
ACAD9	Acyl-CoA dehydrogenase family member 9, mitochondrial (ACAD-9) (EC 1.3.99.-)
ACP2	Lysosomal acid phosphatase (LAP) (EC 3.1.3.2)
ACTB	Actin, cytoplasmic 1 (Beta-actin) (Cleaved into: Actin, cytoplasmic 1, *N*-terminally processed)
ACTBL2	Beta-actin-like protein 2 (Kappa-actin)
ACTN1	Alpha-actinin-1 (Alpha-actinin cytoskeletal isoform) (F-actin cross-linking protein) (Non-muscle alpha-actinin-1)
ALB, GIG20, GIG42, PRO0903, PRO1708, PRO2044, PRO2619, PRO2675, UNQ696/PRO1341	Serum albumin
ALDH1B1, ALDH5, ALDHX	Aldehyde dehydrogenase X, mitochondrial (EC 1.2.1.3) (Aldehyde dehydrogenase 5) (Aldehyde dehydrogenase family 1 member B1)
ALDOA, ALDA	Fructose-bisphosphate aldolase A (EC 4.1.2.13) (Lung cancer antigen NY-LU-1) (Muscle-type aldolase)
ANXA2, ANX2, ANX2L4, CAL1H LPC2D	Annexin A2 (Annexin II) (Annexin-2) (Calpactin I heavy chain) (Calpactin-1 heavy chain) (Chromobindin-8) (Lipocortin II) (Placental anticoagulant protein IV) (PAP-IV) (Protein I) (p36)
APOA1	Apolipoprotein A-I (Apo-AI) (ApoA-I) (Apolipoprotein A1) (Cleaved into: Proapolipoprotein A-I (Proapo A-I); Truncated apolipoprotein A-I (Apolipoprotein A-I(1-242)))
ATP5A1, ATP5A, ATP5AL2, ATPM	ATP synthase subunit alpha, mitochondrial
ATP5B, ATPMB, ATPSB,	ATP synthase subunit beta, mitochondrial (EC 3.6.3.14)
ATP5H, My032	ATP synthase subunit d, mitochondrial (ATPase subunit d)
ATP5I, ATP5K	ATP synthase subunit e, mitochondrial (ATPase subunit e) (Cleaved into: ATP synthase subunit e, mitochondrial, *N*-terminally processed)
BCAP31, BAP31, DXS1357E	B-cell receptor-associated protein 31 (BCR-associated protein 31) (Bap31) (6C6-AG tumor-associated antigen) (Protein CDM) (p28)
C1QBP, GC1QBP, HABP1, SF2P32	Complement component 1 Q subcomponent-binding protein, mitochondrial (ASF/SF2-associated protein p32) (Glycoprotein gC1qBP) (C1qBP) (Hyaluronan-binding protein 1) (Mitochondrial matrix protein p32) (gC1q-R protein) (p33)
CALR, CRTC	Calreticulin (CRP55) (Calregulin) (Endoplasmic reticulum resident protein 60) (ERp60) (HACBP) (grp60)
CCT5, CCTE, KIAA0098	T-complex protein 1 subunit epsilon (TCP-1-epsilon) (CCT-epsilon)
COX4I1, COX4	Cytochrome c oxidase subunit 4 isoform 1, mitochondrial (Cytochrome c oxidase polypeptide IV) (Cytochrome c oxidase subunit IV isoform 1) (COX IV-1)
COX5A	Cytochrome c oxidase subunit 5A, mitochondrial (Cytochrome c oxidase polypeptide Va)
COX6C	Cytochrome c oxidase subunit 6C (Cytochrome c oxidase polypeptide VIc)
DDAH1, DDAH	N(G),N(G)-dimethylarginine dimethylaminohydrolase 1 (DDAH-1) (Dimethylarginine dimethylaminohydrolase 1) (EC 3.5.3.18) (DDAHI) (Dimethylargininase-1)
DDOST, KIAA0115, OST48 OK/SW-cl.45	Dolichyl-diphosphooligosaccharide—protein glycosyltransferase 48 kDa subunit (DDOST 48 kDa subunit) (Oligosaccharyl transferase 48 kDa subunit)
DNM1L, DLP1, DRP1	Dynamin-1-like protein (EC 3.6.5.5) (Dnm1p/Vps1p-like protein) (DVLP) (Dynamin family member proline-rich carboxyl-terminal domain less) (Dymple) (Dynamin-like protein) (Dynamin-like protein 4) (Dynamin-like protein IV) (HdynIV) (Dynamin-related protein 1)
DYNC1H1, DHC1, DNCH1, DNCL, DNECL, DYHC, KIAA0325	Cytoplasmic dynein 1 heavy chain 1 (Cytoplasmic dynein heavy chain 1) (Dynein heavy chain, cytosolic)
EEF1A1, EEF1A, EF1A, LENG7	Elongation factor 1-alpha 1 (EF-1-alpha-1) (Elongation factor Tu) (EF-Tu) (Eukaryotic elongation factor 1 A-1) (eEF1A-1) (Leukocyte receptor cluster member 7)
EEF1B2, EEF1B, EF1B	Elongation factor 1-beta (EF-1-beta)
EIF5A	Eukaryotic translation initiation factor 5A-1 (eIF-5A-1) (eIF-5A1) (Eukaryotic initiation factor 5A isoform 1) (eIF-5A) (Rev-binding factor) (eIF-4D)

Table 3. *Cont.*

Gene Names	Protein Names
FKBP4, FKBP52	Peptidyl-prolyl cis-trans isomerase FKBP4 (PPIase FKBP4) (EC 5.2.1.8) (51 kDa FK506-binding protein) (FKBP51) (52 kDa FK506-binding protein) (52 kDa FKBP) (FKBP-52) (59 kDa immunophilin) (p59) (FK506-binding protein 4) (FKBP-4) (FKBP59) (HSP-binding immunophilin) (HBI) (Immunophilin FKBP52) (Rotamase) (Cleaved into: Peptidyl-prolyl cis-trans isomerase FKBP4, *N*-terminally processed)
FLNC, ABPL, FLN2	Filamin-C (FLN-C) (FLNc) (ABP-280-like protein) (ABP-L) (Actin-binding-like protein) (Filamin-2) (Gamma-filamin)
FLOT1	Flotillin-1
FUBP1	Far upstream element-binding protein 1 (FBP) (FUSE-binding protein 1) (DNA helicase V) (hDH V)
GARS	Glycine-tRNA ligase (EC 3.6.1.17) (EC 6.1.1.14) (Diadenosine tetraphosphate synthetase) (AP-4-A synthetase) (Glycyl-tRNA synthetase) (GlyRS)
GSTK1, HDCMD47P	Glutathione S-transferase kappa 1 (EC 2.5.1.18) (GST 13-13) (GST class-kappa) (GSTK1-1) (hGSTK1) (Glutathione S-transferase subunit 13)
GSTO1, GSTTLP28	Glutathione S-transferase omega-1 (GSTO-1) (EC 2.5.1.18) (Glutathione S-transferase omega 1-1) (GSTO 1-1) (Glutathione-dependent dehydroascorbate reductase) (EC 1.8.5.1) (Monomethylarsonic acid reductase) (MMA(V) reductase) (EC 1.20.4.2) (S-(Phenacyl)glutathione reductase) (SPG-R)
HSP90AB1, HSP90B HSPC2, HSPCB	Heat shock protein HSP 90-beta (HSP 90) (Heat shock 84 kDa) (HSP 84) (HSP84)
HSPA1L	Heat shock 70 kDa protein 1-like (Heat shock 70 kDa protein 1L) (Heat shock 70 kDa protein 1-Hom) (HSP70-Hom)
HSPA5, GRP78	78 kDa glucose-regulated protein (GRP-78) (Endoplasmic reticulum lumenal Ca(2+)-binding protein grp78) (Heat shock 70 kDa protein 5) (Immunoglobulin heavy chain-binding protein) (BiP)
HSPA8, HSC70, HSP73, HSPA10	Heat shock cognate 71 kDa protein (Heat shock 70 kDa protein 8) (Lipopolysaccharide-associated protein 1) (LAP-1) (LPS-associated protein 1)
HSPA9, GRP75, HSPA9B, mt-HSP70	Stress-70 protein, mitochondrial (75 kDa glucose-regulated protein) (GRP-75) (Heat shock 70 kDa protein 9) (Mortalin) (MOT) (Peptide-binding protein 74) (PBP74)
HSPB1, HSP27, HSP28	Heat shock protein beta-1 (HspB1) (28 kDa heat shock protein) (Estrogen-regulated 24 kDa protein) (Heat shock 27 kDa protein) (HSP 27) (Stress-responsive protein 27) (SRP27)
HSPD1, HSP60	60 kDa heat shock protein, mitochondrial (EC 3.6.4.9) (60 kDa chaperonin) (Chaperonin 60) (CPN60) (Heat shock protein 60) (HSP-60) (Hsp60) (HuCHA60) (Mitochondrial matrix protein P1) (P60 lymphocyte protein)
ILVBL, AHAS	Acetolactate synthase-like protein (EC 2.2.1.-) (IlvB-like protein)
IMMT, HMP, MIC60, MINOS2, PIG4, PIG52	MICOS Complex subunit MIC60 (Cell proliferation-inducing gene 4/52 protein) (Inner mitochondrial membrane protein) (Mitofilin) (p87/89)
LDHB	L-lactate dehydrogenase B chain (LDH-B) (EC 1.1.1.27) (LDH heart subunit) (LDH-H) (Renal carcinoma antigen NY-REN-46)
LGALS1	Galectin-1 (Gal-1) (14 kDa laminin-binding protein) (HLBP14) (14 kDa lectin) (Beta-galactoside-binding lectin L-14-I) (Galaptin) (HBL) (HPL) (Lactose-binding lectin 1) (Lectin galactoside-binding soluble 1) (Putative MAPK-activating protein PM12) (S-Lac lectin 1)
LMNA, LMN1	Prelamin-A/C (Cleaved into: Lamin-A/C (70 kDa lamin) (Renal carcinoma antigen NY-REN-32))
MDH2	Malate dehydrogenase, mitochondrial (EC 1.1.1.37)
MFN2, CPRP1, KIAA0214	Mitofusin-2 (EC 3.6.5.-) (Transmembrane GTPase MFN2)
MYL6	Myosin light polypeptide 6 (17 kDa myosin light chain) (LC17) (Myosin light chain 3) (MLC-3) (Myosin light chain alkali 3) (Myosin light chain A3) (Smooth muscle and non-muscle myosin light chain alkali 6)
NDUFA10	NADH dehydrogenase (ubiquinone) 1 alpha subcomplex subunit 10, mitochondrial (Complex I-42kD) (CI-42kD) (NADH-ubiquinone oxidoreductase 42 kDa subunit)
NDUFA11	NADH dehydrogenase [ubiquinone] 1 alpha subcomplex subunit 11 (Complex I-B14.7) (CI-B14.7) (NADH-ubiquinone oxidoreductase subunit B14.7)
NDUFA4	Cytochrome c oxidase subunit NDUFA4 (Complex I-MLRQ) (CI-MLRQ) (NADH-ubiquinone oxidoreductase MLRQ subunit)

Table 3. *Cont.*

Gene Names	Protein Names
NDUFS1	NADH-ubiquinone oxidoreductase 75 kDa subunit, mitochondrial (EC 1.6.5.3) (EC 1.6.99.3) (Complex I-75kD) (CI-75kD)
NDUFS3	NADH dehydrogenase (ubiquinone) iron-sulfur protein 3, mitochondrial (EC 1.6.5.3) (EC 1.6.99.3) (Complex I-30kD) (CI-30kD) (NADH-ubiquinone oxidoreductase 30 kDa subunit)
NEDD8	NEDD8 (Neddylin) (Neural precursor cell expressed developmentally downregulated protein 8) (NEDD-8) (Ubiquitin-like protein Nedd8)
NPM1, NPM	Nucleophosmin (NPM) (Nucleolar phosphoprotein B23) (Nucleolar protein NO38) (Numatrin)
OAT	Ornithine aminotransferase, mitochondrial (EC 2.6.1.13) (Ornithine delta-aminotransferase) (Ornithine—oxo-acid aminotransferase) (Cleaved into: Ornithine aminotransferase, hepatic form; Ornithine aminotransferase, renal form)
OGDH	2-oxoglutarate dehydrogenase, mitochondrial (EC 1.2.4.2) (2-oxoglutarate dehydrogenase complex component E1) (OGDC-E1) (Alpha-ketoglutarate dehydrogenase)
OTUB1, OTB1, OTU1, HSPC263	Ubiquitin thioesterase OTUB1 (EC 3.4.19.12) (Deubiquitinating enzyme OTUB1) (OTU domain-containing ubiquitin aldehyde-binding protein 1) (Otubain-1) (hOTU1) (Ubiquitin-specific-processing protease OTUB1)
PDIA3, ERP57, ERP60, GRP58	Protein disulfide-isomerase A3 (EC 5.3.4.1) (58 kDa glucose-regulated protein) (58 kDa microsomal protein) (p58) (Disulfide isomerase ER-60) (Endoplasmic reticulum resident protein 57) (ER protein 57) (ERp57) (Endoplasmic reticulum resident protein 60) (ER protein 60) (ERp60)
PGK1, PGKA, MIG10, OK/SW-cl.110	Phosphoglycerate kinase 1 (EC 2.7.2.3) (Cell migration-inducing gene 10 protein) (Primer recognition protein 2) (PRP 2)
PHB	Prohibitin
PHB2, BAP, REA	Prohibitin-2 (B-cell receptor-associated protein BAP37) (D-prohibitin) (Repressor of estrogen receptor activity)
PIN1	Peptidyl-prolyl cis-trans isomerase NIMA-interacting 1 (EC 5.2.1.8) (Peptidyl-prolyl cis-trans isomerase Pin1) (PPIase Pin1) (Rotamase Pin1)
PPIA, CYPA	Peptidyl-prolyl cis-trans isomerase A (PPIase A) (EC 5.2.1.8) (Cyclophilin A) (Cyclosporin A-binding protein) (Rotamase A) (Cleaved into: Peptidyl-prolyl cis-trans isomerase A, *N*-terminally processed)
PRDX4	Peroxiredoxin-4 (EC 1.11.1.15) (Antioxidant enzyme AOE372) (AOE37-2) (Peroxiredoxin IV) (Prx-IV) (Thioredoxin peroxidase AO372) (Thioredoxin-dependent peroxide reductase A0372)
PSMA3, HC8, PSC8	Proteasome subunit alpha type-3 (EC 3.4.25.1) (Macropain subunit C8) (Multi-catalytic endopeptidase complex subunit C8) (Proteasome component C8)
PTPN5	Tyrosine-protein phosphatase non-receptor type 5 (EC 3.1.3.48) (Neural-specific protein-tyrosine phosphatase) (Striatum-enriched protein-tyrosine phosphatase) (STEP)
RAB14	Ras-related protein Rab-14
RAB2A, RAB2	Ras-related protein Rab-2A
RAC1, TC25, MIG5	Ras-related C3 botulinum toxin substrate 1 (Cell migration-inducing gene 5 protein) (Ras-like protein TC25) (p21-Rac1)
RAPGEF2, KIAA0313, NRAPGEP, PDZGEF1	Rap guanine nucleotide exchange factor 2 (Cyclic nucleotide ras GEF) (CNrasGEF) (Neural RAP guanine nucleotide exchange protein) (nRap GEP) (PDZ domain-containing guanine nucleotide exchange factor 1) (PDZ-GEF1) (RA-GEF-1) (Ras/Rap1-associating GEF-1)
RHOA, ARH12, ARHA, RHO12	Transforming protein RhoA (Rho cDNA clone 12) (h12)
RNH1, PRI, RNH	Ribonuclease inhibitor (Placental ribonuclease inhibitor) (Placental RNase inhibitor) (Ribonuclease/angiogenin inhibitor 1) (RAI)
RPN1	Dolichyl-diphosphooligosaccharide—protein glycosyltransferase subunit 1 (Dolichyl-diphosphooligosaccharide—protein glycosyltransferase 67 kDa subunit) (Ribophorin I) (RPN-I) (Ribophorin-1)
RPN2	Dolichyl-diphosphooligosaccharide—protein glycosyltransferase subunit 2 (Dolichyl-diphosphooligosaccharide—protein glycosyltransferase 63 kDa subunit) (RIBIIR) (Ribophorin II) (RPN-II) (Ribophorin-2)
RPS15A, OK/SW-cl.82	40S ribosomal protein S15a (Small ribosomal subunit protein uS8)
RPS3, OK/SW-cl.26	40S ribosomal protein S3 (EC 4.2.99.18) (Small ribosomal subunit protein uS3)
S100A10, ANX2LG CAL1L CLP11	Protein S100-A10 (Calpactin I light chain) (Calpactin-1 light chain) (Cellular ligand of annexin II) (S100 calcium-binding protein A10) (p10 protein) (p11)

Table 3. *Cont.*

Gene Names	Protein Names
SAMM50, SAM50 CGI-51 TRG3	Sorting and assembly machinery component 50 homolog (Transformation-related gene 3 protein) (TRG-3)
SELENBP1, SBP	Selenium-binding protein 1 (56 kDa selenium-binding protein) (SBP56) (SP56)
SFXN1	Sideroflexin-1 (Tricarboxylate carrier protein) (TCC)
SH3GLB2, KIAA1848, PP578	Endophilin-B2 (SH3 domain-containing GRB2-like protein B2)
SIRT2, SIR2L, SIR2L2	NAD-dependent protein deacetylase sirtuin-2 (EC 3.5.1.-) (Regulatory protein SIR2 homolog 2) (SIR2-like protein 2)
SLC25A13, ARALAR2	Calcium-binding mitochondrial carrier protein Aralar2 (Citrin) (Mitochondrial aspartate glutamate carrier 2) (Solute carrier family 25 member 13)
SLC25A18, GC2	Mitochondrial glutamate carrier 2 (GC-2) (Glutamate/H(+) symporter 2) (Solute carrier family 25 member 18)
SLC25A5, ANT2	ADP/ATP translocase 2 (ADP, ATP carrier protein 2) (ADP, ATP carrier protein, fibroblast isoform) (Adenine nucleotide translocator 2) (ANT 2) (Solute carrier family 25 member 5) (Cleaved into: ADP/ATP translocase 2, *N*-terminally processed)
SLC9A3R1, NHERF, NHERF1	Na(+)/H(+) exchange regulatory cofactor NHE-RF1 (NHERF-1) (Ezrin-radixin-moesin-binding phosphoprotein 50) (EBP50) (Regulatory cofactor of Na(+)/H(+) exchanger) (Sodium-hydrogen exchanger regulatory factor 1) (Solute carrier family 9 isoform A3 regulatory factor 1)
SSBP1, SSBP	Single-stranded DNA-binding protein, mitochondrial (Mt-SSB) (MtSSB) (PWP1-interacting protein 17)
TPD52	Tumor protein D52 (Protein N8)
TPM1, C15orf13, TMSA	Tropomyosin alpha-1 chain (Alpha-tropomyosin) (Tropomyosin-1)
TPM2, TMSB	Tropomyosin beta chain (Beta-tropomyosin) (Tropomyosin-2)
TPM3	Tropomyosin alpha-3 chain (Gamma-tropomyosin) (Tropomyosin-3) (Tropomyosin-5) (hTM5)
TPM4	Tropomyosin alpha-4 chain (TM30p1) (Tropomyosin-4)
TUBA1A, TUBA3	Tubulin alpha-1A chain (Alpha-tubulin 3) (Tubulin B-alpha-1) (Tubulin alpha-3 chain) (Cleaved into: Detyrosinated tubulin alpha-1A chain)
TUBB, TUBB5, OK/SW-cl.56	Tubulin beta chain (Tubulin beta-5 chain)
TUBB4B, TUBB2C	Tubulin beta-4B chain (Tubulin beta-2 chain) (Tubulin beta-2C chain)
TUFM	Elongation factor Tu, mitochondrial (EF-Tu) (P43)
UQCRB, UQBP	Cytochrome b-c1 complex subunit 7 (Complex III subunit 7) (Complex III subunit VII) (QP-C) (Ubiquinol-cytochrome c reductase complex 14 kDa protein)
UQCRFS1	Cytochrome b-c1 complex subunit Rieske, mitochondrial (EC 1.10.2.2) (Complex III subunit 5) (Cytochrome b-c1 complex subunit 5) (Rieske iron-sulfur protein) (RISP) (Ubiquinol-cytochrome c reductase iron-sulfur subunit) (Cleaved into: Cytochrome b-c1 complex subunit 11 (Complex III subunit IX) (Ubiquinol-cytochrome c reductase 8 kDa protein))
UQCRFS1P1, UQCRFSL1	Putative cytochrome b-c1 complex subunit Rieske-like protein 1 (Ubiquinol-cytochrome c reductase Rieske iron-sulfur subunit pseudogene 1)
UQCRH	Cytochrome b-c1 complex subunit 6, mitochondrial (Complex III subunit 6) (Complex III subunit VIII) (Cytochrome c1 non-heme 11 kDa protein) (Mitochondrial hinge protein) (Ubiquinol-cytochrome c reductase complex 11 kDa protein)
USMG5, DAPIT, HCVFTP2, PD04912	Upregulated during skeletal muscle growth protein 5 (Diabetes-associated protein in insulin-sensitive tissues) (HCV F-transactivated protein 2)
VCP	Transitional endoplasmic reticulum ATPase (TER ATPase) (EC 3.6.4.6) (15S Mg(2+)-ATPase p97 subunit) (Valosin-containing protein) (VCP)
VDAC1, VDAC	Voltage-dependent anion-selective channel protein 1 (VDAC-1) (hVDAC1) (Outer mitochondrial membrane protein porin 1) (Plasmalemmal porin) (Porin 31HL) (Porin 31HM)
VDAC2	Voltage-dependent anion-selective channel protein 2 (VDAC-2) (hVDAC2) (Outer mitochondrial membrane protein porin 2)
VDAC3	Voltage-dependent anion-selective channel protein 3 (VDAC-3) (hVDAC3) (Outer mitochondrial membrane protein porin 3)
VIM	Vimentin
YWHAE	14-3-3 protein epsilon (14-3-3E)
YWHAZ	14-3-3 protein zeta/delta (Factor activating exoenzyme S) (FAS) (Protein kinase C inhibitor protein 1) (KCIP-1)

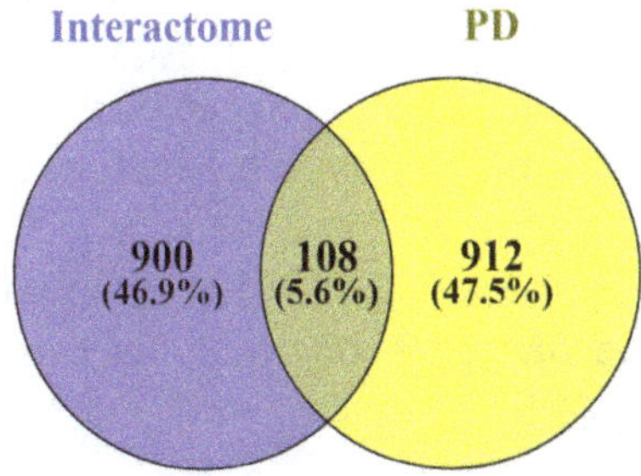

Figure 3. Venn diagram displaying the comparison of the number of the binding partners of the mitochondrial-shaping proteins affected in Parkinson's disease (Table 2) and the proteins found to be differentially expressed in the context of Parkinson's disease (Supplementary Table S1). The Venn diagram was constructed using the Venny 2.1 software [71]. PD—Parkinson's disease.

The proteins used to search for the binding partners were mitochondrial proteins, thus alterations in the mitochondrial cellular components were expected. In this regard, the downregulation of the inner mitochondrial membrane and the mitochondrial proton-transporting ATP synthase complex was anticipated. Several of the proteins found to be altered in the context of Parkinson's disease (Table 2) are proteins located at the inner mitochondrial membrane, and the alteration of these components has also previously been described in the pathology [7].

Interestingly, it has been shown that the ubiquitin-proteasome system regulates the level of proteins targeted to the mitochondrial intermembrane space, and this process depends on the mitochondrial intermembrane space import machinery [102]. Additionally, it has been shown that the ubiquitin-proteasome system acts on the regulation of the mitochondrial biogenesis [103]. In this study, we found an upregulation of the proteasome, which corroborates the evidence of its dysfunction in Parkinson's disease [103,104]. ROS levels are increased in Parkinson's disease and are responsible for the oxidative modification of lipids, DNA, and proteins [105]. These modifications might lead to misfolded proteins and aggregation [106]. Mitochondrial proteins might be dysfunctional due to the harmful effects of ROS, which not only might modify the folded proteins, but also affect the incorporation of newly synthetized mitochondrial proteins since they are translated in the cytosol and must be transported unfolded into the mitochondria [103]. In an oxidative stress scenario, as in Parkinson's disease, the risk of the alteration of unfolded proteins and consequent removal by the proteasome is higher, reducing the amount of mitochondrial proteins available. Besides, it is known that outer mitochondrial membrane proteins involved in mitochondrial fusion are regulated by ubiquitination and that this process is induced by stress [19].

Mitochondrial dynamics not only relies on mitochondrial fusion and fission proteins, but also on the contact sites between mitochondria and the ER, which are fundamental for the initial fission process [107]. It has been described that the shape-forming proteins control mitochondrial morphology by mediating the attachment of the mitochondria to the cytoskeleton and the ER [107,108], and they can also connect the inner and outer mitochondrial membranes, hence influencing the import and assembly of mitochondrial proteins [109]. Regarding the upregulation of the melanosome as a cellular component, although it is an organelle not present in neuronal cells, when we look closely at the proteins contributing to this node, we find that three of the proteins are heat shock proteins. These proteins are key components in ensuring proper protein function and are expressed in response to stress, controlling the subsequent degradation of misfolded proteins, which is also in line with the upregulation of the proteasome complex and the occurrence of the oxidative stress characteristic of the disorder.

The mitochondrial cytochrome bc1 complex from the respiratory chain (Complex III) is one of the main producers of ROS, together with the Complex I [110]. Although Complex I release superoxide into the mitochondrial matrix, Complex III does it into the intermembrane space and the cytosol [111]. In the pathobiology of Parkinson's disease, it is well accepted that there is an increase in ROS leading to oxidative stress [105], which is in agreement with the upregulation of the cellular mitochondria component of the respiratory chain Complex III found in our analysis. This complex is localized in the inner mitochondrial membrane, at the cristae, and has three transmembrane subunits in which the prosthetic groups involved in the redox reactions are located. They must be dimerized for proper functioning, which is also dependent on the mitochondrial membrane potential [110], suggesting that alterations in the organization of the inner mitochondrial membrane might affect their function.

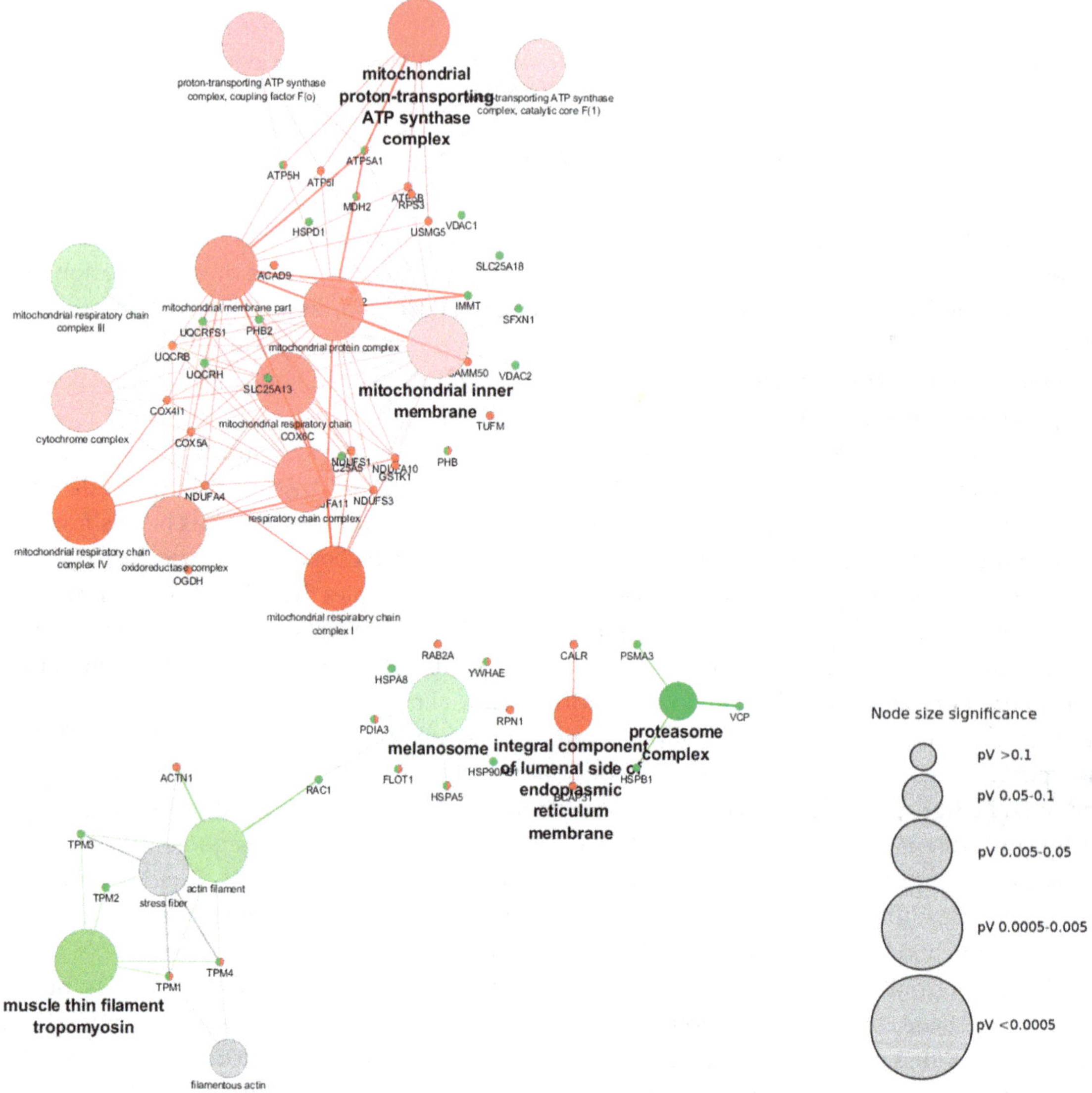

Figure 4. Cytoscape network of the main cellular components associated with mitochondrial-shaping proteins in the context of Parkinson's disease. The binding partners of the mitochondrial-shaping proteins found to be modified in different proteomics-based approaches in the context of Parkinson's disease according to the Human Integrated Protein-Protein Interaction rEference (HIPPIE) and appearing as modified in proteomics-based studies on Parkinson's disease were subjected to network analysis using the plugin ClueGo from the software Cytoscape to analyze the cellular components represented by the proteins from the list. Gray scale nodes correspond to cellular components that were found to be equally up- and downregulated in different studies, while green and red nodes are representative of upregulated and downregulated cellular components respectively, in the context of Parkinson's disease. The increase in green and red color gradient represents higher amounts of the contribution of up- and downregulated proteins, respectively. The size of the nodes is indicative of their statistical significance.

A closer look at the network shows that "muscle thin filament tropomyosin" is connected to cellular components related to the actin cytoskeleton ("actin filament", "stress fiber", and "filamentous actin"). As described above, the cytoskeleton also plays a role in the dynamics and movement of the mitochondria [108]. Interestingly, in the context of Parkinson's disease some models (both genetic and drug-based) showed a negative impact on the dynamics of the actin cytoskeleton and the formation of stress fibers [108,112,113].

3.3. Biological Processes Associated with Mitochondrial-Shaping Proteins Affected in Parkinson's Disease

To obtain information on the biological processes related to the mitochondrial-shaping proteins affected in Parkinson's disease, we undertook a bioinformatic approach using the plugin ClueGo from the Cystoscope software (Figure 5 and Table 4). This plugin allows the extraction of the biological meaning of large lists of proteins [114]. Overall, around 44% altered processes are related to energy production by the mitochondria. This contribution was expected since the dysfunction of this organelle is a hallmark of the disease.

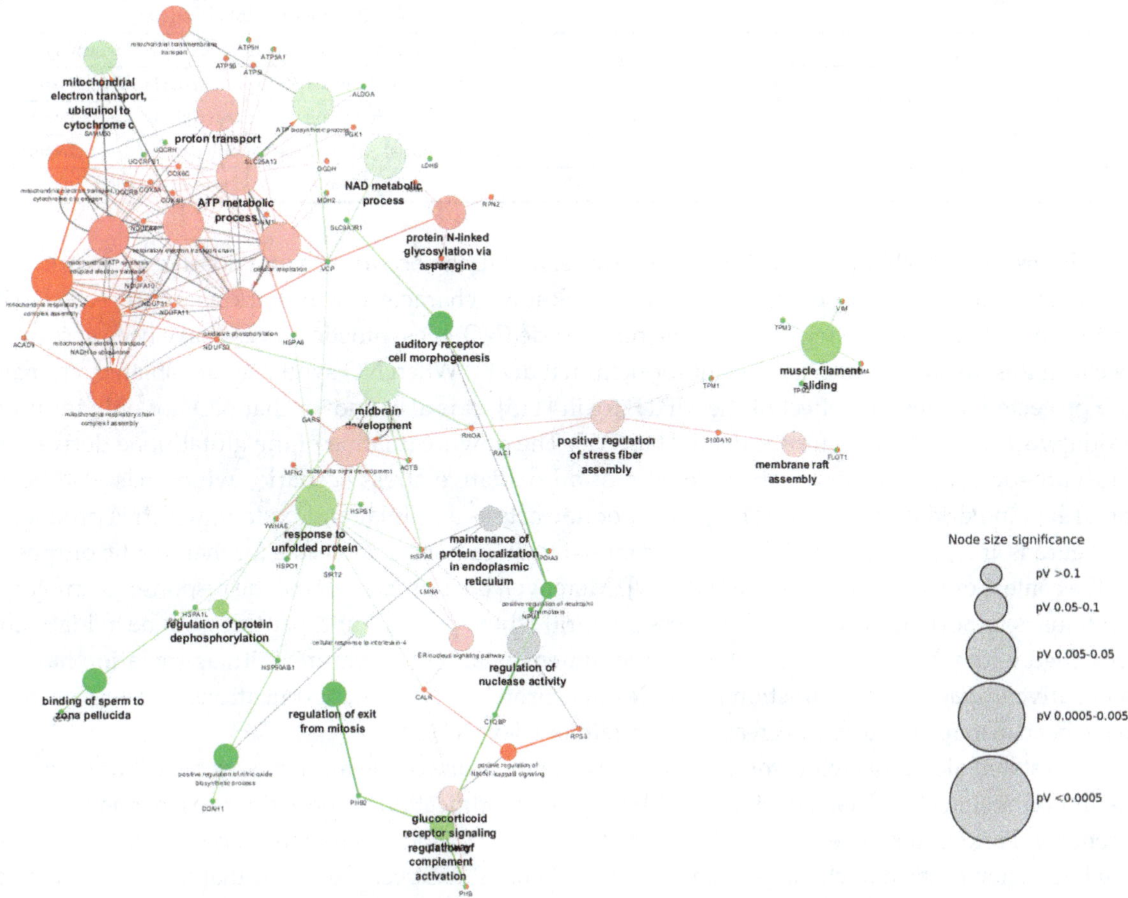

Figure 5. Cytoscape network of the main biological processes associated with mitochondrial-shaping proteins in the context of Parkinson's disease. The binding partners of the mitochondrial-shaping proteins found modified in different proteomics-based approaches in the context of Parkinson's disease were subjected to network analysis using the plugin ClueGo from the software Cytoscape to analyze the biological processes affected in the disease. Gray scale nodes correspond to biological pathways that were found to be equally up- and downregulated in different studies, while green and red nodes are representative of upregulated and downregulated biological pathways, respectively, in the context of Parkinson's disease. The increase in green and red color gradient represents higher amounts of the contribution of up- and downregulated proteins, respectively. The size of the nodes is indicative of their statistical significance.

Table 4. List of biological processes related to the mitochondrial-shaping proteins affected in Parkinson's disease.

Upregulated	Downregulated
ATP biosynthetic process	ATP metabolic process
Positive regulation of nitric oxide biosynthetic process	Membrane raft assembly
Response to unfolded protein	Positive regulation of stress fiber assembly
Auditory receptor cell morphogenesis	Gluthatione derivative biosynthetic process
Binding of sperm to zona pellucida	Protein N-linked glycosylation via asparagine
Regulation of protein dephosphorylation	Glucocorticoid receptor signaling pathway
Mitochondrial electron transport ubiquinol to cytochrome c	ER-nucleus signaling pathway
Regulation of exit from mitosis	Substantia nigra development
NAD metabolic process	Positive regulation of NFkB signaling
Muscle filament sliding	Mitochondrial transmembrane transport
Regulation of complement activation	Mitochondrial electron transport cytochrome c to oxygen
Midbrain development and positive regulation of neutrophil chemotaxis	Respiratory electron transport chain
	Oxidative phosphorylation
	Mitochondrial respiratory chain Complex I assembly
	Mitochondrial electron transport NADH to ubiquinone
	Mitochondria respiratory chain complex assembly
	Mitochondrial ATP synthesis coupled to electron transport
	Cellular respiration and proton transport

Interestingly, other biological processes are related to the occurrence of oxidative stress and the respective alterations in proteins, which is also a known characteristic of Parkinson's disease [105]. In this regard, the positive regulation of the nitric oxide (NO) biosynthetic process have been shown to occur in this disorder, which is relevant for neuronal death. When NO synthases are ablated, animals are protected against the effect of the MPTP toxin [115]. It is also known that NO not only induces oxidative stress but also neuronal death [116,117]. The downregulation of the glutathione derivative biosynthetic process is also a characteristic of an oxidative stress scenario, which has also been described in Parkinson's disease [118]. This peptide acts as a cellular antioxidant, which is produced by neurons and glial cells, and it has been proposed as an important molecule for therapeutic purposes in the context of Parkinson's disease [118,119]. Moreover, the upregulation of the response to unfolded proteins is important in an oxidative stress scenario where proteins and peptides can be oxidatively modified with a harmful effect on their three-dimensional (3D) structure, with aggregation having a negative impact on their function [106]. Besides, protein oxidative modifications and aggregation have been also related to the decreased in glutathione levels [120].

As stated along this work, the cellular cytoskeleton is one of the mechanisms contributing to the definition of mitochondrial morphology [108]. In fact, modification of the actin cytoskeleton has been probed in Parkinson's disease [108,112,113]. Mitochondrial fusion and fission processes are affected by the interaction of the mitochondria with the cytoskeleton. It has been described that the fusion process can be delayed when actin filaments are depolymerized [121]. The actin cytoskeleton is also involved in the fission process [38]. In our network, several processes are related to the actin cytoskeleton, such as the upregulation of the process of "muscle filament sliding" and the downregulation of the "positive regulation of stress fiber assembly". Interestingly, after a closer look at the modified biological process of "binding of sperm to zona pellucida", we observed that the proteins connected to this process are molecular chaperones and, remarkably, TCP-1-epsilon is known to play a role in the folding of actin and tubulin [122].

Regarding the "auditory receptor cell morphogenesis" biological processes, it is important to note that the protein Rac1 contributes to this pathway and is involved in the regulation of secretory processes, the phagocytosis of death cells, cell polarization, and the formation of membrane ruffles. In the context of Parkinson's disease, it has been shown to contribute to a ROS generating pathway acting with Nox1, causing neuronal death [123]. Interestingly, the other component of this node is the NHERF-1 protein, which has been shown to act as a scaffold for connecting plasma membrane proteins with members of the ERM (ezrin/moesin/radixin) family, aiding in their link to the actin cytoskeleton for the regulation of their surface expression [124].

Within the highlighted process of "regulation of protein dephosphorylation" involved in the regulation of protein function, we found an interesting protein contribution to this pathway: the Peptidyl-prolyl cis-trans isomerase (Pin1). This protein has been shown to be involved in the disease, being upregulated in cellular and animal models as well as in SN in patients [125]. The alteration of this biological process might have an impact on stress responses, immune function, and neuronal survival [126]. Also, this pathway is fundamental for proper mitochondrial functioning and signaling since, in response to the metabolic state of the cell, mitochondrial proteins from the import machinery might be regulated by phosphorylation [127].

In the "regulation of exit from mitosis" process, two interesting proteins emerge: Prohibitin-2 and the NAD-dependent protein deacetylase sirtuin-2. The latter deacetylates lysines on histones, alpha-tubulin, and other proteins [128]. By acting on tubulin it has a direct impact on microtubule function. Tubulin can be subjected to different post-translational modifications with influence on the microtubule polymerization state and its function, such as acetylation [129]. This modification on the residue K40 has been reported to alter the interaction of proteins with the cytoskeleton, with subsequent impact on the intracellular transport along the microtubules [129]. As described in this work, this may affect mitochondria morphology and dynamics.

Parkinson's disease has long been linked to increased inflammatory response [130]. In our analysis we found that the processes related to the inflammatory response were upregulated: "positive regulation of neutrophil chemotaxis" and "regulation of complement activation". Interestingly, from the last process, two of the implicated proteins belong to the Prohibitin family, which have been described to be involved in the regulation of mitochondrial respiration [131]. Regarding the downregulation of the process of the "glucocorticoid receptor signaling pathway" it is important to note that a decrease in the levels of the glucocorticoid receptor in both the SN of patients and in animal models of the disease has been reported [132,133]. These receptors regulate inflammation and are dysregulated in microglia in the context of Parkinson's disease. Dysregulation has been proposed to sustain the chronic inflammatory state observed in this disorder as well as the increased permeability of the blood brain barrier, which might increase neuronal vulnerability [132,133]. Another pathway related to the inflammatory process is downregulated: "positive regulation of NF-kB signaling", in which the protein ribosomal protein S3 stands out. Interestingly, this protein has been proposed to protect the dopaminergic neurons from apoptosis [134].

Within the network, the biological processes of "midbrain development" and "substantia nigra development" share three proteins: Actin, Complex I 30 kD from the mitochondrial respiratory chain, and the 14-3-3 protein epsilon. As described previously, the dysfunction of Complex I from the mitochondrial respiratory chain was the first indication of the mitochondria involvement in the pathobiology of Parkinson's disease [7,8]. The contribution of the cytoskeleton has also been shown, in which actin has a key role in the secretion of the synaptic vesicles content that might be then translated into a decrease in the content of neurotransmitters in the synaptic cleft [135]. Although the 14-3-3 protein is ubiquitously expressed and participates in the regulation of many signaling pathways, it has also been found to be a constituent of the Lewy bodies of Parkinson's disease patients [136].

In Parkinson's disease there is a critical modification in the lipid rafts composition, and increasing evidence shows their contribution to the disorder [137–139]. Lipid rafts have a role in diverse cellular processes such as membrane trafficking, signal transduction, and cytoskeletal organization. Their alteration can also have a negative impact on protein-protein interactions, which are fundamental processes for the formation of protein supercomplexes [138]. Interestingly, we found the process of "membrane raft assembly" to be downregulated. Not only was the protein Flotillin-1, a well-known component of the lipid rafts, found to contribute to this node, but also the protein

S100A10. The S100 family of proteins are involved in several cellular processes such as the regulation of cell proliferation and differentiation, apoptosis, calcium homeostasis, energy metabolism, and inflammation. Interestingly, they also interact with cytoskeletal and other cellular proteins [140]. Some of the membrane proteins that interact with the S100A10 are: Annexin 2, ion channels, actin binding proteins, and the serotonin receptor [140]. This protein has been proposed to function on membrane repair and was shown to be downregulated in depressive-like states in mice, with its expression being regulated by neurotrophins [141,142].

N-glycosylation is a post-translational modification that is found in membrane proteins and secreted proteins; amongst them are growth factors and their receptors [143]. In our analysis, we found that the process of "protein N-linked glycosylation via asparagine" was downregulated. This modification takes places in the ER and in the Golgi, having an effect on protein function. Evidence show that *N*-glycosylation is important for proper neuronal function and has a role in synaptic transmission [144], hence having a profound impact on the disease [145].

The occurrence of a role of the ER stress in the context of Parkinson's disease [146] is supported through new evidence, and the process of the "ER-nucleus signaling pathway" was found to be downregulated in our analysis. In this node, we found the LMNA. Lamins are filamentous proteins that contribute to the nucleus architecture and gene expression [147,148]. These proteins also interact with the actin cytoskeleton, which is known to be affected in Parkinson's disease [108,112,113,149]. The other proteins (calreticulin and the heat shock 70 kDa protein 5) are chaperones involved in protein folding and the formation of multimeric complexes [150,151], playing a crucial role in an oxidative stress scenario. Additionally, in the case of fission, not only actin but also the ER is involved in the process of mitochondrial preconstruction and DRP1 assembly [107].

4. Discussion

Mitochondria are fundamental organelles for cells, working mainly on energy production, calcium homeostasis, and apoptosis. Defects in the mitochondrial respiratory chain have received much of the attention as a key player in the pathobiology of Parkinson's disease [8,152]. However, additional modifications of the mitochondria are being increasingly reported [153,154]. Besides, it is now known that the inhibition of Complex I from the mitochondrial respiratory chain by MPP+ and rotenone does not directly trigger cytochrome c release but, instead, increases the amount of cytochrome c within the mitochondrial intermembrane space [155], indicating that there are other processes required to trigger neuronal death. Amongst them are changes in mitochondrial dynamics (i.e., alterations in the fusion and fission processes, alteration of cristae morphology) [85,156].

Increasing evidence shows that for proper mitochondrial function, processes like mitochondrial fusion, fission, and turnover are fundamental, and their dysfunction has been linked to different diseases [1,3]. In the context of Parkinson's disease, an increase in mitochondrial fission has been reported [73,157,158], suggesting that this excessive fragmentation might then enhance cytochrome c release from mitochondria and subsequently triggering apoptosis [159]. However, we found the process of cristae remodeling to be more highlighted in our analysis regarding the alteration of the mitochondrial-shaping proteins in Parkinson's disease. Notably, the alteration of the mitochondria cristae and membrane might affect the proper binding of cytochrome c, favoring its release to the cytosol and initiating the apoptotic process [155]. Some evidence of mitochondrial cristae remodeling exists in the context of Parkinson's disease. One study using a cybrid cell line constructed with mitochondria DNA isolated from cells from Parkinson's disease patients showed that there were deficiencies in both complexes of the mitochondrial respiratory chain I and IV, and cells contained a non-homogenous mitochondrial population with different morphologies ranging from enlarged to swollen and rounded in shape, which also displayed different mitochondrial membrane potential values [160]. At the ultrastructural level, some mitochondria from this cybrid displayed a decreased in the matrix density and contained a reduced number of cristae and a discontinuous outer mitochondrial membrane [160]. Similarly, in a study using transgenic mice for mutated α-synuclein, morphological alterations on the cristae were also observed, showing a disordered inner membrane and swollen matrix [34]. However, this type of study with samples from human patients is insufficient, and an increasing number of studies aiming at deciphering the ultrastructure of the mitochondria in Parkinson's disease by electron and super-resolution microscopy are required.

It is known that cristae remodeling is fundamental during apoptosis for the proper release of cytochrome c [27], and that the cristae are the sites were the OXPHOS components are located (94% of Complex II and ATP synthase [161], and 85% of cytochrome c [27]). Compelling data indicate that the shape of the cristae is crucial for the modulation of the OXPHOS function [18], and relies on the cellular state [162,163]. Disruption of the cristae junctions is a result of the release of apoptotic factors from the mitochondria [27]. Remarkably, in our analysis most of the proteins involved in mitochondrial dynamics that were found to be altered in the context of Parkinson's disease have been previously reported to play a role in the morphology of the cristae.

When imaging mitochondria, four main components can be distinguished at the ultrastructure level: the outer mitochondrial membrane (OMM), important for regulating membrane permeability and the import/export of mitochondrial proteins; the inner mitochondrial membrane (IMM), where the mitochondrial respiratory chain is placed (the invaginations of the IMM into the matrix are the so-called mitochondria cristae); the intermembrane space (IMS), which is the space between the two mitochondrial membranes; and the matrix, where the components of the tricarboxylic acid (TCA) cycle are located. The inner mitochondrial membrane is organized into three specialized zones: the inner boundary membrane, where the inner and outer membranes are associated, containing proteins of the protein import machinery; the cristae, which are the inner membrane invaginations that are enriched in proteins involved in protein translocation and synthesis as well as proteins involved in iron-sulfur biogenesis; and the cristae junctions, which are the portion of the cristae that are constricted and where the MICOS Complex is located [3].

Fundamental to cell survival is the implication of the mitochondria in the regulation of apoptosis. Within this organelle several pro-apoptotic proteins reside, triggering the apoptotic process when released into the cytosol. The permeabilization of the OMM constitutes a point of no return in the activation of this process, where the Bcl2 family of proteins participates in its regulation [164]. Interestingly, our network analysis highlighted the alteration on the permeability of membranes, supporting the apoptotic activation [165].

The OMM morphology is influenced by its interaction with the ER, ribosomes, the nucleus, and the cellular cytoskeleton [3]. Fundamental to the regulation of multiple cellular processes are the mitochondrial-ER contact sites [164]. In our network analysis, this intraorganellar interaction was highlighted as being altered in Parkinson's disease. Amongst the cellular processes are: the regulation of the intracellular calcium levels, mitochondrial fission, the endowment of membranes to phagosomes, and the formation of the inflammasome [166]. It is now clear how the ER participates in the initiation of the mitochondrial fission process. The ER enwraps the mitochondria at the constriction site where the dynamin-like protein Drp1 responsible for the fission process localizes [107,167]. Additionally, actin polymerization and the ER protein inverted formin 2 (INF2) are involved in this process [38]. Interestingly, actin filaments polymerized around the constriction sites might constitute the pulling force for the fission process [38], and several processes related to the actin cytoskeleton were found to be altered in our analysis. Additionally, the actin cytoskeleton plays a fundamental role in synaptic vesicle secretion. The alteration of this process affects synaptic transmission in the disease. Not only actin but also calcium is involved in this process.

The regulation of calcium levels is also dependent on the mitochondria-ER crosstalk, and a modification of its homeostasis has been reported in Parkinson's disease [168]. Mitochondrial calcium channels display low affinity for this ion, and for correct calcium entry into the mitochondria for the formation of the ER-mitochondrial contact sites is fundamental [169]. The relevance of this interaction has been shown by its involvement in the progression of Alzheimer's disease, where it is upregulated [170]. When calcium accumulates within the mitochondria, oxidative phosphorylation and ATP production are enhanced [171]. In addition, different chaperones are involved in the stabilization of these contact sites and could coordinate signaling between mitochondria and the ER [166]. In this direction, we also found that the expression of the chaperone grp78 was altered [172]. The ER-mitochondria contact sites are also related with the ER-stress response, which might trigger apoptosis [173]. This pathway has also been shown to be active in the context of Parkinson's disease [174]. Additionally, the calcium released by the ER at these contact sites might act as an amplifier of the apoptotic pathway [166]. Besides, the fission protein Fis1 has also been shown to facilitate the cleavage of the pro-apoptotic protein Bap31 [175]. Interestingly, these contact sites are not only relevant to the regulation of calcium levels, but also to ROS-mediating signaling [176].

Moreover, the ER contacts with the phagosomes and non-functional mitochondria degraded by mitophagy are recognized by specific OMM proteins [166]. MFN2 has also been indicated as critical to autophagosome formation, and the ER-mitochondria interaction is important for autophagosome formation [166,177]. Accumulating evidence shows that the ER might also be involved in the mitochondrial fusion process, since it was shown that mitofusin2 (MFN2) is necessary for the tethering of both organelles [178].

Relevant to proper neuronal function is the appropriate localization of the mitochondria within the synaptic terminals, where they can provide ATP for exocytosis and regulate calcium levels during synaptic transmission [179]. Mitochondria positioning within these terminals relies not only on mitochondrial fission [180], since only small mitochondria might fit into the terminals, but also in correct mitochondrial movement along microtubules and the actin cytoskeleton [164]. In this work, the network analysis of cellular components and biological pathways indicated that in the context of Parkinson's disease actin filaments are affected [108,112,113]. In addition, dysregulation of the cellular microtubules has been reported, namely in the alteration of proteins involved in tubulin acetylation. Most of the drugs used to induce Parkinson's disease modify microtubules, and specifically, acetylation has been shown to affect the interaction of proteins with the cytoskeleton [129]. Alteration of the cellular cytoskeleton might have an impact not only on mitochondrial fission but also distribution within neurons [181–184]. The modification of the actin cytoskeleton might also have an impact on the regulation of surface receptor distribution [124], which was highlighted in the present work.

The ATP produced by the mitochondria reaches the cytosol by its active transport through the adenine nucleotide translocator. To produce ATP, the processes of the TCA cycle and the respiratory chain/oxidative phosphorylation system act in conjunction. The last is located at the IMM. As a result of the mitochondrial respiratory chain deficiency, ATP production is reduced and ROS are increased, which leads to oxidative stress. This increase leads to modifications in protein, lipids, and DNA within the cells [185]. Amongst the modified lipids, the oxidation of cardiolipin from the IMM has been reported in the context of Parkinson's disease [155], and its oxidation disrupts the normal binding of cytochrome c to the membrane [155]. Furthermore, ER is fundamental for providing membrane lipids to the mitochondria [186], highlighting again the importance of this crosstalk. Phosphatidic acid is considered a fusogenic lipid required for the fusion mediated by mitofusins [187]. Cardiolipin have been reported to control mitochondrial fission [188,189]. Interestingly, in the present work we found the expression of several cardiolipin binding proteins to be modified, which might impact the proper assembly of the mitochondrial membranes. Moreover, synaptic mitochondria present lower levels of cardiolipin, which has been pointed out as a lower threshold for the release of cytochrome c in the apoptotic process [164,190]. It has also been reported that synaptic mitochondria present higher sensitivity to the inhibition of the mitochondrial respiratory chain Complex I [191]. Detachment of cytochrome c from the membrane is necessary for cytochrome c release for apoptotic activation and cristae remodeling [27]. As discussed above, these fundamental processes have been emphasized by the high percentage of mitochondrial-shaping proteins found to be altered in the context of Parkinson's disease in contrast with the proteins involved in fusion and fission.

The ER-mitochondrial connection is also important for the inflammatory response [192]. The activation of the inflammasome might occur under an oxidative stress scenario, i.e., Parkinson's disease, where there is an increase in ROS production by the mitochondria [192]. Specific receptors are translocated to the ER-mitochondrial contact sites in response to inflammation [192]. Besides, relevant to the activation of this inflammasome is the VDAC channel located at the mitochondria. Knockdown of both VDAC1 and -2 abolishes the inflammasome formation [192]. Both channels were found to be downregulated in our study. Furthermore, these channels interact with Bcl-2 proteins, therefore enabling cell survival [192,193].

5. Conclusions

The DA neuron loss from the SN constitutes a hallmark of Parkinson's disease. These neurons are known to be more susceptible than other DA neurons in the brain, and some of the referred sources for this vulnerability are associated with mitochondria. A more complex picture of the alterations of the mitochondria in Parkinson's disease is arising in addition to the widely known deficit in the mitochondrial Complex I dysfunction. Through the so-called "mitochondrial life cycle", these organelles can modulate their function and perform quality control. Accumulating evidence shows that there is a correlation between the morphology of these organelles and the cellular energy status. Increasing efforts have been made to associate the morphology of the mitochondria to its function. Importantly for a neurodegenerative disease such as Parkinson's disease, in which the causes have been linked to mitochondrial dysfunction, this type of analysis will aid in advancing the field, both in the pathobiology of the disease and the search for new therapies.

By network analysis we have correlated the changes in differentially expressed mitochondrial-shaping proteins in the context of Parkinson's disease with the corresponding biological pathways affected in the disease. One of the most striking findings is related to the process of cristae remodeling, since most of the mitochondrial-shaping proteins found to be altered in the context of Parkinson's disease participate in the maintenance of cristae shape. Remarkably, this alteration is evident in different human disorders, including Parkinson's disease. Since these structures regulate protein and lipid distribution as well as soluble molecules (i.e., ADP and cytochrome c), their alteration might have a direct impact on neuronal physiology and survival.

In our opinion, although it is clear in the cellular and animal models of the disease that mitochondrial morphology is altered, more studies from post mortem tissue from patients are needed, aiming at unravelling the alterations of the mitochondrial morphology more specifically related to the cristae shape in the context of Parkinson's disease. These studies would provide new insights into the development of new therapies or aid in biomarkers discovery. Identification of the mitochondrial components that play a role in the process of cristae remodeling might also be fundamental for these purposes.

Acknowledgments: This work was financed by FEDER—*Fundo Europeu de Desenvolvimento Regional* funds through the COMPETE 2020—Operacional Programme for Competitiveness and Internationalisation (POCI), Portugal 2020, and by Portuguese funds through FCT—Fundação para a Ciência e a Tecnologia/ Ministério da Ciência, Tecnologia e Inovação in the framework of the projects "Institute for Research and Innovation in Health Sciences" (POCI-01-0145-FEDER-007274), iBiMED (UID/BIM/04501/2013) and UnIC (UID/IC/00051/2013) research units, the COST ACTION CA15203, and the Investigator Grant to Rui Vitorino (IF/00286/2015). Ana Freitas acknowledges FCT for her Ph.D. scholarship (SFRH/BD/111423/2015), as does Sofia C. Guimaraes (SFRH/BPD/122920/2016), and Miguel Aroso (SFRH/BPD/123261/2016). Sara Rocha was founded by the project Norte-01-0145-FEDER-000008 -Porto Neurosciences and Neurologic Disease Research Initiative at I3S, supported by Norte Portugal Regional Operational Programme (NORTE 2020), under the PORTUGAL 2020 Partnership Agreement, through the European Regional Development Fund (FEDER)".

Author Contributions: Maria Gomez-Lazaro, Miguel Aroso, and Rui Vitorino conceived and designed the workflow of the paper; Maria Gomez-Lazaro, Sara Rocha, Sofia C. Guimaraes, Miguel Aroso, and Ana Freitas performed the literature search, collected the data meeting the criteria, performed the bioinformatics analysis and figures, and analyzed the data; Maria Gomez-Lazaro, Sara Rocha, Sofia C. Guimaraes, and Miguel Aroso wrote the paper; all authors revised the manuscript.

Conflicts of Interest: The authors declare no conflict of interest.

Abbreviations

ABPL	actin-binding-like protein
ACAD9	acyl-CoA dehydrogenase family member 9
ACP2	acid phosphatase 2, lysosomal
ACTB	actin beta
ACTBL2	actin, beta like 2
ACTN1	actinin alpha 1
AD030	ORF name for Mitochondrial Fission Factor
AD033	ORF name for mitochondrial Fission Factor
ADP	adenosine diphosphate
AHAS	acetolactate synthase-like protein
ALB	albumin
ALDA	aldolase, fructose-bisphosphate A
ALDH1B1	aldehyde dehydrogenase 1 family member B1
ALDH5	Aldehyde dehydrogenase 5
ALDHX	Aldehyde dehydrogenase X
ALDOA	aldolase, fructose-bisphosphate A
ALS2CR3	Amyotrophic lateral sclerosis 2 chromosomal region candidate gene 3 protein
ANT2	Adenine nucleotide translocator 2
ANX2	annexin 2
ANX2L4	annexin A2
ANX2LG	annexin A2 ligand
ANXA2	annexin A2
APOA1	apolipoprotein A1
APOO	apolipoprotein O
APOOL	apolipoprotein O like
ARALAR1/AGC1	aspartate-glutamate carrier 1
ARALAR2/AGC2	aspartate-glutamate carrier 2
ARH12	Aplysia ras-related homolog 12
ARHA	Ras Homolog Gene Family, Member A
ATP	adenosine triphosphate
ATP5A	ATP synthase subunit alpha
ATP5A1	ATP synthase subunit alpha subunit 1
ATP5AL2	ATP synthase subunit alpha
ATP5B	ATP synthase subunit beta
ATP5C1	ATP synthase subunit gamma subunit 1
ATP5D	ATP synthase subunit delta
ATP5E	ATP synthase subunit epsilon
ATP5F1	ATP synthase F(0) complex subunit B1
ATP5G1	ATP synthase F(0) complex subunit C1
ATP5G2	ATP synthase F(0) complex subunit C2
ATP5G3	ATP synthase F(0) complex subunit C3
ATP5H	ATP synthase subunit d
ATP5I	ATP synthase subunit e
ATP5J	ATP synthase-coupling factor 6
ATP5J2	ATP synthase subunit f
ATP5K	ATP synthase subunit e
ATP5L	ATP synthase subunit g
ATP5O	ATP synthase subunit O

ATPI	ATP synthase inhibitory factor
ATPIF1	ATP synthase inhibitory factor subunit 1
ATPM	ATP synthase subunit alpha, mitochondrial
ATPMB	ATP synthase subunit beta, mitochondrial
ATPSB	ATP synthase subunit beta
BHAK	Bcl-2 homologous antagonist killer
BAK	BCL2 antagonist killer 1
BAP	B-cell receptor-associated protein
BAP31	B cell receptor associated protein 31
BAX	BCL2 associated X, apoptosis regulator
BCAP31	B cell receptor associated protein 31
BCL2	B-cell lymphoma 2, apoptosis regulator
BCL2A1	BCL2 related protein A1
BCL2L11	BCL2 like protein 11
BCL2L3	BCL2 like protein 3
BCL2L4	BCL2 like protein 4
BCL2L5	BCL2 like protein 5
BCL2L7	BCL2 like protein 7
BCR	Breakpoint cluster region protein
BFL1	Bcl-2-related gene expressed in fetal liver
BID	BH3 interacting domain death agonist
BIK	BCL2 interacting killer
BIM	Bcl-2 Interacting Mediator of cell death
C11orf83	chromosome 11 open reading frame 83
C14orf151	chromosome 14 open reading frame 151
C14orf173	chromosome 14 open reading frame 73
C15orf13	chromosome 15 open reading frame 13
C19orf70	chromosome 19 open reading frame 70
C1orf151	chromosome 1 open reading frame 151
C1orf166	chromosome 1 open reading frame 166
C1QBP	complement C1q binding protein
C20orf52	chromosome 20 open reading frame 52
C2orf33	chromosome 2 open reading frame 33
C9orf54	chromosome 9 open reading frame 54
CAL1H	Calpactin I heavy polypeptide Protein
LPC2D	Lipocortin II
CAL1L	Calpactin-1 light chain
CALR	calreticulin
CCDC56	Cytochrome c oxidase assembly factor 3 homolog
CCT5	Chaperonin Containing TCP1 Subunit 5
CCTE	Chaperonin Containing TCP1, Subunit epsilon
CDM	Caldesmon
CDN1	synonym for Bcl-2 homologous antagonist/killer
CGI-106	comparative gene identification 106
CGI-135	comparative gene identification 135
CGI-51	comparative gene identification 51
CGI-61	comparative gene identification 61
CHCHD3	coiled-coil-helix-coiled-coil-helix domain containing 3
CLP11	human gene encoding p11
CMAR	Cell matrix adhesion regulator
COA3	cytochrome c oxidase assembly factor 3
COX4	Cytochrome c oxidase subunit 4 isoform 1
COX4I1	cytochrome c oxidase subunit 4I1
COX4I2	Cytochrome c oxidase subunit 4 isoform 2

COX5A	Cytochrome c oxidase subunit 5A
COX5B	Cytochrome c oxidase subunit 5B
COX6A1	Cytochrome c oxidase subunit 6A1
COX6A2	Cytochrome c oxidase subunit 6A2
COX6B1	Cytochrome c oxidase subunit 6B1
COX6B2	Cytochrome c oxidase subunit 6B2
COX6C	Cytochrome c oxidase subunit 6C
COX7A1	Cytochrome c oxidase subunit 7A1
COX7A2	Cytochrome c oxidase subunit 7A2
COX7B	Cytochrome c oxidase subunit 7B
COX7B2	Cytochrome c oxidase subunit 7B2
COX7C	Cytochrome c oxidase subunit 7C
COX8A	Cytochrome c oxidase subunit 8A
COX8C	cytochrome c oxidase subunit 8C
CPRP1	synonym of Mitofusin 2
CRTC	Calreticulin
CXorf33	Chromosome X open reading frame 33
CYC1	Ubiquinol-Cytochrome-C Reductase Complex Cytochrome C1 Subunit
CYPA	Peptidyl-prolyl cis-trans isomerase A
DA	dopaminergic
DAPIT	Diabetes-associated protein in insulin-sensitive tissues
DDAH	dimethylarginine dimethylaminohydrolase
DDAH1	dimethylarginine dimethylaminohydrolase 1
DDOST	dolichyl-diphosphooligosaccharide–protein glycosyltransferase non-catalytic subunit
DHC1	Cytoplasmic dynein 1 heavy chain 1
DIC	Mitochondrial dicarboxylate carrier
DJ-1	Protein/nucleic acid deglycase DJ-1
DLP1	dynamin like protein 1
DNA	Deoxyribonucleic acid
DNAJC19	DnaJ heat shock protein family (Hsp40) member C19
DNCH1	Cytoplasmic dynein 1 heavy chain 1
DNCL	Dynein light chain 1
DNECL	Cytoplasmic dynein 1 heavy chain 1
DNM1L	dynamin 1 like
DNM2	dynamin 2
DRP1	dynamin related protein 1
DXS1357E	p28 synonym
DYHC	Cytoplasmic dynein 1 heavy chain 1
DYN2	dynamin 2
DYNC1H1	dynein cytoplasmic 1 heavy chain 1
EC	Enzyme Commission number
EEF1A	eukaryotic translation elongation factor 1 alpha 1
EEF1A1	eukaryotic translation elongation factor 1 alpha 1
EEF1B	Elongation factor 1-beta
EEF1B2	Elongation factor 1-beta
EF1A	Elongation factor 1-alpha 1
EF1B	Elongation factor 1-beta
EFE2	endomyocardial fibroelastosis
EIF5A	eukaryotic translation initiation factor 5A
ER	endoplasmic reticulum
ERM	ezrin/moesin/radixin
ERP57	Endoplasmic reticulum resident protein 57
ERP60	Endoplasmic reticulum resident protein 60
FAM121A	Family With Sequence Similarity 121A
FAM121B	Family With Sequence Similarity 121A

FAM73A	Family With Sequence Similarity 73A
FAM73B	Family With Sequence Similarity 73B
FIS1	fission, mitochondrial 1
FKBP4	FK506 binding protein 4
FKBP52	Peptidyl-prolyl cis-trans isomerase FKBP4
FLN2	filamin 2
FLNC	filamin C
FLOT1	flotillin 1
FTSH1	ATP-dependent zinc metalloprotease YME1L1
FUBP1	far upstream element binding protein 1
FUNDC1	FUN14 domain containing 1
G4.5	synonym of Tafazzin
GARS	glycyl-tRNA synthetase
GC1QBP	complement C1q binding protein
GC2 B415	Glutamate carrier 2
GDAP1	ganglioside induced differentiation associated protein 1
GIDE	Mitochondrial ubiquitin ligase activator of NFKB 1
GIG20	growth-inhibiting gene 20
GIG42	growth-inhibiting gene 42
GL004	synonym of MFF
GRP58	58 kDa glucose-regulated protein
GRP75	75 kDa glucose-regulated protein
GRP78	78 kDa glucose-regulated protein
GRS	Glasgow rearranged sequence
GSTK1	glutathione S-transferase kappa 1
GSTO1	glutathione S-transferase omega 1
GSTTLP28	Glutathione S-transferase omega-1
HABP1	Hyaluronan Binding Protein 1
HACBP	High Affinity Calcium-Binding Protein
HBEBP2	HBEAG-binding protein 2
HBPA1	hematopoietic BCL2-related protein A1
HC8	human proteasome alpha-subunit C8
HCVFTP2	HCV F-Transactivated Protein 2
HDCMD47P	synonym of Glutathione S-transferase Subunit 13
hfzo1	human fuzzy onions 1
HIPPIE	Human Integrated Protein-Protein Interaction rEference web tool
HMP	synonym for inner membrane mitochondrial protein
HSC70	Heat shock cognate 71 kDa protein
HSP27	Heat shock protein beta-1
HSP28	Heat shock protein beta-1
HSP60	heat shock protein family D (Hsp60)
HSP73	Heat shock cognate 71 kDa protein
HSP90AB1	heat shock protein 90 alpha family class B member 1
HSP90B	heat shock protein 90 alpha family class B
HSPA10	Heat shock cognate 71 kDa protein
HSPA1L	heat shock protein family A (Hsp70) member 1 like
HSPA5	heat shock protein family A (Hsp70) member 5
HSPA8	heat shock protein family A (Hsp70) member 8
HSPA9	heat shock protein family A (Hsp70) member 9
HSPA9B	heat shock protein family A (Hsp70) member 9
HSPB1	heat shock protein family B (small) member 1
HSPC009	ORF name for Cytochrome c oxidase assembly factor 3 homolog
HSPC108	ORF name for Stomatin-like protein 2
HSPC2	Heat shock protein HSP 90-beta
HSPC242	ORF name for Mitochondrial fission process protein 1

HSPC263	ORF name for Ubiquitin thioesterase OTUB1
HSPCB	Heat shock protein HSP 90-beta
HSPD1	heat shock protein family D (Hsp60) member 1
IF(1)	Inhibitor Of F(1)F(O)-ATPase
ILVBL	gene ilvB acetolactate synthase like
IMM	inner mitochondrial membrane
IMMT	inner membrane mitochondrial protein
IMS	intermembrane space
INF2	protein inverted formin 2
IPS1	Interferon beta promoter stimulator protein 1
KIAA0098	synonym of CCT5
KIAA0115	synonym of DDOST
KIAA0214	synonym of Mitofusin-2
KIAA0313	synonym of RAPGEF2
KIAA0325	synonym of DYNC1H1
KIAA0348	synonym of SYNJ2
KIAA0491	synonym of SH3GLB1
KIAA0549	synonym of TRAK2
KIAA0567	synonym of Dynamin-like 120 kDa protein
KIAA1042	synonym of TRAK1
KIAA1271	synonym of MAVS
KIAA1848	synonym of SH3GLB2
LDHB	lactate dehydrogenase B
LEM6	Ligand effect modulator 6
LENG7	Elongation factor 1-alpha 1
LETM1	leucine zipper and EF-hand containing transmembrane protein 1
LGALS1	Lectin galactoside-binding soluble 1
LMN1	Prelamin-A/C
LMNA	Lamin A
MADH2	Mothers against decapentaplegic homolog 2
MADR2	Mad-related protein 2 Protein
MAP3K5	Mitogen-activated protein kinase kinase kinase 5
MAPL	Mitochondrial ubiquitin ligase activator of NFKB 1
MARCH5	membrane associated ring-CH-type finger 5
MAVS	mitochondrial antiviral signaling protein
MCL1	Induced myeloid leukemia cell differentiation protein Mcl-1
MDH2	malate dehydrogenase 2
MFF	mitochondrial fission factor
MFN1	mitofusin 1
MFN2	mitofusin 2
MIC 27	synonym for MICOS complex subunit MIC27
MIC10	synonym for MICOS complex subunit MI10
MIC13	synonym for MICOS complex subunit MIC13
MIC19	synonym for MICOS complex subunit MIC19
MIC23	synonym for MICOS complex subunit MIC23
MIC26	synonym for MICOS complex subunit MIC26
MIC60	synonym for MICOS complex subunit MIC60
MICOS	mitochondrial contact site and cristae organizing system
MID49	Mitochondrial dynamics protein MID49
MID51	Mitochondrial dynamics protein MID51
MIEF1	mitochondrial elongation factor 1
MIEF2	mitochondrial elongation factor 2
MIG10	Abnormal cell migration protein 10
MIG5	Abnormal cell migration protein 5

MIGA1	mitoguardin 1
MIGA2	mitoguardin 2
MINOS1	mitochondrial inner membrane organizing system 1
MINOS2	Mitochondrial Inner Membrane Organizing System 2
MINOS3	Mitochondrial Inner Membrane Organizing System 3
Mito_shape	Mitochondrial shaping proteins
MITRAC12	Cytochrome c oxidase assembly factor 3 homolog
MPP+	1-methyl-4-phenylpyridinium
MPRP1	multidrug resistance protein 1
MPTP	1-methyl-4-phenyl-1,2,3,6-tetrahydropyridine
MT-ATP6	Mitochondrially Encoded ATP Synthase 6
MT-ATP8	Mitochondrially Encoded ATP Synthase 8
MT-CO1	Mitochondrially Encoded Cytochrome C Oxidase I
MT-CO2	Mitochondrially Encoded Cytochrome C Oxidase II
MT-CO3	Mitochondrially Encoded Cytochrome C Oxidase III
MT-CYB	Mitochondrially Encoded Cytochrome B
MTFP1	mitochondrial fission process 1
mt-HSP70	mitochondrial heat shock protein family A (Hsp70)
MTP18	Mitochondrial fission process protein 1
MUL1	mitochondrial E3 ubiquitin protein ligase 1
MULAN	Mitochondrial ubiquitin ligase activator of NFKB 1
My022	ORF name for Mitochondrial fission process protein 1
My025	ORF name for MICOS complex subunit MIC26
My032	ORF name for ATP synthase subunit d
MYL6	myosin light chain 6
NAD	nicotinamide adenine dinucleotide oxidized
NADH	nicotinamide adenine dinucleotide reduced
NBK	Bcl-2-interacting killer
NDUFA10	NADH:ubiquinone oxidoreductase subunit A10
NDUFA11	NADH:ubiquinone oxidoreductase subunit A11
NDUFA4	NADH Dehydrogenase (Ubiquinone) 1 Alpha Subcomplex, 4
NDUFS1	NADH:ubiquinone oxidoreductase core subunit S1
NDUFS3	NADH:ubiquinone oxidoreductase core subunit S3
NEDD8	neural precursor cell expressed, developmentally down-regulated 8
NFE2L2	nuclear factor, erythroid 2 like 2
NFKB	nuclear factor kappa-light-chain-enhancer of activated B cells
NHERF	Na(+)/H(+) exchange regulatory cofactor NHE-RF1
NHERF1	Na(+)/H(+) exchange regulatory cofactor NHE-RF1
NHERF-1 protein	Na(+)/H(+) exchange regulatory cofactor NHE-RF1
NIMA	never in mitosis gene a
NO	nitric oxide
Nox1	NADPH oxidase 1
NPM	nucleophosmin
NPM1	nucleophosmin 1
NRAPGEP	Rap guanine nucleotide exchange factor 2
NRF1	nuclear respiratory factor 1
NRF2	Nuclear factor erythroid 2-related factor 2
OAT	ornithine aminotransferase
OGDH	oxoglutarate dehydrogenase
OIP106	O-linked *N*-acetylglucosamine transferase interacting protein 106
OK/SW-cl.110	ORF name for Phosphoglycerate kinase 1
OK/SW-cl.56	ORF name for Tubulin beta chain
OK/SW-cl.82	ORF name for 40S ribosomal protein S15a
OMA1	Overlapping Activity With M-AAA Protease

OMM	outer mitochondrial membrane
OPA1	Optic Atrophy Protein 1
OST48 OK/SW-cl.45	synomym for Dolichyl-diphosphooligosaccharide–protein glycosyltransferase 48 kDa subunit
OTB1	Ubiquitin thioesterase OTUB1
OTU1	Ubiquitin thioesterase OTUB1
OTUB1	OTU deubiquitinase, ubiquitin aldehyde binding 1
OXPHOS	oxidative phosphorylation
PARK2	E3 ubiquitin-protein ligase parkin
PARL	presenilin associated rhomboid like
PD	Parkinson's disease
PD04912	ORF name for Up-regulated during skeletal muscle growth protein 5
PDIA3	protein disulfide isomerase family A member 3
PDZGEF1	Rap guanine nucleotide exchange factor 2
PERC	Peroxisome proliferator-activated receptor gamma coactivator 1-beta
PGAM5	Serine/threonine-protein phosphatase PGAM5
PGC1	Peroxisome proliferator-activated receptor gamma coactivator 1-alpha
PGC1A	Peroxisome proliferator-activated receptor gamma coactivator 1-alpha
PGC1B	Peroxisome proliferator-activated receptor gamma coactivator 1-beta
PGK1	phosphoglycerate kinase 1
PGKA	Phosphoglycerate kinase 1
PGN	paraplegin
PHB	prohibitin
PHB2	prohibitin 2
PIG4	ORF name for MICOS complex subunit MIC60
PIG52	ORF name for MICOS complex subunit MIC60
PIN1	peptidylprolyl cis/trans isomerase, NIMA-interacting 1
PINK1	PTEN-induced putative kinase 1
PLD6	phospholipase D family member 6
PP578	ORF name for Endophilin-B2
PPARGC1	Peroxisome proliferator-activated receptor gamma coactivator 1-alpha
PPARGC1A	Peroxisome proliferator-activated receptor gamma coactivator 1-alpha
PPARGC1B	Peroxisome proliferator-activated receptor gamma coactivator 1-beta
PPIA	peptidylprolyl isomerase A
PRDX4	peroxiredoxin 4
PRELI	Protein Of Relevant Evolutionary And Lymphoid Interest
PRELID1	PRELI domain-containing protein 1
PRI	synonym for Ribonuclease inhibitor
PRKN	parkin RBR E3 ubiquitin protein ligase
PRO0903	ORF name for Serum albumin
PRO1708	ORF name for Serum albumin
PRO2044	ORF name for Serum albumin
PRO2207	ORF name for Presenilins-associated rhomboid-like protein
PRO2619	ORF name for Serum albumin
PRO2675	ORF name for Serum albumin
PSARL	Presenilins-associated rhomboid-like protein
PSC8	Proteasome component C8
PSEC0112	ORF name for Mitoguardin 2
PSMA3	proteasome subunit alpha 3
PTPN5	protein tyrosine phosphatase, non-receptor type 5
QIL1	synonym for Chromosome 19 Open Reading Frame 70
RAB14	Ras-related protein Rab-14
RAB2	Ras-related protein Rab2
RAB2A	Ras-related protein Rab-2A

RAC1	Ras-related C3 botulinum toxin substrate 1
RAPGEF2	Rap guanine nucleotide exchange factor 2
REA	synonym for Prohibitin-2
RHO12	ras homolog family member
RHOA	ras homolog family member A
RING-type E3	really interesting new gene type E3
RNF153	Ring Finger Protein 153
RNF218	Ring Finger Protein 218
RNH	Ribonuclease inhibitor
RNH1	ribonuclease/angiogenin inhibitor 1
ROMO1	reactive oxygen species modulator 1
ROS	reactive oxygen species
RPN1	Ribophorin I
RPN2	ribophorin II
RPS15A	ribosomal protein S15a
RPS3, OK/SW-cl.26	symbol and ORF name for 40S ribosomal protein S3
S100A10	S100 calcium binding protein A10
SAM50	Sorting and assembly machinery component 50 homolog
SAMM50	Sorting and assembly machinery component 50 homolog
SBBI12	ORF name for PRELI domain-containing protein 1
SBP	selenium binding protein
SELENBP1	selenium binding protein 1
SF2P32	nuclear splicing factor
SFXN1	sideroflexin 1
SH3	SRC Homology 3 Domain
SH3GLB1	SH3 domain containing GRB2 like, endophilin B1
SH3GLB2	SH3 domain containing GRB2 like, endophilin B2
SIR2L	SIR2-like protein
SIR2L2	SIR2-like protein 2
SIRT2	sirtuin 2
SLC20A4	solute carrier family 20 member 4
Slc25A	solute carrier family 25
SLC25A10	solute carrier family 25 member 10
SLC25A11	solute carrier family 25 member 11
SLC25A12	solute carrier family 25 member 12
SLC25A13	solute carrier family 25 member 13
SLC25A18	solute carrier family 25 member 18
SLC25A38	solute carrier family 25 member 38
SLC9A3R1	solute carrier family 9 (sodium/hydrogen exchanger), member 3 regulator 1
SLP2	Stomatin-like protein 2
SMAD2	Mothers against decapentaplegic homolog 2
SMCR7	Smith-Magenis Syndrome Chromosomal Region Candidate Gene 7 Protein
SMCR7L	Smith-Magenis Syndrome Chromosomal Region Candidate Gene 7 Protein-like
SN	Substantia nigra
SPG7	Paraplegin
SSBP	single stranded DNA binding protein
SSBP1	single stranded DNA binding protein 1
STOML2	stomatin like 2
SYNJ2	synaptojanin 2
TAZ	tafazzin
TC25	Ras-Like Protein TC25
TCA	tricarboxylic acid cycle
TCF6	Transcription factor
TCF6L2	Transcription Factor 6-Like 2

TCP-1-epsilon	T-complex protein 1 subunit epsilon
TFAM	transcription factor A, mitochondrial
TIM14	Mitochondrial Import Inner Membrane Translocase Subunit TIM14
TIMM14	Translocase Of Inner Mitochondrial Membrane 14
TMSA	Tropomyosin alpha-1 chain
TMSB	tropomyosin Beta
TPD52	tumor protein D52
TPM1	tropomyosin 1
TPM2	tropomyosin 2
TPM3	tropomyosin 3
TPM4	tropomyosin 4
TRAK1	trafficking kinesin protein 1
TRAK2	trafficking kinesin protein 2
TRG3	transformation-related gene 3
TTC11	tetratricopeptide Repeat Domain 11
TUBA1A	tubulin alpha 1a
TUBA3	tubulin alpha-3 chain
TUBB	tubulin beta class I
TUBB2C	Tubulin beta-4B chain
TUBB4B	tubulin beta 4B class IVb
TUBB5	Tubulin beta chain
TUFM	Tu translation elongation factor, mitochondrial
UniProt	Universal Protein Resource
UNQ1866/PRO4302	ORF name for MICOS complex subunit MIC26
UNQ1868/PRO4304	ORF name for ATP-dependent zinc metalloprotease YME1L1
UNQ655/PRO1286	ORF name for Ubiquinol-cytochrome-c reductase complex assembly factor 3
UNQ696/PRO1341	ORF name for Serum albumin
UNQ8193/PRO23204	ORF for MICOS complex subunit MIC27
UQBP	Ubiquinol-cytochrome c reductase complex 14 kDa protein
UQCC3	ubiquinol-cytochrome c reductase complex assembly factor 3
UQCR10	Ubiquinol-Cytochrome C Reductase, Complex III Subunit X
UQCR11	Ubiquinol-Cytochrome C Reductase, Complex III Subunit XI
UQCRB	ubiquinol-cytochrome c reductase binding protein
UQCRC1	ubiquinol-cytochrome c reductase core protein 1
UQCRC2	ubiquinol-cytochrome c reductase core protein 2
UQCRFS1	ubiquinol-cytochrome c reductase, Rieske iron-sulfur polypeptide 1
UQCRFS1	ubiquinol-cytochrome c reductase, Rieske iron-sulfur polypeptide 1
UQCRFS1P1	ubiquinol-cytochrome c reductase, Rieske iron-sulfur polypeptide 1 pseudogene 1
UQCRFSL1	Ubiquinol-cytochrome c reductase Rieske iron-sulfur subunit pseudogene 1
UQCRH	ubiquinol-cytochrome c reductase hinge protein
UQCRQ	ubiquinol-cytochrome c reductase complex ubiquinone-binding protein QP-C
USMG5	Up-regulated during skeletal muscle growth protein 5
VAT1	vesicle amine transport 1
VCP	valosin containing protein
VDAC1	Voltage-dependent anion-selective channel protein 1
VDAC2	voltage dependent anion channel 2
VDAC3	voltage dependent anion channel 3
VDAC	Voltage-dependent anion-selective channel
VIM	vimentin
VISA	Virus-induced-signaling adapter
YME1L	YME1-like protein 1
YME1L1	YME1-like protein 1
YWHAE	tyrosine 3-monooxygenase/tryptophan 5-monooxygenase activation protein epsilon
YWHAZ	tyrosine 3-monooxygenase/tryptophan 5-monooxygenase activation protein zeta

References

1. Kasahara, A.; Scorrano, L. Mitochondria: From cell death executioners to regulators of cell differentiation. *Trends Cell Biol.* **2014**, *24*, 761–770. [CrossRef] [PubMed]
2. Anesti, V.; Scorrano, L. The relationship between mitochondrial shape and function and the cytoskeleton. *Biochim. Biophys. Acta* **2006**, *1757*, 692–699. [CrossRef] [PubMed]
3. Pernas, L.; Scorrano, L. Mito-morphosis: Mitochondrial fusion, fission, and cristae remodeling as key mediators of cellular function. *Annu. Rev. Physiol.* **2016**, *78*, 505–531. [CrossRef] [PubMed]
4. Gao, J.; Wang, L.; Liu, J.; Xie, F.; Su, B.; Wang, X. Abnormalities of mitochondrial dynamics in neurodegenerative diseases. *Antioxidants* **2017**, *6*, 25. [CrossRef] [PubMed]
5. Muangpaisan, W.; Mathews, A.; Hori, H.; Seidel, D. A systematic review of the worldwide prevalence and incidence of Parkinson's disease. *J. Med. Assoc. Thail.* **2011**, *94*, 749–755.
6. Antony, P.M.; Diederich, N.J.; Kruger, R.; Balling, R. The hallmarks of Parkinson's disease. *FEBS J.* **2013**, *280*, 5981–5993. [CrossRef] [PubMed]
7. Schapira, A.H.; Cooper, J.M.; Dexter, D.; Jenner, P.; Clark, J.B.; Marsden, C.D. Mitochondrial complex I deficiency in Parkinson's disease. *Lancet* **1989**, *1*, 1269. [CrossRef]
8. Schapira, A.H.; Cooper, J.M.; Dexter, D.; Clark, J.B.; Jenner, P.; Marsden, C.D. Mitochondrial complex I deficiency in Parkinson's disease. *J. Neurochem.* **1990**, *54*, 823–827. [CrossRef] [PubMed]
9. Haylett, W.; Swart, C.; van der Westhuizen, F.; van Dyk, H.; van der Merwe, L.; van der Merwe, C.; Loos, B.; Carr, J.; Kinnear, C.; Bardien, S. Altered mitochondrial respiration and other features of mitochondrial function in parkin-mutant fibroblasts from Parkinson's disease patients. *Parkinson's Dis.* **2016**, *2016*, 1819209.
10. Hao, L.Y.; Giasson, B.I.; Bonini, N.M. Dj-1 is critical for mitochondrial function and rescues pink1 loss of function. *Proc. Natl. Acad. Sci. USA* **2010**, *107*, 9747–9752. [CrossRef] [PubMed]
11. Ahmad, T.; Aggarwal, K.; Pattnaik, B.; Mukherjee, S.; Sethi, T.; Tiwari, B.K.; Kumar, M.; Micheal, A.; Mabalirajan, U.; Ghosh, B.; et al. Computational classification of mitochondrial shapes reflects stress and redox state. *Cell Death Dis.* **2013**, *4*, e461. [CrossRef] [PubMed]
12. Haddad, D.; Nakamura, K. Understanding the susceptibility of dopamine neurons to mitochondrial stressors in Parkinson's disease. *FEBS Lett.* **2015**, *589*, 3702–3713. [CrossRef] [PubMed]
13. Apweiler, R.; Bairoch, A.; Wu, C.H.; Barker, W.C.; Boeckmann, B.; Ferro, S.; Gasteiger, E.; Huang, H.; Lopez, R.; Magrane, M.; et al. Uniprot: The universal protein knowledgebase. *Nucleic Acids Res.* **2017**, *45*, D158–D169. [CrossRef] [PubMed]
14. Friedman, J.R.; Mourier, A.; Yamada, J.; McCaffery, J.M.; Nunnari, J. MICOS coordinates with respiratory complexes and lipids to establish inner mitochondrial membrane architecture. *eLife* **2015**, *4*. [CrossRef] [PubMed]
15. Ikon, N.; Ryan, R.O. Cardiolipin and mitochondrial cristae organization. *Biochim. Biophys. Acta* **2017**, *1859*, 1156–1163. [CrossRef] [PubMed]
16. Koob, S.; Barrera, M.; Anand, R.; Reichert, A.S. The non-glycosylated isoform of MIC26 is a constituent of the mammalian MICOS complex and promotes formation of crista junctions. *Biochimi. Biophys. Acta* **2015**, *1853*, 1551–1563. [CrossRef] [PubMed]
17. Wilkens, V.; Kohl, W.; Busch, K. Restricted diffusion of OXPHOS complexes in dynamic mitochondria delays their exchange between cristae and engenders a transitory mosaic distribution. *J. Cell Sci.* **2013**, *126*, 103–116. [CrossRef] [PubMed]
18. Cogliati, S.; Enriquez, J.A.; Scorrano, L. Mitochondrial cristae: Where beauty meets functionality. *Trends Biochem. Sci.* **2016**, *41*, 261–273. [CrossRef] [PubMed]
19. van der Bliek, A.M.; Shen, Q.; Kawajiri, S. Mechanisms of mitochondrial fission and fusion. *Cold Spring Harb. Perspect. Biol.* **2013**, *5*, a011072. [CrossRef] [PubMed]
20. Faccenda, D.; Tan, C.H.; Seraphim, A.; Duchen, M.R.; Campanella, M. IF1 limits the apoptotic-signalling cascade by preventing mitochondrial remodelling. *Cell Death Differ.* **2013**, *20*, 686–697. [CrossRef] [PubMed]
21. Luna-Vargas, M.P.; Chipuk, J.E. Physiological and pharmacological control of BAK, BAX, and beyond. *Trends Cell Biol.* **2016**, *26*, 906–917. [CrossRef] [PubMed]
22. Campello, S.; Scorrano, L. Mitochondrial shape changes: Orchestrating cell pathophysiology. *EMBO Rep.* **2010**, *11*, 678–684. [CrossRef] [PubMed]

23. Scorrano, L. Opening the doors to cytochrome c: Changes in mitochondrial shape and apoptosis. *Int. J. Biochem. Cell Biol.* **2009**, *41*, 1875–1883. [CrossRef] [PubMed]
24. Valero, J.G.; Cornut-Thibaut, A.; Juge, R.; Debaud, A.L.; Gimenez, D.; Gillet, G.; Bonnefoy-Berard, N.; Salgado, J.; Salles, G.; Aouacheria, A.; et al. Micro-calpain conversion of antiapoptotic Bfl-1 (BCL2A1) into a prodeath factor reveals two distinct alpha-helices inducing mitochondria-mediated apoptosis. *PLoS ONE* **2012**, *7*, e38620. [CrossRef] [PubMed]
25. Wasilewski, M.; Scorrano, L. The changing shape of mitochondrial apoptosis. *Trends Endocrinol. Metab.* **2009**, *20*, 287–294. [CrossRef] [PubMed]
26. Yamaguchi, R.; Lartigue, L.; Perkins, G.; Scott, R.T.; Dixit, A.; Kushnareva, Y.; Kuwana, T.; Ellisman, M.H.; Newmeyer, D.D. Opa1-mediated cristae opening is Bax/Bak and BH3 dependent, required for apoptosis, and independent of Bak oligomerization. *Mol. Cell* **2008**, *31*, 557–569. [CrossRef] [PubMed]
27. Scorrano, L.; Ashiya, M.; Buttle, K.; Weiler, S.; Oakes, S.A.; Mannella, C.A.; Korsmeyer, S.J. A distinct pathway remodels mitochondrial cristae and mobilizes cytochrome *c* during apoptosis. *Dev. Cell* **2002**, *2*, 55–67. [CrossRef]
28. Germain, M.; Mathai, J.P.; McBride, H.M.; Shore, G.C. Endoplasmic reticulum Bik initiates DRP1-regulated remodelling of mitochondrial cristae during apoptosis. *EMBO J.* **2005**, *24*, 1546–1556. [CrossRef] [PubMed]
29. Ong, S.B.; Kalkhoran, S.B.; Hernandez-Resendiz, S.; Samangouei, P.; Ong, S.G.; Hausenloy, D.J. Mitochondrial-shaping proteins in cardiac health and disease—The long and the short of it! *Cardiovasc. Drugs Ther. Spons. Int. Soc. Cardiovasc. Pharmacother.* **2017**, *31*, 87–107. [CrossRef] [PubMed]
30. Ban-Ishihara, R.; Tomohiro-Takamiya, S.; Tani, M.; Baudier, J.; Ishihara, N.; Kuge, O. COX assembly factor ccdc56 regulates mitochondrial morphology by affecting mitochondrial recruitment of Drp1. *FEBS Lett.* **2015**, *589*, 3126–3132. [CrossRef] [PubMed]
31. Richter-Dennerlein, R.; Korwitz, A.; Haag, M.; Tatsuta, T.; Dargazanli, S.; Baker, M.; Decker, T.; Lamkemeyer, T.; Rugarli, E.I.; Langer, T. DNAJC19, a mitochondrial cochaperone associated with cardiomyopathy, forms a complex with prohibitins to regulate cardiolipin remodeling. *Cell Metab.* **2014**, *20*, 158–171. [CrossRef] [PubMed]
32. Davey, K.M.; Parboosingh, J.S.; McLeod, D.R.; Chan, A.; Casey, R.; Ferreira, P.; Snyder, F.F.; Bridge, P.J.; Bernier, F.P. Mutation of DNAJC19, a human homologue of yeast inner mitochondrial membrane co-chaperones, causes DCMA syndrome, a novel autosomal recessive Barth syndrome-like condition. *J. Med. Genet.* **2006**, *43*, 385–393. [CrossRef] [PubMed]
33. Lee, J.E.; Westrate, L.M.; Wu, H.; Page, C.; Voeltz, G.K. Multiple dynamin family members collaborate to drive mitochondrial division. *Nature* **2016**, *540*, 139–143. [CrossRef] [PubMed]
34. Chen, M.; Chen, Z.; Wang, Y.; Tan, Z.; Zhu, C.; Li, Y.; Han, Z.; Chen, L.; Gao, R.; Liu, L.; et al. Mitophagy receptor FUNDC1 regulates mitochondrial dynamics and mitophagy. *Autophagy* **2016**, *12*, 689–702. [CrossRef] [PubMed]
35. Liu, L.; Feng, D.; Chen, G.; Chen, M.; Zheng, Q.; Song, P.; Ma, Q.; Zhu, C.; Wang, R.; Qi, W.; et al. Mitochondrial outer-membrane protein FUNDC1 mediates hypoxia-induced mitophagy in mammalian cells. *Nat. Cell Biol.* **2012**, *14*, 177–185. [CrossRef] [PubMed]
36. Gomes, L.C.; Scorrano, L. Mitochondrial morphology in mitophagy and macroautophagy. *Biochim. Biophys. Acta* **2013**, *1833*, 205–212. [CrossRef] [PubMed]
37. John, G.B.; Shang, Y.; Li, L.; Renken, C.; Mannella, C.A.; Selker, J.M.; Rangell, L.; Bennett, M.J.; Zha, J. The inner mitochondrial membrane protein mitofilin controls cristae morphology. *Mol. Biol. Cell* **2005**, *16*, 1543–1554. [CrossRef] [PubMed]
38. Korobova, F.; Ramabhadran, V.; Higgs, H.N. An actin-dependent step in mitochondrial fission mediated by the ER-associated formin INF2. *Science* **2013**, *339*, 464–467. [CrossRef] [PubMed]
39. Dimmer, K.S.; Navoni, F.; Casarin, A.; Trevisson, E.; Endele, S.; Winterpacht, A.; Salviati, L.; Scorrano, L. *LETM1*, deleted in Wolf-Hirschhorn syndrome is required for normal mitochondrial morphology and cellular viability. *Hum. Mol. Genet.* **2008**, *17*, 201–214. [CrossRef] [PubMed]
40. Koshiba, T. Mitochondrial-mediated antiviral immunity. *Biochim. Biophys. Acta* **2013**, *1833*, 225–232. [CrossRef] [PubMed]
41. Perciavalle, R.M.; Stewart, D.P.; Koss, B.; Lynch, J.; Milasta, S.; Bathina, M.; Temirov, J.; Cleland, M.M.; Pelletier, S.; Schuetz, J.D.; et al. Anti-apoptotic MCL-1 localizes to the mitochondrial matrix and couples mitochondrial fusion to respiration. *Nat. Cell Biol.* **2012**, *14*, 575–583. [CrossRef] [PubMed]

42. Morciano, G.; Giorgi, C.; Balestra, D.; Marchi, S.; Perrone, D.; Pinotti, M.; Pinton, P. MCL-1 involvement in mitochondrial dynamics is associated with apoptotic cell death. *Mol. Biol. Cell* **2016**, *27*, 20–34. [CrossRef] [PubMed]
43. Chen, H.; Detmer, S.A.; Ewald, A.J.; Griffin, E.E.; Fraser, S.E.; Chan, D.C. Mitofusins Mfn1 and Mfn2 coordinately regulate mitochondrial fusion and are essential for embryonic development. *J. Cell Biol.* **2003**, *160*, 189–200. [CrossRef] [PubMed]
44. Zhang, Y.; Liu, X.; Bai, J.; Tian, X.; Zhao, X.; Liu, W.; Duan, X.; Shang, W.; Fan, H.Y.; Tong, C. Mitoguardin regulates mitochondrial fusion through mitopld and is required for neuronal homeostasis. *Mol. Cell* **2016**, *61*, 111–124. [CrossRef] [PubMed]
45. Wai, T.; Langer, T. Mitochondrial dynamics and metabolic regulation. *Trends Endocrinol. Metab.* **2016**, *27*, 105–117. [CrossRef] [PubMed]
46. Yin, X.; Manczak, M.; Reddy, P.H. Mitochondria-targeted molecules MitoQ and SS31 reduce mutant huntingtin-induced mitochondrial toxicity and synaptic damage in Huntington's disease. *Hum. Mol. Genet.* **2016**, *25*, 1739–1753. [CrossRef] [PubMed]
47. Dinkova-Kostova, A.T.; Abramov, A.Y. The emerging role of Nrf2 in mitochondrial function. *Free Radic. Biol. Med.* **2015**, *88*, 179–188. [CrossRef] [PubMed]
48. Bereiter-Hahn, J.; Jendrach, M. Mitochondrial dynamics. *Int. Rev. Cell Mol. Biol.* **2010**, *284*, 1–65. [PubMed]
49. Dabrowska, A.; Venero, J.L.; Iwasawa, R.; Hankir, M.K.; Rahman, S.; Boobis, A.; Hajji, N. PGC-1alpha controls mitochondrial biogenesis and dynamics in lead-induced neurotoxicity. *Aging* **2015**, *7*, 629–647. [CrossRef] [PubMed]
50. Patten, D.A.; Wong, J.; Khacho, M.; Soubannier, V.; Mailloux, R.J.; Pilon-Larose, K.; MacLaurin, J.G.; Park, D.S.; McBride, H.M.; Trinkle-Mulcahy, L.; et al. Opa1-dependent cristae modulation is essential for cellular adaptation to metabolic demand. *EMBO J.* **2014**, *33*, 2676–2691. [CrossRef] [PubMed]
51. Hall, A.R.; Burke, N.; Dongworth, R.K.; Hausenloy, D.J. Mitochondrial fusion and fission proteins: Novel therapeutic targets for combating cardiovascular disease. *Br. J. Pharmacol.* **2014**, *171*, 1890–1906. [CrossRef] [PubMed]
52. Wang, Z.; Jiang, H.; Chen, S.; Du, F.; Wang, X. The mitochondrial phosphatase PGAM5 functions at the convergence point of multiple necrotic death pathways. *Cell* **2012**, *148*, 228–243. [CrossRef] [PubMed]
53. Merkwirth, C.; Dargazanli, S.; Tatsuta, T.; Geimer, S.; Lower, B.; Wunderlich, F.T.; von Kleist-Retzow, J.C.; Waisman, A.; Westermann, B.; Langer, T. Prohibitins control cell proliferation and apoptosis by regulating opa1-dependent cristae morphogenesis in mitochondria. *Genes Dev.* **2008**, *22*, 476–488. [CrossRef] [PubMed]
54. Buhlman, L.; Damiano, M.; Bertolin, G.; Ferrando-Miguel, R.; Lombes, A.; Brice, A.; Corti, O. Functional interplay between parkin and Drp1 in mitochondrial fission and clearance. *Biochim. Biophys. Acta* **2014**, *1843*, 2012–2026. [CrossRef] [PubMed]
55. LeBleu, V.S.; O'Connell, J.T.; Gonzalez Herrera, K.N.; Wikman, H.; Pantel, K.; Haigis, M.C.; de Carvalho, F.M.; Damascena, A.; Domingos Chinen, L.T.; Rocha, R.M.; et al. PGC-1alpha mediates mitochondrial biogenesis and oxidative phosphorylation in cancer cells to promote metastasis. *Nat. Cell Biol.* **2014**, *16*, 992–1003. [CrossRef] [PubMed]
56. Shao, D.; Liu, Y.; Liu, X.; Zhu, L.; Cui, Y.; Cui, A.; Qiao, A.; Kong, X.; Chen, Q.; Gupta, N.; et al. PGC-1 beta-regulated mitochondrial biogenesis and function in myotubes is mediated by Nrf-1 and ERR alpha. *Mitochondrion* **2010**, *10*, 516–527. [CrossRef] [PubMed]
57. Sesaki, H.; Dunn, C.D.; Iijima, M.; Shepard, K.A.; Yaffe, M.P.; Machamer, C.E.; Jensen, R.E. Ups1p, a conserved intermembrane space protein, regulates mitochondrial shape and alternative topogenesis of Mgm1p. *J. Cell Biol.* **2006**, *173*, 651–658. [CrossRef] [PubMed]
58. Hartmann, B.; Wai, T.; Hu, H.; MacVicar, T.; Musante, L.; Fischer-Zirnsak, B.; Stenzel, W.; Graf, R.; van den Heuvel, L.; Ropers, H.H.; et al. Homozygous YME1L1 mutation causes mitochondriopathy with optic atrophy and mitochondrial network fragmentation. *eLife* **2016**, *5*, e16078. [CrossRef] [PubMed]
59. Gomes, L.C.; Di Benedetto, G.; Scorrano, L. During autophagy mitochondria elongate, are spared from degradation and sustain cell viability. *Nat. Cell Biol.* **2011**, *13*, 589–598. [CrossRef] [PubMed]
60. Shaltouki, A.; Sivapatham, R.; Pei, Y.; Gerencser, A.A.; Momcilovic, O.; Rao, M.S.; Zeng, X. Mitochondrial alterations by PARKIN in dopaminergic neurons using PARK2 patient-specific and *PARK2* knockout isogenic IPSC lines. *Stem Cell Rep.* **2015**, *4*, 847–859. [CrossRef] [PubMed]

61. Norton, M.; Ng, A.C.; Baird, S.; Dumoulin, A.; Shutt, T.; Mah, N.; Andrade-Navarro, M.A.; McBride, H.M.; Screaton, R.A. ROMO1 is an essential redox-dependent regulator of mitochondrial dynamics. *Sci. Signal.* **2014**, *7*, ra10. [CrossRef] [PubMed]
62. Karbowski, M.; Jeong, S.Y.; Youle, R.J. Endophilin B1 is required for the maintenance of mitochondrial morphology. *J. Cell Biol.* **2004**, *166*, 1027–1039. [CrossRef] [PubMed]
63. Wang, Y.H.; Wang, J.Q.; Wang, Q.; Wang, Y.; Guo, C.; Chen, Q.; Chai, T.; Tang, T.S. Endophilin B2 promotes inner mitochondrial membrane degradation by forming heterodimers with endophilin B1 during mitophagy. *Sci. Rep.* **2016**, *6*, 25153. [CrossRef] [PubMed]
64. Zhang, C.; Shi, Z.; Zhang, L.; Zhou, Z.; Zheng, X.; Liu, G.; Bu, G.; Fraser, P.E.; Xu, H.; Zhang, Y.W. Appoptosin interacts with mitochondrial outer-membrane fusion proteins and regulates mitochondrial morphology. *J. Cell Sci.* **2016**, *129*, 994–1002. [CrossRef] [PubMed]
65. Kumar, S.; Pan, C.C.; Shah, N.; Wheeler, S.E.; Hoyt, K.R.; Hempel, N.; Mythreye, K.; Lee, N.Y. Activation of mitofusin2 by smad2-RIN1 complex during mitochondrial fusion. *Mol. Cell* **2016**, *62*, 520–531. [CrossRef] [PubMed]
66. Nemoto, Y.; De Camilli, P. Recruitment of an alternatively spliced form of synaptojanin 2 to mitochondria by the interaction with the PDZ domain of a outer mitochondrial membrane protein. *EMBO J.* **1999**, *18*, 2991–3006. [CrossRef] [PubMed]
67. Gonzalvez, F.; D'Aurelio, M.; Boutant, M.; Moustapha, A.; Puech, J.P.; Landes, T.; Arnaune-Pelloquin, L.; Vial, G.; Taleux, N.; Slomianny, C.; et al. Barth syndrome: Cellular compensation of mitochondrial dysfunction and apoptosis inhibition due to changes in cardiolipin remodeling linked to *tafazzin* (TAZ) gene mutation. *Biochim. Biophys. Acta* **2013**, *1832*, 1194–1206. [CrossRef] [PubMed]
68. Acehan, D.; Xu, Y.; Stokes, D.L.; Schlame, M. Comparison of lymphoblast mitochondria from normal subjects and patients with barth syndrome using electron microscopic tomography. *Lab. Investig. J. Tech. Methods Pathol.* **2007**, *87*, 40–48. [CrossRef] [PubMed]
69. Desmurs, M.; Foti, M.; Raemy, E.; Vaz, F.M.; Martinou, J.C.; Bairoch, A.; Lane, L. C11orf83, a mitochondrial cardiolipin-binding protein involved in *bc1* complex assembly and supercomplex stabilization. *Mol. Cell. Biol.* **2015**, *35*, 1139–1156. [CrossRef] [PubMed]
70. Eura, Y.; Ishihara, N.; Oka, T.; Mihara, K. Identification of a novel protein that regulates mitochondrial fusion by modulating mitofusin (Mfn) protein function. *J. Cell Sci.* **2006**, *119*, 4913–4925. [CrossRef] [PubMed]
71. Oliveros, J.C. Venny. An Interactive Tool for Comparing Lists with Venn's Diagrams. Available online: http://bioinfogp.cnb.csic.es/tools/venny/index.html (accessed on 29 August 2017).
72. Alanis-Lobato, G.; Andrade-Navarro, M.A.; Schaefer, M.H. Hippie v2.0: Enhancing meaningfulness and reliability of protein-protein interaction networks. *Nucleic Acids Res.* **2017**, *45*, D408–D414. [CrossRef] [PubMed]
73. Gomez-Lazaro, M.; Bonekamp, N.A.; Galindo, M.F.; Jordan, J.; Schrader, M. 6-hydroxydopamine (6-OHDA) induces Drp1-dependent mitochondrial fragmentation in SH-SY5Y cells. *Free Radic. Biol. Med.* **2008**, *44*, 1960–1969. [CrossRef] [PubMed]
74. Yang, Y.; Lu, B. Mitochondrial morphogenesis, distribution, and Parkinson disease: Insights from pink1. *J. Neuropathol. Exp. Neurol.* **2009**, *68*, 953–963. [CrossRef] [PubMed]
75. Winklhofer, K.F.; Haass, C. Mitochondrial dysfunction in Parkinson's disease. *Biochim. Biophys. Acta* **2010**, *1802*, 29–44. [CrossRef] [PubMed]
76. Wiemerslage, L.; Ismael, S.; Lee, D. Early alterations of mitochondrial morphology in dopaminergic neurons from Parkinson's disease-like pathology and time-dependent neuroprotection with D2 receptor activation. *Mitochondrion* **2016**, *30*, 138–147. [CrossRef] [PubMed]
77. Van Laar, V.S.; Berman, S.B. Mitochondrial dynamics in Parkinson's disease. *Exp. Neurol.* **2009**, *218*, 247–256. [CrossRef] [PubMed]
78. Lee, H.J.; Khoshaghideh, F.; Lee, S.; Lee, S.J. Impairment of microtubule-dependent trafficking by overexpression of alpha-synuclein. *Eur. J. Neurosci.* **2006**, *24*, 3153–3162. [CrossRef] [PubMed]
79. Gillardon, F. Leucine-rich repeat kinase 2 phosphorylates brain tubulin-beta isoforms and modulates microtubule stability—A point of convergence in Parkinsonian neurodegeneration? *J. Neurochem.* **2009**, *110*, 1514–1522. [CrossRef] [PubMed]

80. Lutz, A.K.; Exner, N.; Fett, M.E.; Schlehe, J.S.; Kloos, K.; Lammermann, K.; Brunner, B.; Kurz-Drexler, A.; Vogel, F.; Reichert, A.S.; et al. Loss of parkin or PINK1 function increases Drp1-dependent mitochondrial fragmentation. *J. Biol. Chem.* **2009**, *284*, 22938–22951. [CrossRef] [PubMed]
81. Sandebring, A.; Thomas, K.J.; Beilina, A.; van der Brug, M.; Cleland, M.M.; Ahmad, R.; Miller, D.W.; Zambrano, I.; Cowburn, R.F.; Behbahani, H.; et al. Mitochondrial alterations in PINK1 deficient cells are influenced by calcineurin-dependent dephosphorylation of dynamin-related protein 1. *PLoS ONE* **2009**, *4*, e5701. [CrossRef] [PubMed]
82. Dagda, R.K.; Gusdon, A.M.; Pien, I.; Strack, S.; Green, S.; Li, C.; Van Houten, B.; Cherra, S.J., 3rd; Chu, C.T. Mitochondrially localized PKA reverses mitochondrial pathology and dysfunction in a cellular model of Parkinson's disease. *Cell Death Differ.* **2011**, *18*, 1914–1923. [CrossRef] [PubMed]
83. Van Laar, V.S.; Arnold, B.; Cassady, S.J.; Chu, C.T.; Burton, E.A.; Berman, S.B. Bioenergetics of neurons inhibit the translocation response of parkin following rapid mitochondrial depolarization. *Hum. Mol. Genet.* **2011**, *20*, 927–940. [CrossRef] [PubMed]
84. Chen, Y.; Csordas, G.; Jowdy, C.; Schneider, T.G.; Csordas, N.; Wang, W.; Liu, Y.; Kohlhaas, M.; Meiser, M.; Bergem, S.; et al. Mitofusin 2-containing mitochondrial-reticular microdomains direct rapid cardiomyocyte bioenergetic responses via interorganelle Ca(2+) crosstalk. *Circ. Res.* **2012**, *111*, 863–875. [CrossRef] [PubMed]
85. Zuchner, S.; Mersiyanova, I.V.; Muglia, M.; Bissar-Tadmouri, N.; Rochelle, J.; Dadali, E.L.; Zappia, M.; Nelis, E.; Patitucci, A.; Senderek, J.; et al. Mutations in the mitochondrial GTPase mitofusin 2 cause charcot-marie-tooth neuropathy type 2A. *Nat. Genet.* **2004**, *36*, 449–451. [CrossRef] [PubMed]
86. Hoekstra, J.G.; Cook, T.J.; Stewart, T.; Mattison, H.; Dreisbach, M.T.; Hoffer, Z.S.; Zhang, J. Astrocytic dynamin-like protein 1 regulates neuronal protection against excitotoxicity in Parkinson disease. *Am. J. Pathol.* **2015**, *185*, 536–549. [CrossRef] [PubMed]
87. Jin, J.; Hulette, C.; Wang, Y.; Zhang, T.; Pan, C.; Wadhwa, R.; Zhang, J. Proteomic identification of a stress protein, mortalin/mthsp70/GRP75: Relevance to Parkinson disease. *Mol. Cell. Proteom.* **2006**, *5*, 1193–1204. [CrossRef] [PubMed]
88. Jakobs, S.; Wurm, C.A. Super-resolution microscopy of mitochondria. *Curr. Opin. Chem. Biol.* **2014**, *20*, 9–15. [CrossRef] [PubMed]
89. Jans, D.C.; Wurm, C.A.; Riedel, D.; Wenzel, D.; Stagge, F.; Deckers, M.; Rehling, P.; Jakobs, S. Sted super-resolution microscopy reveals an array of minos clusters along human mitochondria. *Proc. Natl. Acad. Sci. USA* **2013**, *110*, 8936–8941. [CrossRef] [PubMed]
90. Pfanner, N.; van der Laan, M.; Amati, P.; Capaldi, R.A.; Caudy, A.A.; Chacinska, A.; Darshi, M.; Deckers, M.; Hoppins, S.; Icho, T.; et al. Uniform nomenclature for the mitochondrial contact site and cristae organizing system. *J. Cell Biol.* **2014**, *204*, 1083–1086. [CrossRef] [PubMed]
91. Ott, C.; Ross, K.; Straub, S.; Thiede, B.; Gotz, M.; Goosmann, C.; Krischke, M.; Mueller, M.J.; Krohne, G.; Rudel, T.; et al. Sam50 functions in mitochondrial intermembrane space bridging and biogenesis of respiratory complexes. *Mol. Cell. Biol.* **2012**, *32*, 1173–1188. [CrossRef] [PubMed]
92. Tondera, D.; Grandemange, S.; Jourdain, A.; Karbowski, M.; Mattenberger, Y.; Herzig, S.; Da Cruz, S.; Clerc, P.; Raschke, I.; Merkwirth, C.; et al. SLP-2 is required for stress-induced mitochondrial hyperfusion. *EMBO J.* **2009**, *28*, 1589–1600. [CrossRef] [PubMed]
93. Steglich, G.; Neupert, W.; Langer, T. Prohibitins regulate membrane protein degradation by the m-AAA protease in mitochondria. *Mol. Cell. Biol.* **1999**, *19*, 3435–3442. [CrossRef] [PubMed]
94. Nijtmans, L.G.; de Jong, L.; Artal Sanz, M.; Coates, P.J.; Berden, J.A.; Back, J.W.; Muijsers, A.O.; van der Spek, H.; Grivell, L.A. Prohibitins act as a membrane-bound chaperone for the stabilization of mitochondrial proteins. *EMBO J.* **2000**, *19*, 2444–2451. [CrossRef] [PubMed]
95. Paumard, P.; Vaillier, J.; Coulary, B.; Schaeffer, J.; Soubannier, V.; Mueller, D.M.; Brethes, D.; di Rago, J.P.; Velours, J. The ATP synthase is involved in generating mitochondrial cristae morphology. *EMBO J.* **2002**, *21*, 221–230. [CrossRef] [PubMed]
96. Habersetzer, J.; Larrieu, I.; Priault, M.; Salin, B.; Rossignol, R.; Brethes, D.; Paumard, P. Human F1F0 ATP synthase, mitochondrial ultrastructure and OXPHOS impairment: A (super-) complex matter? *PLoS ONE* **2013**, *8*, e75429. [CrossRef] [PubMed]
97. Strauss, M.; Hofhaus, G.; Schroder, R.R.; Kuhlbrandt, W. Dimer ribbons of ATP synthase shape the inner mitochondrial membrane. *EMBO J.* **2008**, *27*, 1154–1160. [CrossRef] [PubMed]

98. Cereghetti, G.M.; Stangherlin, A.; Martins de Brito, O.; Chang, C.R.; Blackstone, C.; Bernardi, P.; Scorrano, L. Dephosphorylation by calcineurin regulates translocation of Drp1 to mitochondria. *Proc. Natl. Acad. Sci. USA* **2008**, *105*, 15803–15808. [CrossRef] [PubMed]
99. Schaefer, M.H.; Fontaine, J.F.; Vinayagam, A.; Porras, P.; Wanker, E.E.; Andrade-Navarro, M.A. Hippie: Integrating protein interaction networks with experiment based quality scores. *PLoS ONE* **2012**, *7*, e31826. [CrossRef] [PubMed]
100. Schaefer, M.H.; Lopes, T.J.; Mah, N.; Shoemaker, J.E.; Matsuoka, Y.; Fontaine, J.F.; Louis-Jeune, C.; Eisfeld, A.J.; Neumann, G.; Perez-Iratxeta, C.; et al. Adding protein context to the human protein-protein interaction network to reveal meaningful interactions. *PLoS Comput. Biol.* **2013**, *9*, e1002860. [CrossRef] [PubMed]
101. Suratanee, A.; Schaefer, M.H.; Betts, M.J.; Soons, Z.; Mannsperger, H.; Harder, N.; Oswald, M.; Gipp, M.; Ramminger, E.; Marcus, G.; et al. Characterizing protein interactions employing a genome-wide sirna cellular phenotyping screen. *PLoS Comput. Biol.* **2014**, *10*, e1003814. [CrossRef] [PubMed]
102. Bragoszewski, P.; Gornicka, A.; Sztolsztener, M.E.; Chacinska, A. The ubiquitin-proteasome system regulates mitochondrial intermembrane space proteins. *Mol. Cell. Biol.* **2013**, *33*, 2136–2148. [CrossRef] [PubMed]
103. Bragoszewski, P.; Turek, M.; Chacinska, A. Control of mitochondrial biogenesis and function by the ubiquitin-proteasome system. *Open Biol.* **2017**, *7*, 170007. [CrossRef] [PubMed]
104. Cook, C.; Petrucelli, L. A critical evaluation of the ubiquitin-proteasome system in Parkinson's disease. *Biochim. Biophys. Acta* **2009**, *1792*, 664–675. [CrossRef] [PubMed]
105. Hwang, O. Role of oxidative stress in Parkinson's disease. *Exp. Neurobiol.* **2013**, *22*, 11–17. [CrossRef] [PubMed]
106. Danielson, S.R.; Andersen, J.K. Oxidative and nitrative protein modifications in Parkinson's disease. *Free Radic. Biol. Med.* **2008**, *44*, 1787–1794. [CrossRef] [PubMed]
107. Friedman, J.R.; Lackner, L.L.; West, M.; DiBenedetto, J.R.; Nunnari, J.; Voeltz, G.K. ER tubules mark sites of mitochondrial division. *Science* **2011**, *334*, 358–362. [CrossRef] [PubMed]
108. Cartelli, D.; Casagrande, F.; Busceti, C.L.; Bucci, D.; Molinaro, G.; Traficante, A.; Passarella, D.; Giavini, E.; Pezzoli, G.; Battaglia, G.; et al. Microtubule alterations occur early in experimental Parkinsonism and the microtubule stabilizer epothilone D is neuroprotective. *Sci. Rep.* **2013**, *3*, 1837. [CrossRef] [PubMed]
109. Jensen, R.E. Control of mitochondrial shape. *Curr. Opin. Cell Biol.* **2005**, *17*, 384–388. [CrossRef] [PubMed]
110. Bleier, L.; Drose, S. Superoxide generation by complex III: From mechanistic rationales to functional consequences. *Biochim. Biophys. Acta* **2013**, *1827*, 1320–1331. [CrossRef] [PubMed]
111. Muller, F.L.; Liu, Y.; Van Remmen, H. Complex III releases superoxide to both sides of the inner mitochondrial membrane. *J. Biol. Chem.* **2004**, *279*, 49064–49073. [CrossRef] [PubMed]
112. Cartelli, D.; Goldwurm, S.; Casagrande, F.; Pezzoli, G.; Cappelletti, G. Microtubule destabilization is shared by genetic and idiopathic Parkinson's disease patient fibroblasts. *PLoS ONE* **2012**, *7*, e37467. [CrossRef]
113. Passmore, J.B.; Pinho, S.; Gomez-Lazaro, M.; Schrader, M. The respiratory chain inhibitor rotenone affects peroxisomal dynamics via its microtubule-destabilising activity. *Histochem. Cell Biol.* **2017**, *148*, 331–341. [CrossRef] [PubMed]
114. Bindea, G.; Mlecnik, B.; Hackl, H.; Charoentong, P.; Tosolini, M.; Kirilovsky, A.; Fridman, W.H.; Pages, F.; Trajanoski, Z.; Galon, J. ClueGo: A cytoscape plug-in to decipher functionally grouped gene ontology and pathway annotation networks. *Bioinformatics* **2009**, *25*, 1091–1093. [CrossRef] [PubMed]
115. Tieu, K.; Ischiropoulos, H.; Przedborski, S. Nitric oxide and reactive oxygen species in Parkinson's disease. *IUBMB Life* **2003**, *55*, 329–335. [CrossRef] [PubMed]
116. Wei, T.; Chen, C.; Hou, J.; Xin, W.; Mori, A. Nitric oxide induces oxidative stress and apoptosis in neuronal cells. *Biochim. Biophys. Acta* **2000**, *1498*, 72–79. [CrossRef]
117. Pierini, D.; Bryan, N.S. Nitric oxide availability as a marker of oxidative stress. *Methods Mol. Biol.* **2015**, *1208*, 63–71. [PubMed]
118. Smeyne, M.; Smeyne, R.J. Glutathione metabolism and Parkinson's disease. *Free Radic. Biol. Med.* **2013**, *62*, 13–25. [CrossRef] [PubMed]
119. Baraibar, M.A.; Liu, L.; Ahmed, E.K.; Friguet, B. Protein oxidative damage at the crossroads of cellular senescence, aging, and age-related diseases. *Oxid. Med. Cell. Longev.* **2012**, *2012*, 919832. [CrossRef] [PubMed]
120. Dasgupta, A.; Zheng, J.; Bizzozero, O.A. Protein carbonylation and aggregation precede neuronal apoptosis induced by partial glutathione depletion. *ASN Neuro* **2012**, *4*, e00084. [CrossRef] [PubMed]

121. Mattenberger, Y.; James, D.I.; Martinou, J.C. Fusion of mitochondria in mammalian cells is dependent on the inner mitochondrial membrane potential and independent of microtubules or actin. *FEBS Lett.* **2003**, *538*, 53–59. [CrossRef]
122. Brackley, K.I.; Grantham, J. Activities of the chaperonin containing TCP-1 (CCT): Implications for cell cycle progression and cytoskeletal organisation. *Cell Stress Chaperones* **2009**, *14*, 23–31. [CrossRef] [PubMed]
123. Choi, D.H.; Cristovao, A.C.; Guhathakurta, S.; Lee, J.; Joh, T.H.; Beal, M.F.; Kim, Y.S. NADPH oxidase 1-mediated oxidative stress leads to dopamine neuron death in Parkinson's disease. *Antioxid. Redox Signal.* **2012**, *16*, 1033–1045. [CrossRef] [PubMed]
124. Murthy, A.; Gonzalez-Agosti, C.; Cordero, E.; Pinney, D.; Candia, C.; Solomon, F.; Gusella, J.; Ramesh, V. NHE-RF, a regulatory cofactor for Na(+)-H+ exchange, is a common interactor for merlin and ERM (MERM) proteins. *J. Biol. Chem.* **1998**, *273*, 1273–1276. [CrossRef] [PubMed]
125. Ghosh, A.; Saminathan, H.; Kanthasamy, A.; Anantharam, V.; Jin, H.; Sondarva, G.; Harischandra, D.S.; Qian, Z.; Rana, A.; Kanthasamy, A.G. The Peptidyl-prolyl Isomerase Pin1 Up-regulation and Proapoptotic Function in Dopaminergic Neurons: Relevance to the pathogenesis of Parkinson disease. *J. Biol. Chem.* **2013**, *288*, 21955–21971. [CrossRef] [PubMed]
126. Braithwaite, A.W.; Del Sal, G.; Lu, X. Some p53-binding proteins that can function as arbiters of life and death. *Cell Death Differ.* **2006**, *13*, 984–993. [CrossRef] [PubMed]
127. Schmidt, O.; Harbauer, A.B.; Rao, S.; Eyrich, B.; Zahedi, R.P.; Stojanovski, D.; Schonfisch, B.; Guiard, B.; Sickmann, A.; Pfanner, N.; et al. Regulation of mitochondrial protein import by cytosolic kinases. *Cell* **2011**, *144*, 227–239. [CrossRef] [PubMed]
128. North, B.J.; Marshall, B.L.; Borra, M.T.; Denu, J.M.; Verdin, E. The human Sir2 ortholog, Sirt2, is an NAD+-dependent tubulin deacetylase. *Mol. Cell* **2003**, *11*, 437–444. [CrossRef]
129. Janke, C. The tubulin code: Molecular components, readout mechanisms, and functions. *J. Cell Biol.* **2014**, *206*, 461–472. [CrossRef] [PubMed]
130. Loeffler, D.A.; Camp, D.M.; Conant, S.B. Complement activation in the Parkinson's disease substantia nigra: An immunocytochemical study. *J. Neuroinflamm.* **2006**, *3*, 29. [CrossRef] [PubMed]
131. Coates, P.J.; Nenutil, R.; McGregor, A.; Picksley, S.M.; Crouch, D.H.; Hall, P.A.; Wright, E.G. Mammalian prohibitin proteins respond to mitochondrial stress and decrease during cellular senescence. *Exp. Cell Res.* **2001**, *265*, 262–273. [CrossRef] [PubMed]
132. Ros-Bernal, F.; Hunot, S.; Herrero, M.T.; Parnadeau, S.; Corvol, J.C.; Lu, L.; Alvarez-Fischer, D.; Carrillo-de Sauvage, M.A.; Saurini, F.; Coussieu, C.; et al. Microglial glucocorticoid receptors play a pivotal role in regulating dopaminergic neurodegeneration in Parkinsonism. *Proc. Natl. Acad. Sci. USA* **2011**, *108*, 6632–6637. [CrossRef] [PubMed]
133. Herrero, M.T.; Estrada, C.; Maatouk, L.; Vyas, S. Inflammation in Parkinson's disease: Role of glucocorticoids. *Front. Neuroanat.* **2015**, *9*, 32. [CrossRef] [PubMed]
134. Ahn, E.H.; Kim, D.W.; Shin, M.J.; Kim, Y.N.; Kim, H.R.; Woo, S.J.; Kim, S.M.; Kim, D.S.; Kim, J.; Park, J.; et al. PEP-1-ribosomal protein S3 protects dopaminergic neurons in an MPTP-induced Parkinson's disease mouse model. *Free Radic. Biol. Med.* **2013**, *55*, 36–45. [CrossRef] [PubMed]
135. Morales, M.; Colicos, M.A.; Goda, Y. Actin-dependent regulation of neurotransmitter release at central synapses. *Neuron* **2000**, *27*, 539–550. [CrossRef]
136. Kawamoto, Y.; Akiguchi, I.; Nakamura, S.; Honjyo, Y.; Shibasaki, H.; Budka, H. 14-3-3 proteins in lewy bodies in Parkinson disease and diffuse lewy body disease brains. *J. Neuropathol. Exp. Neurol.* **2002**, *61*, 245–253. [CrossRef] [PubMed]
137. Fabelo, N.; Martin, V.; Santpere, G.; Marin, R.; Torrent, L.; Ferrer, I.; Diaz, M. Severe alterations in lipid composition of frontal cortex lipid rafts from Parkinson's disease and incidental Parkinson's disease. *Mol. Med.* **2011**, *17*, 1107–1118. [CrossRef] [PubMed]
138. Kubo, S.; Hatano, T.; Hattori, N. Lipid rafts involvement in the pathogenesis of Parkinson's disease. *Front. Biosci.* **2015**, *20*, 263–279. [CrossRef]
139. Cha, S.H.; Choi, Y.R.; Heo, C.H.; Kang, S.J.; Joe, E.H.; Jou, I.; Kim, H.M.; Park, S.M. Loss of parkin promotes lipid rafts-dependent endocytosis through accumulating caveolin-1: Implications for Parkinson's disease. *Mol. Neurodegener.* **2015**, *10*, 63. [CrossRef] [PubMed]
140. Donato, R.; Cannon, B.R.; Sorci, G.; Riuzzi, F.; Hsu, K.; Weber, D.J.; Geczy, C.L. Functions of S100 proteins. *Curr. Mol. Med.* **2013**, *13*, 24–57. [CrossRef] [PubMed]

141. Warner-Schmidt, J.L.; Chen, E.Y.; Zhang, X.; Marshall, J.J.; Morozov, A.; Svenningsson, P.; Greengard, P. A role for p11 in the antidepressant action of brain-derived neurotrophic factor. *Biol. Psychiatry* **2010**, *68*, 528–535. [CrossRef] [PubMed]
142. Rezvanpour, A.; Santamaria-Kisiel, L.; Shaw, G.S. The S100A10-annexin A2 complex provides a novel asymmetric platform for membrane repair. *J. Biol. Chem.* **2011**, *286*, 40174–40183. [CrossRef] [PubMed]
143. Bieberich, E. Synthesis, processing, and function of *N*-glycans in *N*-glycoproteins. *Adv. Neurobiol.* **2014**, *9*, 47–70. [PubMed]
144. Scott, H.; Panin, V.M. The role of protein *N*-glycosylation in neural transmission. *Glycobiology* **2014**, *24*, 407–417. [CrossRef] [PubMed]
145. Picconi, B.; Piccoli, G.; Calabresi, P. Synaptic dysfunction in Parkinson's disease. *Adv. Exp. Med. Biol.* **2012**, *970*, 553–572. [PubMed]
146. Mercado, G.; Valdes, P.; Hetz, C. An ercentric view of Parkinson's disease. *Trends Mol. Med.* **2013**, *19*, 165–175. [CrossRef] [PubMed]
147. Broers, J.L.; Ramaekers, F.C.; Bonne, G.; Yaou, R.B.; Hutchison, C.J. Nuclear lamins: Laminopathies and their role in premature ageing. *Physiol. Rev.* **2006**, *86*, 967–1008. [CrossRef] [PubMed]
148. Van de Vosse, D.W.; Wan, Y.; Wozniak, R.W.; Aitchison, J.D. Role of the nuclear envelope in genome organization and gene expression. *Wiley Interdiscip. Rev. Syst. Biol. Med.* **2011**, *3*, 147–166. [CrossRef] [PubMed]
149. Simon, D.N.; Zastrow, M.S.; Wilson, K.L. Direct actin binding to A- and B-type lamin tails and actin filament bundling by the lamin A tail. *Nucleus* **2010**, *1*, 264–272. [CrossRef] [PubMed]
150. Nauseef, W.M.; McCormick, S.J.; Clark, R.A. Calreticulin functions as a molecular chaperone in the biosynthesis of myeloperoxidase. *J. Biol. Chem.* **1995**, *270*, 4741–4747. [CrossRef] [PubMed]
151. Oka, O.B.; Pringle, M.A.; Schopp, I.M.; Braakman, I.; Bulleid, N.J. Erdj5 is the ER reductase that catalyzes the removal of non-native disulfides and correct folding of the LDL receptor. *Mol. Cell* **2013**, *50*, 793–804. [CrossRef] [PubMed]
152. Langston, J.W.; Ballard, P.A., Jr. Parkinson's disease in a chemist working with 1-methyl-4-phenyl-1,2,5,6-tetrahydropyridine. *N. Engl. J. Med.* **1983**, *309*, 310. [PubMed]
153. Gautier, C.A.; Corti, O.; Brice, A. Mitochondrial dysfunctions in Parkinson's disease. *Rev. Neurol.* **2014**, *170*, 339–343. [CrossRef] [PubMed]
154. Aroso, M.; Ferreira, R.; Freitas, A.; Vitorino, R.; Gomez-Lazaro, M. New insights on the mitochondrial proteome plasticity in Parkinson's disease. *Proteom. Clin. Appl.* **2016**, *10*, 416–429. [CrossRef] [PubMed]
155. Perier, C.; Tieu, K.; Guegan, C.; Caspersen, C.; Jackson-Lewis, V.; Carelli, V.; Martinuzzi, A.; Hirano, M.; Przedborski, S.; Vila, M. Complex I deficiency primes Bax-dependent neuronal apoptosis through mitochondrial oxidative damage. *Proc. Natl. Acad. Sci. USA* **2005**, *102*, 19126–19131. [CrossRef] [PubMed]
156. Waterham, H.R.; Koster, J.; van Roermund, C.W.; Mooyer, P.A.; Wanders, R.J.; Leonard, J.V. A lethal defect of mitochondrial and peroxisomal fission. *N. Engl. J. Med.* **2007**, *356*, 1736–1741. [CrossRef] [PubMed]
157. Vila, M.; Przedborski, S. Genetic clues to the pathogenesis of Parkinson's disease. *Nat. Med.* **2004**, *10*, S58–S62. [CrossRef] [PubMed]
158. Barsoum, M.J.; Yuan, H.; Gerencser, A.A.; Liot, G.; Kushnareva, Y.; Graber, S.; Kovacs, I.; Lee, W.D.; Waggoner, J.; Cui, J.; et al. Nitric oxide-induced mitochondrial fission is regulated by dynamin-related GTPases in neurons. *EMBO J.* **2006**, *25*, 3900–3911. [CrossRef] [PubMed]
159. Frank, S.; Gaume, B.; Bergmann-Leitner, E.S.; Leitner, W.W.; Robert, E.G.; Catez, F.; Smith, C.L.; Youle, R.J. The role of dynamin-related protein 1, a mediator of mitochondrial fission, in apoptosis. *Dev. Cell* **2001**, *1*, 515–525. [CrossRef]
160. Trimmer, P.A.; Swerdlow, R.H.; Parks, J.K.; Keeney, P.; Bennett, J.P., Jr.; Miller, S.W.; Davis, R.E.; Parker, W.D., Jr. Abnormal mitochondrial morphology in sporadic Parpkinson's and Alzheimer's disease cybrid cell lines. *Exp. Neurol.* **2000**, *162*, 37–50. [CrossRef] [PubMed]
161. Gilkerson, R.W.; Selker, J.M.; Capaldi, R.A. The cristal membrane of mitochondria is the principal site of oxidative phosphorylation. *FEBS Lett.* **2003**, *546*, 355–358. [CrossRef]
162. Mannella, C.A. Structure and dynamics of the inner mitochondrial membrane cristae. *Biochim. Biophys. Acta* **2006**, *1763*, 542–548. [CrossRef] [PubMed]
163. Zick, M.; Rabl, R.; Reichert, A.S. Cristae formation-linking ultrastructure and function of mitochondria. *Biochim. Biophys. Acta* **2009**, *1793*, 5–19. [CrossRef] [PubMed]

164. Perier, C.; Bove, J.; Vila, M. Mitochondria and programmed cell death in Parkinson's disease: Apoptosis and beyond. *Antioxid. Redox Signal.* **2012**, *16*, 883–895. [CrossRef] [PubMed]
165. Vila, M.; Przedborski, S. Targeting programmed cell death in neurodegenerative diseases. *Nat. Rev. Neurosci.* **2003**, *4*, 365–375. [CrossRef] [PubMed]
166. Marchi, S.; Patergnani, S.; Pinton, P. The endoplasmic reticulum-mitochondria connection: One touch, multiple functions. *Biochim. Biophys. Acta* **2014**, *1837*, 461–469. [CrossRef] [PubMed]
167. Shim, S.H.; Xia, C.; Zhong, G.; Babcock, H.P.; Vaughan, J.C.; Huang, B.; Wang, X.; Xu, C.; Bi, G.Q.; Zhuang, X. Super-resolution fluorescence imaging of organelles in live cells with photoswitchable membrane probes. *Proc. Natl. Acad. Sci. USA* **2012**, *109*, 13978–13983. [CrossRef] [PubMed]
168. Sheehan, J.P.; Swerdlow, R.H.; Parker, W.D.; Miller, S.W.; Davis, R.E.; Tuttle, J.B. Altered calcium homeostasis in cells transformed by mitochondria from individuals with Parkinson's disease. *J. Neurochem.* **1997**, *68*, 1221–1233. [CrossRef] [PubMed]
169. Giacomello, M.; Drago, I.; Pizzo, P.; Pozzan, T. Mitochondrial Ca^{2+} as a key regulator of cell life and death. *Cell Death Differ.* **2007**, *14*, 1267–1274. [CrossRef] [PubMed]
170. Hedskog, L.; Pinho, C.M.; Filadi, R.; Ronnback, A.; Hertwig, L.; Wiehager, B.; Larssen, P.; Gellhaar, S.; Sandebring, A.; Westerlund, M.; et al. Modulation of the endoplasmic reticulum-mitochondria interface in Alzheimer's disease and related models. *Proc. Natl. Acad. Sci. USA* **2013**, *110*, 7916–7921. [CrossRef] [PubMed]
171. Gleichmann, M.; Mattson, M.P. Neuronal calcium homeostasis and dysregulation. *Antioxid. Redox Signal.* **2011**, *14*, 1261–1273. [CrossRef] [PubMed]
172. Szabadkai, G.; Bianchi, K.; Varnai, P.; De Stefani, D.; Wieckowski, M.R.; Cavagna, D.; Nagy, A.I.; Balla, T.; Rizzuto, R. Chaperone-mediated coupling of endoplasmic reticulum and mitochondrial Ca^{2+} channels. *J. Cell Biol.* **2006**, *175*, 901–911. [CrossRef] [PubMed]
173. Hayashi, T.; Su, T.P. Sigma-1 receptor chaperones at the ER-mitochondrion interface regulate Ca^{2+} signaling and cell survival. *Cell* **2007**, *131*, 596–610. [CrossRef] [PubMed]
174. Mercado, G.; Castillo, V.; Soto, P.; Sidhu, A. ER stress and Parkinson's disease: Pathological inputs that converge into the secretory pathway. *Brain Res.* **2016**, *1648*, 626–632. [CrossRef] [PubMed]
175. Iwasawa, R.; Mahul-Mellier, A.L.; Datler, C.; Pazarentzos, E.; Grimm, S. Fis1 and Bap31 bridge the mitochondria-ER interface to establish a platform for apoptosis induction. *EMBO J.* **2011**, *30*, 556–568. [CrossRef] [PubMed]
176. Verfaillie, T.; Rubio, N.; Garg, A.D.; Bultynck, G.; Rizzuto, R.; Decuypere, J.P.; Piette, J.; Linehan, C.; Gupta, S.; Samali, A.; et al. Perk is required at the ER-mitochondrial contact sites to convey apoptosis after ROS-based ER stress. *Cell Death Differ.* **2012**, *19*, 1880–1891. [CrossRef] [PubMed]
177. Hamasaki, M.; Furuta, N.; Matsuda, A.; Nezu, A.; Yamamoto, A.; Fujita, N.; Oomori, H.; Noda, T.; Haraguchi, T.; Hiraoka, Y.; et al. Autophagosomes form at ER-mitochondria contact sites. *Nature* **2013**, *495*, 389–393. [CrossRef] [PubMed]
178. de Brito, O.M.; Scorrano, L. Mitofusin 2 tethers endoplasmic reticulum to mitochondria. *Nature* **2008**, *456*, 605–610. [CrossRef] [PubMed]
179. Keating, D.J. Mitochondrial dysfunction, oxidative stress, regulation of exocytosis and their relevance to neurodegenerative diseases. *J. Neurochem.* **2008**, *104*, 298–305. [CrossRef] [PubMed]
180. Brown, M.R.; Sullivan, P.G.; Geddes, J.W. Synaptic mitochondria are more susceptible to Ca^{2+} overload than nonsynaptic mitochondria. *J. Biol. Chem.* **2006**, *281*, 11658–11668. [CrossRef] [PubMed]
181. Hollenbeck, P.J. The pattern and mechanism of mitochondrial transport in axons. *Front. Biosci. J. Virtual Libr.* **1996**, *1*, d91–d102. [CrossRef]
182. Jung, C.; Chylinski, T.M.; Pimenta, A.; Ortiz, D.; Shea, T.B. Neurofilament transport is dependent on actin and myosin. *J. Neurosci. Off. J. Soc. Neurosci.* **2004**, *24*, 9486–9496. [CrossRef] [PubMed]
183. Schon, E.A.; Przedborski, S. Mitochondria: The next (neurode) generation. *Neuron* **2011**, *70*, 1033–1053. [CrossRef] [PubMed]
184. Kim-Han, J.S.; Antenor-Dorsey, J.A.; O'Malley, K.L. The Parkinsonian mimetic, MPP+, specifically impairs mitochondrial transport in dopamine axons. *J. Neurosci. Off. J. Soc. Neurosci.* **2011**, *31*, 7212–7221. [CrossRef] [PubMed]
185. Dauer, W.; Przedborski, S. Parkinson's disease: Mechanisms and models. *Neuron* **2003**, *39*, 889–909. [CrossRef]

186. Osman, C.; Voelker, D.R.; Langer, T. Making heads or tails of phospholipids in mitochondria. *J. Cell Biol.* **2011**, *192*, 7–16. [CrossRef] [PubMed]
187. Choi, S.Y.; Huang, P.; Jenkins, G.M.; Chan, D.C.; Schiller, J.; Frohman, M.A. A common lipid links mfn-mediated mitochondrial fusion and snare-regulated exocytosis. *Nat. Cell Biol.* **2006**, *8*, 1255–1262. [CrossRef] [PubMed]
188. Montessuit, S.; Somasekharan, S.P.; Terrones, O.; Lucken-Ardjomande, S.; Herzig, S.; Schwarzenbacher, R.; Manstein, D.J.; Bossy-Wetzel, E.; Basanez, G.; Meda, P.; et al. Membrane remodeling induced by the dynamin-related protein Drp1 stimulates Bax oligomerization. *Cell* **2010**, *142*, 889–901. [CrossRef] [PubMed]
189. Macdonald, P.J.; Stepanyants, N.; Mehrotra, N.; Mears, J.A.; Qi, X.; Sesaki, H.; Ramachandran, R. A dimeric equilibrium intermediate nucleates Drp1 reassembly on mitochondrial membranes for fission. *Mol. Biol. Cell* **2014**, *25*, 1905–1915. [CrossRef] [PubMed]
190. Kiebish, M.A.; Han, X.; Cheng, H.; Lunceford, A.; Clarke, C.F.; Moon, H.; Chuang, J.H.; Seyfried, T.N. Lipidomic analysis and electron transport chain activities in c57bl/6j mouse brain mitochondria. *J. Neurochem.* **2008**, *106*, 299–312. [CrossRef] [PubMed]
191. Davey, G.P.; Peuchen, S.; Clark, J.B. Energy thresholds in brain mitochondria. Potential involvement in neurodegeneration. *J. Biol. Chem.* **1998**, *273*, 12753–12757. [CrossRef] [PubMed]
192. Zhou, R.; Yazdi, A.S.; Menu, P.; Tschopp, J. A role for mitochondria in NLRP3 inflammasome activation. *Nature* **2011**, *469*, 221–225. [CrossRef] [PubMed]
193. Arbel, N.; Shoshan-Barmatz, V. Voltage-dependent anion channel 1-based peptides interact with Bcl-2 to prevent antiapoptotic activity. *J. Biol. Chem.* **2010**, *285*, 6053–6062. [CrossRef] [PubMed]

12

Targeting Oxidative Stress and Mitochondrial Dysfunction in the Treatment of Impaired Wound Healing

Mariola Cano Sanchez [1,2], Steve Lancel [3], Eric Boulanger [4,5] and Remi Neviere [1,4,6,*]

[1] Laboratory of Cardiovascular Physiology, Antilles University, P-97200 Fort de France, France; mariola.cano@uvic.cat
[2] Tissue Repair and Regeneration Laboratory (TR2Lab), University of Vic-UCC, Vic P-08500 Barcelone, Spain
[3] INSERM U1011-EGID, Institut Pasteur de Lille, Université Lille, CHU Lille, F-59000 Lille, France; slancel@univ-lille2.fr
[4] INSERM U995-LIRIC Inflammation Research International Centre, Université Lille, F-59000 Lille, France; eric.boulanger@univ-lille.fr
[5] Département de Gériatrie, CHU Lille, F-59000 Lille, France
[6] Département de Physiologie, CHU Lille, F-59000 Lille, France
* Correspondence: remi.neviere@chu-martinique.fr

Abstract: Wound healing is a well-tuned biological process, which is achieved via consecutive and overlapping phases including hemostasis, inflammatory-related events, cell proliferation and tissue remodeling. Several factors can impair wound healing such as oxygenation defects, aging, and stress as well as deleterious health conditions such as infection, diabetes, alcohol overuse, smoking and impaired nutritional status. Growing evidence suggests that reactive oxygen species (ROS) are crucial regulators of several phases of healing processes. ROS are centrally involved in all wound healing processes as low concentrations of ROS generation are required for the fight against invading microorganisms and cell survival signaling. Excessive production of ROS or impaired ROS detoxification causes oxidative damage, which is the main cause of non-healing chronic wounds. In this context, experimental and clinical studies have revealed that antioxidant and anti-inflammatory strategies have proven beneficial in the non-healing state. Among available antioxidant strategies, treatments using mitochondrial-targeted antioxidants are of particular interest. Specifically, mitochondrial-targeted peptides such as elamipretide have the potential to mitigate mitochondrial dysfunction and aberrant inflammatory response through activation of nucleotide-binding oligomerization domain (NOD)-like family receptors, such as the pyrin domain containing 3 (NLRP3) inflammasome, nuclear factor-kappa B (NF-κB) signaling pathway inhibition, and nuclear factor (erythroid-derived 2)-like 2 (Nrf2).

Keywords: wound healing; reactive oxygen species; mitochondria; advanced glycation end products; diabetes; inflammation; antioxidants

---

1. Introduction

Wound healing is a well-tuned biological process, which is achieved via consecutive and overlapping phases including hemostasis, inflammatory-related events, cell proliferation and tissue remodeling [1,2]. Redox signaling and increased oxidative stress play a significant role in regulating normal wound healing by facilitating hemostasis, inflammation, angiogenesis, granulation tissue formation, wound closure, and development and maturation of the extracellular matrix [3]. ROS (reactive oxygen species) are centrally involved in all wound healing processes as low concentrations of ROS generation are required to fight against invading microorganisms and cell surviving signaling [3–6]. Excessive and uncontrolled oxidative stress contribute to sustaining and deregulating inflammation processes, which play a central role in the pathogenesis of chronic non-healing wounds [6,7]. In line, antioxidant and anti-inflammatory properties of several antioxidant strategies have proven beneficial to improve non-healing state [8–10]. This review will examine the role of redox signaling and oxidative stress in the etiology of impaired wound healing, with a particular focus on the development of treatment strategies based on mitochondrial-targeted antioxidants.

2. Normal Wound Healing and Redox Regulation

2.1. Wound Healing Phases

The complex molecular and cellular processes of wound healing occur in overlapping phases consisting of inflammation, formation of the granulation tissue including myofibroblast accumulation, extracellular matrix synthesis, angiogenesis, re-epithelialization, and tissue remodeling [1,2] (Figure 1).

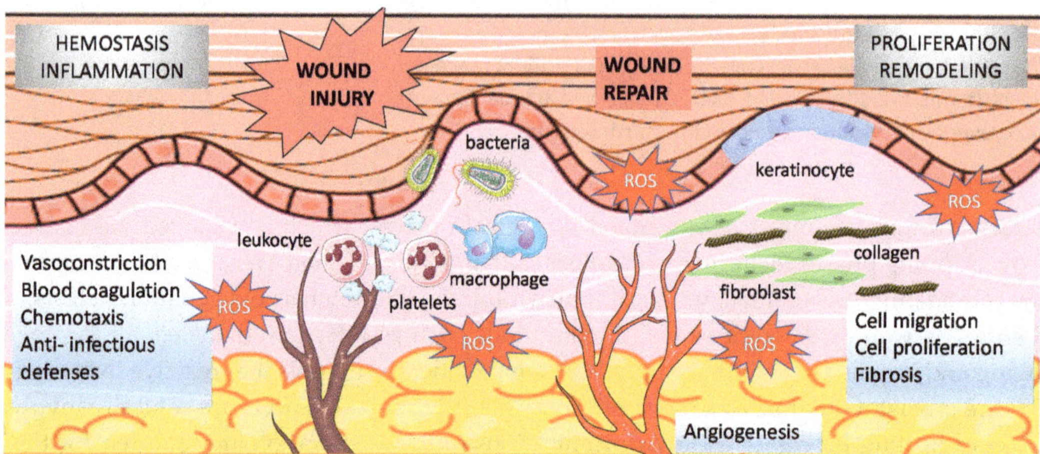

Figure 1. Normal wound healing phases. Relationships between wound healing and reactive oxygen species (ROS) are illustrated. In the hemostatic and inflammatory phase, large amounts of superoxide are generated from molecular oxygen mainly by NADPH oxidase expressed in immune cells. Redox signaling is also critical to modulate key events that occur during cell migration, proliferation, fibrosis and remodeling phases.

Hemostasis typically begins immediately following injury in order to stop bleeding. Platelets are cells that are devoted to sealing off the injured blood vessel. First, platelets are plugged into the injured endothelium to form a clot, so-called primary hemostasis; this process is associated with platelet degranulation leading to the release in the extracellular milieu of cytoplasmic granules containing serotonin and thromboxane A2. These mediators induce vasoconstriction and thus limit blood loss through the disrupted vascular walls [11,12]. Ongoing accumulation of thrombin at the injured vascular site elicits recruitment of platelets to stimulate hemostatic plug growth. This phenomenon is associated with chemotaxis of many cell types such as macrophages, leukocytes, vascular smooth muscle cells and fibroblasts. In this pro-inflammatory milieu, platelets also release cytokines and growth factors, such as platelet-derived growth factor (PDGF), transforming growth factor (TGF)-β, fibroblast growth factor (FGF) and epidermal growth factor (EGF). Release of these growth factors presents potent signaling events for activation and proliferation of smooth muscle cells and fibroblasts concurring to blood vessel repair [13,14].

The inflammatory cells migrate to the injury site to fight infection and prepare the injured site for healing [15,16]. Migration of inflammatory cells at the site of injury participates to microorganism killing, preparing for successful healing [15,16]. In line, macrophages release TGF-β initiating a positive feedback loop as TGF-β further stimulates macrophages to secrete additional cytokines such as FGF,

PDGF, tumor necrosis factor (TNF)-α and interleukin (IL)-1β [17]. Along with immune competent cell recruitment, mast cell activation and degranulation result in the release of prothombotic factors and antithrombotic/fibrinolytic components, histamine and other active amines, which cause increased endothelial permeability and edema allowing further mononuclear cells recruitment [17,18]. Overall, once vascular wall disruption is secured, chemotaxis promotes migration of inflammatory cells and initiate sequential infiltration of neutrophils, macrophages, and lymphocytes within the wound.

The proliferative phase generally follows and overlaps with the inflammatory phase. First, changes in macrophage phenotype allow for the transition of inflammation to proliferation and epithelial migration. As such, macrophages are responsible for initiation of cell apoptosis and clearance, including leukocytes, initiating the resolution of inflammatory processes [16–18]. Along with apoptotic cell clearance, transition of macrophage phenotype also initiates the recruitment of TGF-β released by platelets and macrophages stimulate production of collagen by fibroblasts. Secretions of growth factors (PDGF, FGF) and cytokines (TNF-α, IL-1β) stimulate in turn angiogenesis, fibroblast proliferation, collagen production and wound contraction [16–18]. Cross-talk between fibroblasts and keratinocytes is crucial to stimulate proliferation of keratinocytes which regenerates epithelium integrity. During the last few years, adipocytes from the dermis have been implicated in various physiological and pathological processes, among them hair follicle cycling, wound healing and cutaneous fibrosis. Specifically, adipocyte precursor cells and/or mature adipocytes have been implicated in several regenerative and pathological processes in the skin including hair follicle regeneration and fibroblast regeneration after injury.

During the proliferative stage of wound healing, release of cytokines and growth factors, such as TGF-β, stimulates the migration of keratinocytes and fibroblasts toward the wound area to begin the re-epithelialization and tissue rebuilding process. The proliferative phase involves the conversion of fibroblasts into myofibroblasts that secrete extracelluar matrix ECM proteins, which are required for closure of the wound [19,20]. Myofibroblasts also exhibit contractile properties, due to the expression of α- smooth muscle actin in microfilament bundles or stress fibers, playing a major role in contraction and in maturation of the granulation tissue [19,20]. Depending on experimental or clinical situation, myofibroblasts can also express other smooth muscle related contractile proteins, such as desmin or smooth muscle-myosin heavy chain.

Remodeling and maturation phases allow the termination of wound repair. During these processes, rates of collagen synthesis collagen breakdown equilibrate. During remodeling processes, proteolytic enzymes, essentially matrix metalloproteinases (MMPs), and their inhibitors (tissue inhibitor of metalloproteinases, TIMPs) play a major role. Deposit disorganized collagen in the wound, it is cross-linked and aligned along tissue tension lines. More fibroblasts are gathered in the new connective tissue, so-called granulation tissue, which lay down collagen, eventually resulting in the formation of a scar [17–19]. At this point, synthesis of ECM is considerably reduced. In addition, synthesized components are modified as the matrix is remodeled. Progressively, type I collagen, the main structural component of the dermis, replaces type III collagen which is the major collagenous component of granulation tissue. Finally, elastin which is absent in the granulation tissue and normally contributes to skin elasticity also reappears. During the resolution phase of healing, generally, when the tissue integrity has been sufficiently restored to be mechanically coherent, cellularity is drastically reduced by apoptosis of both myofibroblasts and vascular cells [17–20].

2.2. *Redox Regulation of Normal Wound Healing*

Oxygen is required to disinfect wounds and provide adequate fuel for healing. In addition, oxygen (O_2)-dependent redox signaling is crucial for wound repair [3]. Physiologically, hydrogen peroxide (H_2O_2) and superoxide serve as intracellular messengers stimulating key phases of wound healing including cell recruitment, production of cytokines and angiogenesis [3–6] (Figure 1). Of note, H_2O_2, a reactive species produced by dismutation of superoxide, acts as the principal secondary messenger in wound healing and is present at low concentrations (100–250 μM) in normal wounds [21].

Current understanding of the role of homeostatic levels ROS and redox signaling in wound healing has been well established [3–7]. Physiological levels of ROS are important to reduce local blood flow via vasoconstriction and thrombus formation. Early onset ROS peak levels are related to initial platelet aggregation, which contribute to platelet and inflammatory cell recruitment to the wound by stimulating chemotaxis and adhesion molecule expression [22]. Second, release of ROS within tissue stimulates diapedesis of adherent leukocytes across the vascular wall in order to induce microorganism killing at the injured site. High levels of superoxide and H_2O_2 are thus generated by neutrophils and macrophages via NADPH oxidase [22]. This oxidative burst serves as the primary mechanism of bacterial killing and prevention of wound infection, and is accompanied by a temporary down-regulation of some ROS scavenging enzymes [23]. ROS also provide further signals supporting wound repair as evidenced by their stimulating effects on tumor necrosis factor-α (TNF-α) and platelet-derived growth factor (PDGF) release. Other immune competent cells, including monocytes and macrophages, migrate towards the wound site to help attack invading pathogens [22,23]. Redox signaling is also critical for the proliferation phase. ROS promote fibroblast proliferation and migration, and mediate TGF-β1 signaling, which results in migration, collagen and fibronectin production, and basic fibroblast growth factor (FGF) expression [22,24]. ROS also stimulates angiogenesis, endothelial cell division and migration for blood vessel reformation via VEGF expression. ROS facilitate wound edge and stimulated both proliferation and migration of fibroblasts leading to ECM formation. At the same time, keratinocyte proliferation and migration are promoted, facilitating re-epithelialization [22].

Generation of ROS during the hemostatic phase of wound healing is related to NADPH oxidases (NOX) located in vascular cells, which are activated by tissue factor expression secreted by platelets [22,24,25]. During inflammation, ROS production by NOX enzymes plays a central role in microorganism killing by neutrophil and macrophage oxidative burst [22–24]. Whereas the NOX2 isoform is responsible for the large amounts of ROS produced during the respiratory burst, NOX4 isoform has been implicated in phagocyte recruitment [22,25]. Production of ROS by NOX enzymes is also involved in wound angiogenesis and in the regulation of re-epithelialization processes favoring effective wound closure [22]. Overall, crucial functions of inflammatory cells, vascular endothelial cells, fibroblasts and epithelial cells in wound healing are related to their potent ability to produce ROS via NOX activation [22].

Key events of wound re-epithelialization are dependent on adequate migration, proliferation and differentiation of keratinocytes. Eventually, wound contraction, which guarantees rapid wound closure, is under redox control as ROS produced by NOX4 have shown to be a prerequisite for TGF1-induced myofibroblast differentiation, extracellular matrix production. After wound closure, controlled cell removal and ECM remodeling are dependent upon NOX-mediated ROS production, which is likely to play a direct role during scar maturation [22,25]. ROS generated in wounds is tightly regulated by ROS scavenging enzymes, such as superoxide dismutases (Cu/ZnSOD, MnSOD, SOD3), peroxidases (catalase, phospholipid hydroperoxide glutathione peroxidase) and peroxiredoxins, as well as small molecule antioxidants, such as vitamin E and glutathione [8–10]. Many of the enzymes are up-regulated in healing wounds, while levels of small molecule antioxidants decrease as depleted by ROS [8–10]. Overall, a balance of ROS generation and scavenging is required for efficient and timely wound healing.

3. Definition of Chronic Wound

Several pathologic conditions result in an incomplete and prolonged healing process [2]. Pathogenesis of chronic wounds is difficult to study due to many factors including complexity of the wound repair process and heterogeneity of chronic wounds. Local ischemia and reperfusion injury, type 2 diabetes, chronic inflammation, aging and senescence are the most important factors that may elicit chronic wound states [2–4].

Among these factors, the chronic state of inflammation is present in the majority of cases [16]. Inflammation is associated with persistent macrophages which limit and delay proliferation. Chronic inflammation also induces cell senescence, which is now considered as a critical pathophysiological process in the development of chronic wounds [16,26]. A chronic wound environment is characterized by elevated levels of proteases such as matrix metalloproteinase (MMPs), reduced levels of protease inhibitors such as tissue inhibitors of mMMP (TIMPs), and an abundance of inflammatory cells releasing excessive amounts of proinflammatory cytokines, proteolytic enzymes, and ROS [27]. A combination of these factors elicits accelerated degradation of extracellular matrix and growth factors, deregulation of the inflammatory response, inhibition of cellular proliferation, inadequate vascularization, and accumulation of necrotic tissue due to ischemia. In turn, these effects encourage bacterial colonization and can perpetuate the inflammatory response, inhibiting wound repair.

4. Oxidative Stress in Chronic Wound

As discussed above, a delicate balance between the positive role of ROS and their deleterious effects is important for proper wound healing. Whereas production of ROS is essential to initiate wound repair, excessive amount of ROS generation is deleterious in wound healing. Ongoing oxidative stress, associated with lipid peroxidation, protein modification and DNA damage has been shown to impair wound healing processes via increased cell apoptosis and senescence [3–7]. In physiological conditions, low levels of ROS production by NOX activation in neutrophils and macrophages are responsible for respiratory bursts during phagocytosis of the inflammatory phase [22–24]. In contrast, as chronic inflammation develops in pathological conditions, NOX activation is exacerbated, which may lead to excessive production of ROS production, further accelerating inflammation and oxidative stress cellular damage. Clinical studies suggest that non-healing wounds are maintained in highly oxidizing environment, which lead to impaired wound repair. Clinical conditions such as tissue hypoxia and hyperglycemia are typically associated with highly oxidizing environments.

4.1. Hypoxic Wound

Whereas generation of ROS during the normal wound healing is related to NOX activation [22–24], the presence of hypoxia stimulates oxidant production by the electron transport chain (ETC) of the mitochondria mainly via complexes I and III [28]. This observation is paradoxical, in the sense that superoxide is a product of the one-electron reduction of O_2, which is reduced in hypoxia. ETC-derived ROS are transferred across the inter-membrane space to reach the cytosol where they act as second messengers. During hypoxia, mitochondria augment the release of ROS in the cytosol, which appears counter intuitive as O_2 tension is reduced in the mitochondrial compartment [28,29]. Hypoxia-induced mitochondrial ROS release has been shown to activate cell protection signaling through transcriptional and post-translational mechanisms [28,29].

In line, low oxygen levels leading to mitochondrial ROS production activate prolyl-4-hydroxylases. Prolyl-4-hydroxyases can induce hypoxia-inducible factor 1 (HIF-1) activation, which is involved in regeneration of lost or damaged tissue in mammals [29,30]. In the microenvironment of early wounds, ischemia due to vascular disruption and high O_2 consumption by immune competent cells can favor O_2 depletion and hypoxia [2,6]. Moreover, pathological conditions, such as diabetes, impair microvascular blood flow, thus aggravating tissue oxygenation [2], whereas temporary hypoxia after injury can be beneficial for wound healing, prolonged or chronic hypoxia delays wound healing. Impaired wound repair in hypoxic tissue has been related to the combination of mechanisms that increase ROS production and reduce antioxidant defenses [6].

4.2. Diabetic Chronic Wound

ROS production by several ROS-generating enzymes is elevated in diabetic wounds [10]. Expression and activity of NOX, the major source of ROS in many cell types, are increased in response to hyperglycemia through activation of the receptor for advanced glycation end products (RAGE) [31]. NOX activity is also increased downstream of hyperglycemia-induced protein kinase C (PKC) activation in smooth muscle and endothelial cells [32]. Similarly, hyperglycemia-induced angiotensin II type 1 receptor AT1 activation increases expression of p47phox and enhances ROS production by NADPH oxidase [33]. AT1 is expressed by several cell types in the wound, including myofibroblasts and keratinocytes [34]. Expression and activity of H_2O_2-producing enzyme xanthine oxidase (XO) is also increased in diabetic mouse wounds and in response to high glucose levels [35].

One of the most important sources of ROS in diabetes is the mitochondrial electron transport chain [32]. In line, hyperglycemia increases superoxide production by increasing the amount of pyruvate oxidation in the TCA cycle and consequently the availability of electron donors NADH and FADH2 [32,36]. Increased electron flux then increases the proton gradient across the inner mitochondrial membrane, which at a critical threshold disrupts electron transport through complex III [36]. Electron transport is then largely mediated by coenzyme Q, which transfers only one electron to oxygen, producing excess superoxide [36]. Excessive mitochondrial superoxide production further impacts ROS levels by altering the flux through several intracellular pathways. For example, ROS leads to GAPDH inhibition by poly (ADP-ribose) modification, which increases levels of glycolysis intermediates upstream of GAPDH [32,36]. This provides increased substrate levels for the polyol, protein kinase C, and hexosamine pathways [32,36]. Activation and interaction of these pathways ultimately alters gene expression, depletes antioxidant resources, and favors the production of further ROS and advanced glycation end products. In addition, multiple lines of evidence have emerged showing that intracellular sites of ROS production are functionally connected. So-called ROS-induced ROS release cross talk represents a common mechanism for ROS amplification and regional ROS generation [37]. A large number of mitochondrial pores (mPTP, inner membrane anion channel (IMAC), voltage dependent anion channels VDAC) has been identified as facilitating superoxide escape to the cytosol [37,38].

Hyperglycemia, mitochondrial ROS generation, and oxidative stress are involved in the pathogenesis of several diabetic complications. Deleterious effects of ROS on cellular homeostasis are also related to the reduction in antioxidant defenses, which intensifies the redox imbalance. Analysis of blood collected from diabetes patients showed reduced SOD, CAT, and glutathione peroxidase activity, and an overall decrease in antioxidant status [39]. Of note, signaling through the transcription factor nuclear factor erythroid 2-related factor 2 (Nrf2), a master regulator of antioxidant gene expression, is impaired in diabetes [40]. Expression and nuclear translocation of Nrf2 are decreased in diabetic dermal fibroblasts. In response to oxidative stress, Nrf2 activity decrease was associated with reductions in expression of CAT, NADPH dehydrogenase quinone 1 (NOQ1), glutathione reductase, and glutathione S-transferase [41]. In fibroblasts exposed to high glucose concentrations, Nrf2 is retained in the cytoplasm by its regulator Keap1, and transcription of MnSOD and NOQ1 is reduced [42]. Activation of ATF-3 and NF-κB is involved in antioxidant enzyme regulation is also altered in response to foot ulceration in diabetic patients [43].

5. Glycoxidation and AGE Formation in the Diabetic Chronic Wound

AGEs are produced by the Maillard reaction. A reducing sugar, such as glucose, reacts non-enzymatically with the amino group of proteins to produce a Schiff base that rearranges into Amadori compounds [5]. These Amadori adducts then very slowly undergo irreversible dehydration and condensation reactions, eventually producing AGEs, which are yellowish-brown materials with particular fluorescence.

Advanced glycation end products (AGEs) are a heterogeneous group of compounds produced by the non-enzymatic Maillard reaction. In this reaction, a reducing sugar reacts with the amino group of proteins to form a Schiff base that form Amadori structures. These adducts then slowly transform to eventually produce AGE [44]. Formation of AGE is a physiological process that is part of normal metabolism during lifetime and accumulates slowly in human tissues during ageing [45,46]. However, more rapid and intense accumulation occurs in association with consistent hyperglycemia and enhanced oxidative or carbonyl stress [44]. In addition, glycoxidation, a combinational effect of oxidation and glycation, causes formation of dicarbonyls methyleglyoxal and glyoxal which further fuels AGE formation [44]. Proposed mechanisms of AGE-induced diabetic complications include accumulation of AGE in the extracellular matrix causing aberrant crosslinking and vessel rigidity increase. AGE also bind to AGE-receptors leading to the activation of key cell signaling pathways such as NADPH oxidase and NF-κB activation. Eventually, intracellular formation may impair biomolecule and protein functions including nitric oxide quenching and growth factor effects [45,46] (Figure 2). In line, complications of diabetes such as micro and macrovascular complications, neuropathy and impaired wound healing have attributed to AGE formation and glycoxidation within tissues [45,46].

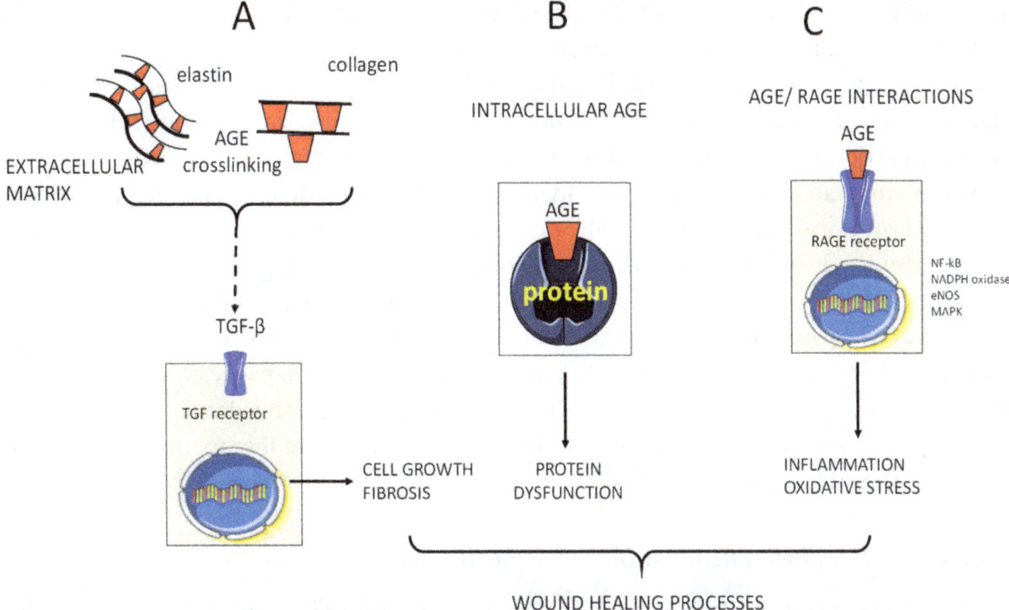

Figure 2. Advanced glycation end products AGE (advanced glycation end products) modulate wound healing. Effects of AGE accumulation in the extracellular (**A**) and intracellular environment (**B**), and interactions with the receptor RAGE (**C**) are illustrated. In extracellular matrix, AGE form on different molecules as collagen, laminin and elastin, increasing matrix stiffness. AGE products upregulate transforming growth factor (TGF)-β that increases the production of extracellular matrix components by binding to TGF β receptor. AGE interact with RAGE on the cell surface leading to transduction of signaling cascade, which activates the ROS generating NADPH oxidase and mitogen-activated protein kinases (MAPK). A main step in AGE/RAGE signaling is activation of NF-κB and its translocation to the nucleus, where it enhances transcription of target genes involved in the inflammatory response. AGE may decrease nitric oxide (NO) availability by reducing endothelial nitric oxide synthase (eNOS) activity and by inactivating NOS elicits ROS production.

An increasing body of in vitro and in vivo experimental diabetic models as well as anti-AGE agents suggest that AGE contribute to the impaired wound healing [47,48]. First, AGE formation may impair micro and macrovascular function leading to vascular flow deficit and poor tissue oxygenation [49]. In addition, increased AGE accumulation, along with expression of their receptors, primarily the RAGE, are associated with formation of atheromatous lesions, impairing blood flow as well as ischemia-induced neovascularization and formation of collateral circulation [50]. Second, either AGE accumulation in diabetic tissues or activation of RAGE have been implicated in the decreased transendothelial migration of neutrophils, which ultimately concurs to wound hypocellularity and delayed inflammatory response [48,51]. In addition, binding of AGE to RAGE induced ROS production from inflammatory and endothelial cells via NADPH activation, which promotes further cellular activation and proinflammatory cytokine expression [52]. Wound AGE accumulation can sustain inflammatory response eliciting ROS production, which further increases AGE formation creating a vicious cycle. Third, a large body of evidence demonstrates that activation of the AGE/RAGE axis alters locomotion, invasiveness, phenotype, behavior, and survival of the cells as well as cell membrane interactions with the extracellular matrix [48]. AGE/RAGE activation in the diabetic skin is associated with extracellular matrix glycation leading to cell cycle arrest of cultured dermal fibroblasts [52]. AGE also activates apoptosis of dermal fibroblasts that would deprive cell proliferative processes necessary for proper behavior. Eventually, accumulation of AGE is associated with derangement in wound contraction and remodeling in diabetic *db/db* mice [53]. In this diabetic mouse model, lowering circulating and tissue accumulating AGE by low AGE diet has been shown to improve wound repair [54]. In addition, delayed epidermal regeneration, thin granulation tissue formation, and impaired neovascularization that led to a significant delay in wound contraction and wound closure were almost reversed by blocking RAGE [55].

In humans, activation of the AGE/RAGE axis has been associated with chronic wound states featured by decreased epithelialization and angiogenesis, deregulation of inflammation, impaired granulation tissue deposition and collagen organization, as well as increased contraction and delayed wound closure [48,50]. Studies in skin of diabetic patients suggest that accumulation of AGEs in fibroblasts is associated with oxidative damage and can alter dermis characteristics of diabetic patients including reduced dermis thickness, disorganization of collagen fibrils, and infiltration of inflammatory cells [52]. In these experiments, RAGE-blocking antibodies prevented glycosylated matrix induced cell cycle arrest and apoptosis of cultured dermal fibroblasts [52]. Interestingly, use of topical soluble RAGE treated wounds also shown increased granulation tissue area and micro-vascular density [55]. Overall, growing evidence suggests that AGE accumulation is involved in dermal wound healing dysfunction and that its prevention could represent a valuable therapeutic option to improve wound healing in diabetic patients.

6. Redox Balance Modules Inflammation in the Healing Wound

Inflammation is a key step to prepare the onset of wound repair [1,7,15,16]. However, resolution of inflammation delay can result in a chronic and deregulated response creating further tissue damage [23]. As previously mentioned, increased and prolonged levels of ROS production in the wound result in chronic inflammation. Interestingly, restoring the redox balance has been shown to improve inflammatory skin conditions.

Excessive presence of ROS in the skin promotes activation of a variety of transcription factors including nuclear factor kappa B (NF-kB), activator protein 1 (AP-1), nuclear factor erythroid-derived 2-like 2 (Nrf2), and mitogen-activated protein kinase (MAPK) pathways [3–6]. Nrf2 is the master regulator of antioxidant gene expression that regulates the transcription of cytoprotective genes by binding to the antioxidant response element (ARE) to activate the transcription of its target genes [39,40]. The main function of Nrf2 during wound healing is protection against the excessive accumulation of endogenous ROS. Growing evidence suggest that overexpression of Nrf2 can limit cellular damage induced by oxidative stress. In addition, Nrf2 expression is essential for the regulation of re-epithelialization processes [39–42]. In the opposite direction, activation of NF-kB and AP-1 has been shown to increase matrix metalloproteinase (MMP) activity in dermal fibroblasts resulting in extracellular matrix (ECM) protein degradation and features of premature aging of the skin. Hence, Nfr2 and NF-κB have reciprocal role in wound healing. On the one hand, Nrf2 controls inflammation and ROS production. On the other hand, Nf-κB can activate the innate immune response, regulate proliferation and migration of many cell types, activate matrix metalloproteinases, and alter cytokines and growth factor cell functions [56]. Interestingly, Nrf2 expression in chronic wounds has been related to major down-regulation of in the diabetic mice as well as increases in protein oxidation in the skin of diabetic patients. Overall, the existing literature supports the contention that Nrf2 activators could improve wound healing in diabetic conditions [40–42].

Deregulation of the inflammatory phase of wound healing and persistence of the pro-inflammatory macrophages in the diabetic wounds has been related to sustained NLRP3 inflammasome activity [57]. NLRP3 inflammasomes are multiprotein complexes with an inherent ability to elicit innate immune responses by sensing pathogen-associated molecular patterns (PAMP) and damage-associated molecular signals (DAMP) through NOD-like receptors (NLR) family pyrin domain containing 3 (NLRP3) binding. Upon activation by PAMPs or DAMPs, NLRP3 interacts with the adapter protein apoptosis associated speck-like protein (ASC). Then, the caspase recruitment domain (CARD) of ASC binds to the CARD domain on procaspase-1, forming the NLRP3 inflammasome. The assembled complexes act as proteolytic cleavers which activate the precursor of interleukin (IL)-1β and IL-18, which are involved in a series of immune and inflammatory processes (Figure 3). Inflammasomes are associated with an antimicrobial response as well as numerous autoimmune, autoinflammatory, metabolic, and infectious diseases.

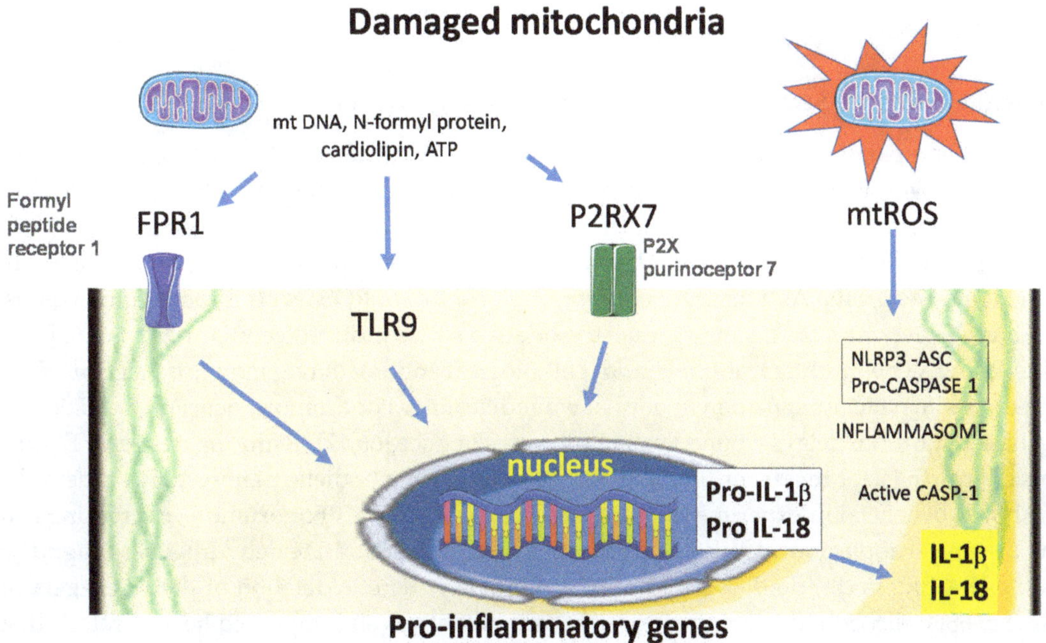

Figure 3. Mitochondria dysfunction elicits inflammasome activation. Injured mitochondria release molecular pattern that are recognized by cell membrane receptors and cytosolic toll-like receptor (TLR) 9. NLRP3 inflammasomes are activated by a myriad of stimuli that include danger-associated molecular patterns (DAMPs). Once activated, NLRP3 forms a multimeric protein complex with associated speck- like protein containing a caspase activation and recruitment domain (CARD; ASC) and caspase-1 (CASP1) termed the inflammasome. Caspase-1 is activated in the inflammasome complex, which cleaves pro-IL-1β (pro-interleukin-1β) and pro-IL-18 into their bioactive mature forms. Mitochondrial DNA (mtDNA), N-formyl proteins, ATP and mitochondrial reactive oxygen species (mtROS), have all been shown to promote NLRP3 inflammasome activation either directly or via specific receptor such as formyl peptide receptor 1 (FPR1) and P2X purinoceptor 7 (P2RX7). TLR9 preferentially binds DNA motifs present in mitochondria and triggers signaling cascades that lead to a pro-inflammatory cytokine response.

In vitro and preclinical studies suggest that the NLRP-3 inflammasome is a key regulatory pathway in wound healing [58,59]. In vitro and experimental studies indicated that the NLRP3 inflammasome may be activated via a ROS-mediated pathway in the diabetic wound environment [60]. In these studies, downstream targets of NLRP3, namely IL-1β and IL-18 contribute to the sustained inflammatory response. Strategies aimed to inhibit NLRP3 inflammasome in vivo, such as topical application of pharmacological inhibitors, NLRP-3 bone marrow transfer and deletion of caspase-1 in *db/db* mice, have been shown to beneficially alter wound repair. In these studies, modulation of

NLRP3 inflammasome was associated with an improved healing response and down-regulation of a pro-inflammatory phenotype of macrophages [58–60].

Growing evidence suggests that ROS originating from mitochondria are centrally involved in NLRP3/NALP3 inflammasome activation, which is required to direct the proteolytic maturation of inflammatory cytokines such as IL-1β [61]. One may thus hypothesize that excessive wound inflammation in diabetic patients may be improved by mitochondria-targeted antioxidants in compromised wound healing. This contention is supported by recent studies showing that antioxidant SkQ1 may improve dermal wound healing in genetically diabetic mice [62]. In these experiments, prevention of excessive mitochondrial ROS production by SkQ1 improved resolution of the inflammatory phase, simultaneously decreasing content of neutrophils and increasing content of macrophages [62]. It seems reasonable to suggest that beneficial effects of SkQ1 on the inflamed wound could be attributed, at least in part, to the reduction of NLRP3 inflammasome activity, as these mitochondria-targeted ROS scavengers have been shown to decrease IL-1β and IL-18 production [63,64].

7. Targeting Oxidative Stress in the Treatment of Chronic Wound

In diabetic patients, standard wound care practices include surgical debridement, antibiotic treatment, moisture dressing, and pressure off-loading [1,2]. Recent advances have focused on specific defects in the diabetic wound environment, including topical application of growth factors, introduction of bone marrow-derived endothelial and epithelial cells, and collagen-based tissue-engineered grafts. As a different concept, strict control of ROS levels through antioxidants and antioxidative enzyme systems may reduced oxidative stress-induced cellular damage [65]. In line, studies using gene-modified animals and pathological models have shown beneficial effects of antioxidative enzyme upregulation in normal wound healing. For example, deficiency of SOD1, heme oxygenase (HO)-1 can delays wound healing processes in mice [66,67]. Reducing excessive ROS by the means of growth factor treatment, antioxidant N-acetyl cysteine or dietary antioxidants generation has been shown beneficial in experimental models of chronic wound. For example, decreasing activity of XO by topical application of siRNA targeting its precursor, xanthine dehydrogenase, significantly improves healing in db/db diabetic mice [68]. Similarly, genetic deletion of the H_2O_2-generating enzyme p66Shc elicited reduction of nitrosative oxidative stress and improved healing rate in diabetic mice [69]. Increasing antioxidant capacity via in vivo MnSOD transfer expression has also proven to be effective in diabetic mice [70]. Activation of Nrf2-mediated antioxidant defenses has been clearly associated in the recent literature with protection against diabetic wound healing in mice [39–41]. In human cells, inducers of Nrf2 have been suggested as a promising pharmacological strategy for skin photoprotection [71].

The next step in the evaluation of antioxidant-based therapy of chronic wound in humans may be clinical use of strategies targeting mitochondria ROS production. Mitochondria-targeted antioxidants have been initially designed to deliver treatments to mitochondria in cardiovascular and neurodegenerative diseases in order to reduce ROS and mitochondrial dysfunction [72,73]. Mitochondria-targeted antioxidants include triphenylphosphonium lipophilic cation-based molecules such as MitoQ Mito-αlipoic acid and 10-(6′-plastoquinonyl) SkQ1, small-cell permeable tetra peptide molecules such as elamipretide choline esters of glutathione and N-acetylL-cysteine [72,73]. As mentioned above, 10-(6′-plastoquinonyl) SkQ1 antioxidant may improve dermal wound healing via better resolution of inflammation in genetically diabetic mice [62]. Mitochondrial-targeted antioxidant elamipretide can bind to cardiolipin, reduce ROS production and stabilize mitochondrial function. Human studies have already shown that elamipretide improves heart failure and mitochondrial myopathy [74,75]. It is likely that elamipretide would also improve chronic wounds, thanks to effects of this compound on mitochondrial ROS production, NLRP3 inflammasome activity as well as NF-κB and Nrf2-ARE signaling pathways.

8. Conclusions

When combined with the successful pre-clinical models described above, promising clinical data suggest the value of redox-based therapeutics for wound healing in diabetic and hypoxic environments. There must be further development of current antioxidant treatment strategies and evaluation of new targets to address imbalances in redox signaling in these clinical situations. Rationale for the use of mitochondrial-targeted antioxidant strategies came from their beneficial effects on oxidative damage, exaggerated inflammatory response, apoptosis and senescence, all of which are implicated in chronic wounds.

Author Contributions: The project idea was developed by M.C.S. and R.N., R.N. wrote the first draft of the manuscript. M.C.S. and S.L conducted the literature search and R.N., M.C.S., and E.B. revised the manuscript. All authors have approved the submitted version.

Acknowledgments: This work was supported by a grant from the Délégation Régionale à la Recherche Clinique des Hôpitaux de Martinique 2016 and from the Inflammation Research International Centre (LIRIC) INSERM U995, Université Lille, France.

Conflicts of Interest: The authors declare no conflict of interest.

References

1. Janis, J.E.; Harrison, B. Wound healing: Part I. Basic science. *Plast. Reconstr. Surg.* **2016**, *138*, 9S–17S. [CrossRef] [PubMed]
2. Guo, S.; Dipietro, L.A. Factors affecting wound healing. *J. Dent. Res.* **2010**, *89*, 219–229. [CrossRef] [PubMed]
3. Sen, C.K.; Roy, S. Redox signals in wound healing. *Biochim. Biophys. Acta* **2008**, *1780*, 1348–1361. [CrossRef] [PubMed]
4. Schafer, M.; Werner, S. Oxidative stress in normal and impaired wound repair. *Pharmacol. Res.* **2008**, *58*, 165–171. [CrossRef] [PubMed]
5. Dunnill, C.; Patton, T.; Brennan, J.; Barrett, J.; Dryden, M.; Cooke, J.; Leaper, D.; Georgopoulos, N.T. Reactive oxygen species (ROS) and wound healing: The functional role of ROS and emerging ROS-modulating technologies for augmentation of the healing process. *Int. Wound J.* **2017**, *14*, 89–96. [CrossRef] [PubMed]
6. Sen, C.K. Wound healing essentials: Let there be oxygen. *Wound Repair Regen.* **2009**, *17*, 1–18. [CrossRef] [PubMed]
7. Bryan, N.; Ahswin, H.; Smart, N.; Bayon, Y.; Wohlert, S.; Hunt, J.A. Reactive oxygen species (ROS)—A family of fate deciding molecules pivotal in constructive inflammation and wound healing. *Eur. Cells Mater.* **2012**, *24*, 249–265. [CrossRef]
8. Fitzmaurice, S.D.; Sivamani, R.K.; Isseroff, R.R. Antioxidant therapies for wound healing: A clinical guide to currently commercially available products. *Skin Pharmacol. Physiol.* **2011**, *24*, 113–126. [CrossRef] [PubMed]
9. Kunkemoeller, B.; Kyriakides, T.R. Redox signaling in diabetic wound healing regulates extracellular matrix deposition. *Antioxid. Redox Signal.* **2017**, *27*, 823–838. [CrossRef] [PubMed]
10. Golebiewska, E.M.; Poole, A.W. Platelet secretion: From haemostasis to wound healing and beyond. *Blood Rev.* **2015**, *29*, 153–162. [CrossRef] [PubMed]
11. Berna-Erro, A.; Redondo, P.C.; Lopez, E.; Albarran, L.; Rosado, J.A. Molecular interplay between platelets and the vascular wall in thrombosis and hemostasis. *Curr. Vasc. Pharmacol.* **2013**, *11*, 409–430. [CrossRef] [PubMed]
12. Kaltalioglu, K.; Coskun-Cevher, S. A bioactive molecule in a complex wound healing process: Platelet-derived growth factor. *Int. J. Dermatol.* **2015**, *54*, 972–977. [CrossRef] [PubMed]
13. Demidova-Rice, T.N.; Hamblin, M.R.; Herman, I.M. Acute and impaired wound healing: Pathophysiology and current methods for drug delivery, part 2: Role of growth factors in normal and pathological wound healing: Therapeutic potential and methods of delivery. *Adv. Skin Wound Care* **2012**, *25*, 349–370. [CrossRef] [PubMed]
14. Nurden, A.T. The biology of the platelet with special reference to inflammation, wound healing and immunity. *Front. Biosci. (Landmark Ed.)* **2018**, *23*, 726–751. [CrossRef] [PubMed]
15. Portou, M.J.; Baker, D.; Abraham, D.; Tsui, J. The innate immune system, toll-like receptors and dermal wound healing: A review. *Vasc. Pharmacol.* **2015**, *71*, 31–36. [CrossRef] [PubMed]

16. Kasuya, A.; Tokura, Y. Attempts to accelerate wound healing. *J. Dermatol. Sci.* **2014**, *76*, 169–172. [CrossRef] [PubMed]
17. Landen, N.X.; Li, D.; Stahle, M. Transition from inflammation to proliferation: A critical step during wound healing. *Cell. Mol. Life Sci.* **2016**, *73*, 3861–3885. [CrossRef] [PubMed]
18. Tracy, L.E.; Minasian, R.A.; Caterson, E.J. Extracellular matrix and dermal fibroblast function in the healing wound. *Adv. Wound Care (New Rochelle)* **2016**, *5*, 119–136. [CrossRef] [PubMed]
19. Bainbridge, P. Wound healing and the role of fibroblasts. *J. Wound Care* **2013**, *22*, 407–412. [CrossRef] [PubMed]
20. Zhu, G.; Wang, Q.; Lu, S.; Niu, Y. Hydrogen peroxide: A potential wound therapeutic target? *Med. Princ. Pract.* **2017**, *26*, 301–308. [CrossRef] [PubMed]
21. Andre-Levigne, D.; Modarressi, A.; Pepper, M.S.; Pittet-Cuenod, B. Reactive oxygen species and nox enzymes are emerging as key players in cutaneous wound repair. *Int. J. Mol. Sci.* **2017**, *18*, 2149. [CrossRef] [PubMed]
22. Hoffmann, M.H.; Griffiths, H.R. The dual role of ROS in autoimmune and inflammatory diseases: Evidence from preclinical models. *Free Radic. Biol. Med.* **2018**. [CrossRef] [PubMed]
23. Jiang, F.; Zhang, Y.; Dusting, G.J. Nadph oxidase-mediated redox signaling: Roles in cellular stress response, stress tolerance, and tissue repair. *Pharmacol. Rev.* **2011**, *63*, 218–242. [CrossRef] [PubMed]
24. Levigne, D.; Modarressi, A.; Krause, K.H.; Pittet-Cuenod, B. Nadph oxidase 4 deficiency leads to impaired wound repair and reduced dityrosine-crosslinking, but does not affect myofibroblast formation. *Free Radic. Biol. Med.* **2016**, *96*, 374–384. [CrossRef] [PubMed]
25. Hesketh, M.; Sahin, K.B.; West, Z.E.; Murray, R.Z. Macrophage phenotypes regulate scar formation and chronic wound healing. *Int. J. Mol. Sci.* **2017**, *18*, 1545. [CrossRef] [PubMed]
26. Patel, S.; Maheshwari, A.; Chandra, A. Biomarkers for wound healing and their evaluation. *J. Wound Care* **2016**, *25*, 46–55. [CrossRef] [PubMed]
27. Smith, K.A.; Waypa, G.B.; Schumacker, P.T. Redox signaling during hypoxia in mammalian cells. *Redox Biol.* **2017**, *13*, 228–234. [CrossRef] [PubMed]
28. Waypa, G.B.; Smith, K.A.; Schumacker, P.T. O2 sensing, mitochondria and ROS signaling: The fog is lifting. *Mol. Asp. Med.* **2016**, *47–48*, 76–89. [CrossRef] [PubMed]
29. Fuhrmann, D.C.; Brune, B. Mitochondrial composition and function under the control of hypoxia. *Redox Biol.* **2017**, *12*, 208–215. [CrossRef] [PubMed]
30. Wautier, M.P.; Guillausseau, P.J.; Wautier, J.L. Activation of the receptor for advanced glycation end products and consequences on health. *Diabetes Metab. Syndr.* **2017**, *11*, 305–309. [CrossRef] [PubMed]
31. Shah, M.S.; Brownlee, M. Molecular and cellular mechanisms of cardiovascular disorders in diabetes. *Circ. Res.* **2016**, *118*, 1808–1829. [CrossRef] [PubMed]
32. Schramm, A.; Matusik, P.; Osmenda, G.; Guzik, T.J. Targeting nadph oxidases in vascular pharmacology. *Vasc. Pharmacol.* **2012**, *56*, 216–231. [CrossRef] [PubMed]
33. Kurosaka, M.; Suzuki, T.; Hosono, K.; Kamata, Y.; Fukamizu, A.; Kitasato, H.; Fujita, Y.; Majima, M. Reduced angiogenesis and delay in wound healing in angiotensin ii type 1a receptor-deficient mice. *Biomed. Pharmacother.* **2009**, *63*, 627–634. [CrossRef] [PubMed]
34. Fernandez, M.L.; Stupar, D.; Croll, T.; Leavesley, D.; Upton, Z. Xanthine oxidoreductase: A novel therapeutic target for the treatment of chronic wounds? *Adv. Wound Care (New Rochelle)* **2018**, *7*, 95–104. [CrossRef] [PubMed]
35. Forrester, S.J.; Kikuchi, D.S.; Hernandes, M.S.; Xu, Q.; Griendling, K.K. Reactive oxygen species in metabolic and inflammatory signaling. *Circ. Res.* **2018**, *122*, 877–902. [CrossRef] [PubMed]
36. Zinkevich, N.S.; Gutterman, D.D. Ros-induced ROS release in vascular biology: Redox-redox signaling. *Am. J. Physiol. Heart Circ. Physiol.* **2011**, *301*, H647–H653. [CrossRef] [PubMed]
37. Zorov, D.B.; Juhaszova, M.; Sollott, S.J. Mitochondrial reactive oxygen species (ROS) and ROS-induced ROS release. *Physiol. Rev.* **2014**, *94*, 909–950. [CrossRef] [PubMed]
38. Banerjee, M.; Vats, P. Reactive metabolites and antioxidant gene polymorphisms in type 2 diabetes mellitus. *Redox Biol.* **2014**, *2*, 170–177. [CrossRef] [PubMed]
39. David, J.A.; Rifkin, W.J.; Rabbani, P.S.; Ceradini, D.J. The Nrf2/Keap1/ARE pathway and oxidative stress as a therapeutic target in type ii diabetes mellitus. *J. Diabetes Res.* **2017**, *2017*, 4826724. [CrossRef] [PubMed]

40. Bitar, M.S.; Al-Mulla, F. A defect in Nrf2 signaling constitutes a mechanism for cellular stress hypersensitivity in a genetic rat model of type 2 diabetes. *Am. J. Physiol. Endocrinol. Metab.* **2011**, *301*, E1119–H1129. [CrossRef] [PubMed]
41. Soares, M.A.; Cohen, O.D.; Low, Y.C.; Sartor, R.A.; Ellison, T.; Anil, U.; Anzai, L.; Chang, J.B.; Saadeh, P.B.; Rabbani, P.S.; et al. Restoration of Nrf2 signaling normalizes the regenerative niche. *Diabetes* **2016**, *65*, 633–646. [CrossRef] [PubMed]
42. Ambrozova, N.; Ulrichova, J.; Galandakova, A. Models for the study of skin wound healing. The role of Nrf2 and NF-kappaB. *Biomed. Pap. Med. Fac. Univ. Palacky Olomouc Czech Repub.* **2017**, *161*, 1–13. [CrossRef] [PubMed]
43. Wang, T.; He, R.; Zhao, J.; Mei, J.C.; Shao, M.Z.; Pan, Y.; Zhang, J.; Wu, H.S.; Yu, M.; Yan, W.C.; et al. Negative pressure wound therapy inhibits inflammation and upregulates activating transcription factor-3 and downregulates nuclear factor-kappab in diabetic patients with foot ulcerations. *Diabetes Metab. Res. Rev.* **2017**, *33*. [CrossRef] [PubMed]
44. Vistoli, G.; De Maddis, D.; Cipak, A.; Zarkovic, N.; Carini, M.; Aldini, G. Advanced glycoxidation and lipoxidation end products (ages and ales): An overview of their mechanisms of formation. *Free Radic. Res.* **2013**, *47* (Suppl. 1), 3–27. [CrossRef] [PubMed]
45. Frimat, M.; Daroux, M.; Litke, R.; Neviere, R.; Tessier, F.J.; Boulanger, E. Kidney, heart and brain: Three organs targeted by ageing and glycation. *Clin. Sci. (Lond.)* **2017**, *131*, 1069–1092. [CrossRef] [PubMed]
46. Neviere, R.; Yu, Y.; Wang, L.; Tessier, F.; Boulanger, E. Implication of advanced glycation end products (AGES) and their receptor (RAGE) on myocardial contractile and mitochondrial functions. *Glycoconj. J.* **2016**, *33*, 607–617. [CrossRef] [PubMed]
47. Van Putte, L.; De Schrijver, S.; Moortgat, P. The effects of advanced glycation end products (ages) on dermal wound healing and scar formation: A systematic review. *Scars Burn Heal.* **2016**, *2*. [CrossRef] [PubMed]
48. Huijberts, M.S.; Schaper, N.C.; Schalkwijk, C.G. Advanced glycation end products and diabetic foot disease. *Diabetes Metab. Res. Rev.* **2008**, *24* (Suppl. 1), S19–S24. [CrossRef] [PubMed]
49. Yamagishi, S.I.; Nakamura, N.; Matsui, T. Glycation and cardiovascular disease in diabetes: A perspective on the concept of metabolic memory. *J. Diabetes* **2017**, *9*, 141–148. [CrossRef] [PubMed]
50. Peppa, M.; Stavroulakis, P.; Raptis, S.A. Advanced glycoxidation products and impaired diabetic wound healing. *Wound Repair Regen.* **2009**, *17*, 461–472. [CrossRef] [PubMed]
51. Koulis, C.; Watson, A.M.; Gray, S.P.; Jandeleit-Dahm, K.A. Linking rage and nox in diabetic micro- and macrovascular complications. *Diabetes Metab.* **2015**, *41*, 272–281. [CrossRef] [PubMed]
52. Niu, Y.; Xie, T.; Ge, K.; Lin, Y.; Lu, S. Effects of extracellular matrix glycosylation on proliferation and apoptosis of human dermal fibroblasts via the receptor for advanced glycosylated end products. *Am. J. Dermatopathol.* **2008**, *30*, 344–351. [CrossRef] [PubMed]
53. Peppa, M.; Brem, H.; Ehrlich, P.; Zhang, J.G.; Cai, W.; Li, Z.; Croitoru, A.; Thung, S.; Vlassara, H. Adverse effects of dietary glycotoxins on wound healing in genetically diabetic mice. *Diabetes* **2003**, *52*, 2805–2813. [CrossRef] [PubMed]
54. Goova, M.T.; Li, J.; Kislinger, T.; Qu, W.; Lu, Y.; Bucciarelli, L.G.; Nowygrod, S.; Wolf, B.M.; Caliste, X.; Yan, S.F.; et al. Blockade of receptor for advanced glycation end-products restores effective wound healing in diabetic mice. *Am. J. Pathol.* **2001**, *159*, 513–525. [CrossRef]
55. Wear-Maggitti, K.; Lee, J.; Conejero, A.; Schmidt, A.M.; Grant, R.; Breitbart, A. Use of topical srage in diabetic wounds increases neovascularization and granulation tissue formation. *Ann. Plast. Surg.* **2004**, *52*, 519–521. [CrossRef] [PubMed]
56. Bigot, N.; Beauchef, G.; Hervieu, M.; Oddos, T.; Demoor, M.; Boumediene, K.; Galera, P. Nf-kappab accumulation associated with col1a1 transactivators defects during chronological aging represses type I collagen expression through a -112/-61-bp region of the col1a1 promoter in human skin fibroblasts. *J. Investig. Dermatol.* **2012**, *132*, 2360–2367. [CrossRef] [PubMed]
57. Artlett, C.M. Inflammasomes in wound healing and fibrosis. *J. Pathol.* **2013**, *229*, 157–167. [CrossRef] [PubMed]
58. Ito, H.; Kanbe, A.; Sakai, H.; Seishima, M. Activation of NLRP3 signalling accelerates skin wound healing. *Exp. Dermatol.* **2018**, *27*, 80–86. [CrossRef] [PubMed]
59. Weinheimer-Haus, E.M.; Mirza, R.E.; Koh, T.J. Nod-like receptor protein-3 inflammasome plays an important role during early stages of wound healing. *PLoS ONE* **2015**, *10*, e0119106. [CrossRef] [PubMed]

60. Zhang, X.; Dai, J.; Li, L.; Chen, H.; Chai, Y. Nlrp3 inflammasome expression and signaling in human diabetic wounds and in high glucose induced macrophages. *J. Diabetes Res.* **2017**, *2017*, 5281358. [CrossRef] [PubMed]
61. Meyer, A.; Laverny, G.; Bernardi, L.; Charles, A.L.; Alsaleh, G.; Pottecher, J.; Sibilia, J.; Geny, B. Mitochondria: An organelle of bacterial origin controlling inflammation. *Front. Immunol.* **2018**, *9*, 536. [CrossRef] [PubMed]
62. Demyanenko, I.A.; Zakharova, V.V.; Ilyinskaya, O.P.; Vasilieva, T.V.; Fedorov, A.V.; Manskikh, V.N.; Zinovkin, R.A.; Pletjushkina, O.Y.; Chernyak, B.V.; Skulachev, V.P.; et al. Mitochondria-targeted antioxidant SkQ1 improves dermal wound healing in genetically diabetic mice. *Oxid. Med. Cell. Longev.* **2017**, *2017*, 6408278. [CrossRef] [PubMed]
63. Dashdorj, A.; Jyothi, K.R.; Lim, S.; Jo, A.; Nguyen, M.N.; Ha, J.; Yoon, K.S.; Kim, H.J.; Park, J.H.; Murphy, M.P.; et al. Mitochondria-targeted antioxidant mitoq ameliorates experimental mouse colitis by suppressing nlrp3 inflammasome-mediated inflammatory cytokines. *BMC Med.* **2013**, *11*, 178. [CrossRef] [PubMed]
64. Jabaut, J.; Ather, J.L.; Taracanova, A.; Poynter, M.E.; Ckless, K. Mitochondria-targeted drugs enhance Nlrp3 inflammasome-dependent IL-1beta secretion in association with alterations in cellular redox and energy status. *Free Radic. Biol. Med.* **2013**, *60*, 233–245. [CrossRef] [PubMed]
65. Zielins, E.R.; Brett, E.A.; Luan, A.; Hu, M.S.; Walmsley, G.G.; Paik, K.; Senarath-Yapa, K.; Atashroo, D.A.; Wearda, T.; Lorenz, H.P.; et al. Emerging drugs for the treatment of wound healing. *Expert Opin. Emerg. Drugs* **2015**, *20*, 235–246. [CrossRef] [PubMed]
66. Iuchi, Y.; Roy, D.; Okada, F.; Kibe, N.; Tsunoda, S.; Suzuki, S.; Takahashi, M.; Yokoyama, H.; Yoshitake, J.; Kondo, S.; et al. Spontaneous skin damage and delayed wound healing in sod1-deficient mice. *Mol. Cell. Biochem.* **2010**, *341*, 181–194. [CrossRef] [PubMed]
67. Deshane, J.; Chen, S.; Caballero, S.; Grochot-Przeczek, A.; Was, H.; Li Calzi, S.; Lach, R.; Hock, T.D.; Chen, B.; Hill-Kapturczak, N.; et al. Stromal cell-derived factor 1 promotes angiogenesis via a heme oxygenase 1-dependent mechanism. *J. Exp. Med.* **2007**, *204*, 605–618. [CrossRef] [PubMed]
68. Weinstein, A.L.; Lalezarzadeh, F.D.; Soares, M.A.; Saadeh, P.B.; Ceradini, D.J. Normalizing dysfunctional purine metabolism accelerates diabetic wound healing. *Wound Repair Regen.* **2015**, *23*, 14–21. [CrossRef] [PubMed]
69. Fadini, G.P.; Albiero, M.; Menegazzo, L.; Boscaro, E.; Pagnin, E.; Iori, E.; Cosma, C.; Lapolla, A.; Pengo, V.; Stendardo, M.; et al. The redox enzyme p66Shc contributes to diabetes and ischemia-induced delay in cutaneous wound healing. *Diabetes* **2010**, *59*, 2306–2314. [CrossRef] [PubMed]
70. Luo, J.D.; Wang, Y.Y.; Fu, W.L.; Wu, J.; Chen, A.F. Gene therapy of endothelial nitric oxide synthase and manganese superoxide dismutase restores delayed wound healing in type 1 diabetic mice. *Circulation* **2004**, *110*, 2484–2493. [CrossRef] [PubMed]
71. Tao, S.; Justiniano, R.; Zhang, D.D.; Wondrak, G.T. The Nrf2-inducers tanshinone I and dihydrotanshinone protect human skin cells and reconstructed human skin against solar simulated Uv. *Redox Biol.* **2013**, *1*, 532–541. [CrossRef] [PubMed]
72. Kim, H.K.; Han, J. Mitochondria-targeted antioxidants for the treatment of cardiovascular disorders. *Adv. Exp. Med. Biol.* **2017**, *982*, 621–646. [CrossRef] [PubMed]
73. Reddy, A.P.; Reddy, P.H. Mitochondria-targeted molecules as potential drugs to treat patients with alzheimer's disease. *Prog. Mol. Biol. Transl. Sci.* **2017**, *146*, 173–201. [CrossRef] [PubMed]
74. Karaa, A.; Haas, R.; Goldstein, A.; Vockley, J.; Weaver, W.D.; Cohen, B.H. Randomized dose-escalation trial of elamipretide in adults with primary mitochondrial myopathy. *Neurology* **2018**, *90*, e1212–e1221. [CrossRef] [PubMed]
75. Daubert, M.A.; Yow, E.; Dunn, G.; Marchev, S.; Barnhart, H.; Douglas, P.S.; O'Connor, C.; Goldstein, S.; Udelson, J.E.; Sabbah, H.N. Novel mitochondria-targeting peptide in heart failure treatment: A randomized, placebo-controlled trial of elamipretide. *Circ. Heart Fail.* **2017**, *10*, e004389. [CrossRef] [PubMed]

13

Antioxidant Tocols as Radiation Countermeasures (Challenges to be Addressed to use Tocols as Radiation Countermeasures in Humans)

Ujwani Nukala [1,2], Shraddha Thakkar [3], Kimberly J. Krager [1], Philip J. Breen [1,4], Cesar M. Compadre [1,4] and Nukhet Aykin-Burns [1,4,*]

1 Department of Pharmaceutical Sciences, College of Pharmacy, University of Arkansas for Medical Sciences, Little Rock, AR 72205, USA; uxnukala@ualr.edu (U.N.); KJKrager@uams.edu (K.J.K.); BreenPhilipJ@uams.edu (P.J.B.); CompadreCesarM@uams.edu (C.M.C.)

2 Joint Bioinformatics Graduate Program, University of Arkansas at Little Rock, Little Rock, AR 72204, USA

3 Division of Bioinformatics and Biostatistics, National Center for Toxicological Research, US Food and Drug Administration, Jefferson, AR 72079, USA; Shraddha.Thakkar@fda.hhs.gov

4 Tocol Pharmaceuticals, LLC, Little Rock, AR 77205, USA

* Correspondence: NAykinBurns@uams.edu

Abstract: Radiation countermeasures fall under three categories, radiation protectors, radiation mitigators, and radiation therapeutics. Radiation protectors are agents that are administered before radiation exposure to protect from radiation-induced injuries by numerous mechanisms, including scavenging free radicals that are generated by initial radiochemical events. Radiation mitigators are agents that are administered after the exposure of radiation but before the onset of symptoms by accelerating the recovery and repair from radiation-induced injuries. Whereas radiation therapeutic agents administered after the onset of symptoms act by regenerating the tissues that are injured by radiation. Vitamin E is an antioxidant that neutralizes free radicals generated by radiation exposure by donating H atoms. The vitamin E family consists of eight different vitamers, including four tocopherols and four tocotrienols. Though alpha-tocopherol was extensively studied in the past, tocotrienols have recently gained attention as radiation countermeasures. Despite several studies performed on tocotrienols, there is no clear evidence on the factors that are responsible for their superior radiation protection properties over tocopherols. Their absorption and bioavailability are also not well understood. In this review, we discuss tocopherol's and tocotrienol's efficacy as radiation countermeasures and identify the challenges to be addressed to develop them into radiation countermeasures for human use in the event of radiological emergencies.

Keywords: tocopherol; tocotrienol; tocols; radioprotectors; radiation countermeasures; radiomitigators; alpha tocopherol transfer protein

---

1. Introduction

The use of ionizing radiation is increasing day by day for various purposes, including its clinical uses for diagnostic purposes and cancer treatment and in non-clinical applications, such as the nuclear generated energy production, engineering, construction, and sterilization of food products [1–3]. With such widespread uses, the likelihood of an intentional or unintentional encounter with radiation is quite high. The risk of radiation exposure has been increasing mainly with increased use of ionizing radiation for nuclear power plants or nuclear weapons, both of which can result in accidental radiological emergencies. There were nearly 105 civilian and military nuclear reactor accidents between 1952 and 2015 that resulted in massive loss of human life and property [1]. Recently, on 24 August 2017 the Pennsylvania Department of Health distributed potassium iodide tablets for free to the residents who live or work within 10 miles of the Peach Bottom and Three Mile Island nuclear plants to be ready in case of an emergency. However, potassium iodide, a specific blocker of thyroid radioactive iodine uptake, only protects the thyroid gland of individuals exposed to radiation.

Exposure to ionizing radiation produces oxygen derived reactive oxygen and nitrogen species (ROS and RNS), including hydroxyl radical (OH•), superoxide ($O_2•^-$), peroxynitrite ($ONOO^-$), and hydrogen peroxide (H_2O_2). Ionizing radiation-induced ROS and RNS damage DNA, proteins, and lipids as well as activate intracellular signaling pathways and stimulate cytochrome C release from mitochondria, leading to apoptosis [4–6].

The Office of Science and Technology Policy and the United States Department of Homeland Security have identified radiation countermeasure development as the highest priority for preparedness against a potential bioterrorism event [1]. As of today, amifostine is the only FDA approved drug for use in patients undergoing radiotherapy. However, because of its adverse side effects, its use is limited and the search for safe and effective radiation countermeasures continues.

Vitamin E and its derivatives have attracted the attention of researchers in recent years for their radioprotective effects, which have been heavily studied against total body irradiation [7–10], as well as partial body irradiation [11–16]. In this review, we outline the research endeavors dedicated to studying the radiation protection efficacy of vitamin E analogs. We also identify the issues that need to be addressed when using vitamin E analogues as safe and effective radiation countermeasures in humans.

2. Radiation Induced Injuries

Ionizing radiation is radiation that carries sufficient energy to liberate electrons from atoms or molecules leaving them with unpaired electrons thereby ionizing them and producing free radicals. These free radicals and ROS/RNS including, OH•, $O_2•^-$, $ONOO^-$, and H_2O_2 can damage nucleic acids, proteins, and membrane lipids. Exposing an individual to ionizing radiation for a brief period can cause severe tissue injuries, referred to as Acute Radiation Syndrome (ARS). ARS can occur with doses higher than 1 Gray (Gy) that are delivered at relatively high rates. The three clinical syndromes of ARS are based on the acute whole-body dose, duration, and dose rate, including hematopoietic or bone marrow sub-syndrome, gastro-intestinal sub-syndrome, and cerebrovascular sub-syndrome. Each of these three sub-syndromes follows a 4-phase clinical pattern according to CDC Emergency Preparedness and Response, as detailed in Table 1 [17]

Table 1. Acute Radiation Syndrome.

Acute Radiation Syndrome			
	Hematopoietic Sub-Syndrome	Gastro-Intestinal Sub-Syndrome	Neuro/Cerebrovascular Sub-Syndrome
Quantity of radiation	>2–3 Gy	5–12 Gy	10–20 Gy
Prodromal stage symptoms	Anorexia, nausea and vomiting	Anorexia, severe nausea, vomiting, cramps and diarrhea	Extreme nervousness and confusion; severe nausea, vomiting, and watery diarrhea; loss of consciousness; and burning sensations of the skin.
Latent Stage symptoms	Stem cells in bone marrow are dying, although patient may appear and feel well.	Stem cells in bone marrow and cells lining GI tract are dying, although patient may appear and feel well.	Patient may return to partial functionality.
Manifest Phase/Illness Phase symptoms	Anorexia, fever, and malaise. Drop in all blood cell counts occurs for several weeks.	Malaise, anorexia, severe diarrhea, fever, dehydration, and electrolyte imbalance.	Watery diarrhea, convulsions, and coma.
Recovery or death	Bone marrow cells will begin to repopulate the marrow.	>10 Gy radiation leads to death due to gastro-intestinal syndrome	No recovery is expected.

3. Radiation Countermeasures

Effective radiation countermeasures should be safe, efficient, stable, easy to administer, and have good bioavailability. Radiation countermeasures fall under three categories, radiation protectors, radiation mitigators, and radiation therapeutics.

Radiation protectors are agents that are administered prior to radiation exposure to protect from radiation-induced injuries by many mechanisms, such as scavenging free radicals that are generated by initial radiochemical events, delaying cell cycle, promoting DNA repair, etc. Radiation protectants are given to personnel that are at risk of exposure to radiation like the military, first responders and civilians during the evacuation of disaster areas. Radiation mitigators are agents that are administered after the exposure of radiation but before the onset of symptoms. They accelerate the recovery and repair from radiation-induced injuries. Whereas radiation therapeutic agents are administered after the onset of symptoms and act by regenerating the tissues that are injured by radiation. Radiation mitigators and radiation therapeutics can be given to people who are victims of nuclear accidents or terrorist attacks or to patients undergoing radiotherapy. One among the various candidates [18–21] that are under development as radiation countermeasures are vitamin E's tocols.

Natural products with health benefits are often attractive targets for research [22]. Among the natural products, vitamins are notably considered beneficial for human health. Vitamin E is a well-known antioxidant that can scavenge free radicals produced by radiation exposure. Vitamin E is found in our diet and has an acceptable toxicity profile [23].

The vitamin E family consists of eight different naturally occurring vitamers, four saturated analogs (α, β, γ, and δ) called tocopherols, and four unsaturated analogs (α, β, γ, and δ) referred to as tocotrienols, which are collectively called tocols. Tocopherols and tocotrienols are structurally similar with the same chromanol head, except that tocotrienols have unsaturated farnesyl isoprenoid side chain at C-3′, C-7′, and C-11′, whereas tocopherols have saturated phytyl isoprenoid side chain (Figure 1).

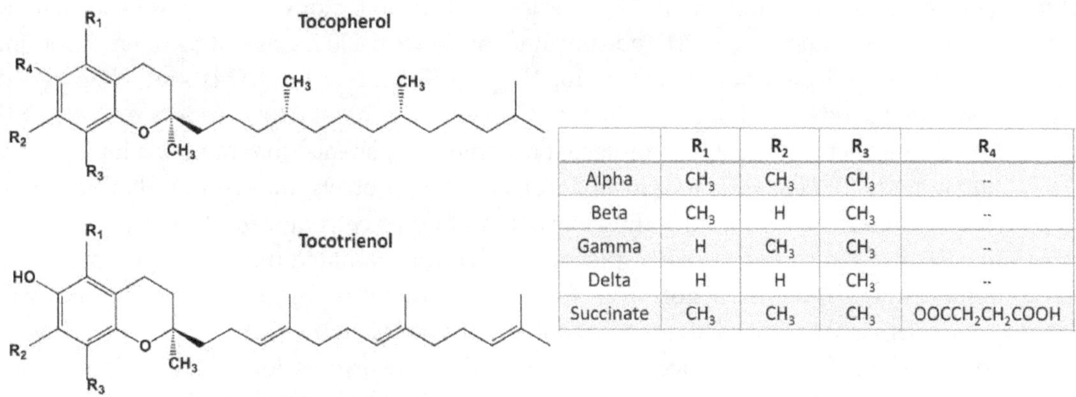

	R_1	R_2	R_3	R_4
Alpha	CH_3	CH_3	CH_3	--
Beta	CH_3	H	CH_3	--
Gamma	H	CH_3	CH_3	--
Delta	H	H	CH_3	--
Succinate	CH_3	CH_3	CH_3	$OOCCH_2CH_2COOH$

Figure 1. Chemical structures of tocopherol and tocotrienol isoforms.

3.1. *Tocopherols and Tocopherol Succinate*

Vitamin E components have been reported to be radioprotective in various studies [24–26]. However, there are several factors that influence the differential radioprotective efficacy of tocol analogs, including the rate of absorption after oral administration, which is found to be greater in tocotrienols than tocopherols due to higher absorption of tocotrienols by the intestinal epithelial cells [27]. Serbinova et al. [28] reported that the antioxidant potential of tocotrienols is 1600 times more than that of α-tocopherol (AT). Studies by Pearce et al. [29] and Qureshi et al. [30] suggest that tocotrienols are better radio-protectants because of their ability to inhibit HMG-CoA reductase.

AT's dose reduction factor was determined to be 1.11 when administered subcutaneously at a dose of 100 IU/kg when administered within 15 m after irradiation of 9 Gy in mice. AT significantly increased the 30-day survival of male CD2F1 mice when given one h before or within 15 m after irradiation. Combination studies of α-tocopherol with WR-3689 showed that the radio-protective efficacy of WR-3689 (150 mg/kg) significantly increased when given in combination with α-tocopherol at 100 IU/kg with a dose reduction factor of 1.49 [31]. AT also reduced the frequency of micronuclei and chromosomal aberrations in bone marrow cells when administered orally either 2 h before, immediately after, or 2 h after irradiation of 1 Gy in mice [32]. The study by Kumar et al. [33], demonstrated that AT has more radio-protective activity when administered subcutaneously than when given orally at a dose of 400 IU/kg 24 h before total body irradiation at 10.5 Gy. AT (20 IU/kg/day) in combination with pentoxifylline (100 mg/kg/day) induced a significant improvement in radiation-induced myocardial fibrosis and left ventricular diastolic dysfunction after irradiation at 9 Gy [34]. A study by Empey et al. [35] showed that AT protects gastrointestinal mucosa against radiation induced absorptive injury when administered before 10 Gy of abdominal radiation. In another study, AT protected mice from radiation injury when administered i.p. after irradiation of <10 Gy, when administered no later than 5 h after irradiation, suggesting enhancement of repair processes and antioxidant scavenging of metabolically produced radicals when produced by irradiation [36].

To study the role of hematopoietic cytokines in the radioprotective activity of tocopherol succinate and other tocols (α-tocopherol, δ-tocopherol, γ-tocopherol, γ-tocotrienol, and tocopherol acetate), Singh et al. [8] measured cytokine levels by Luminex, ELISA, and cytokine array in mice serum after administrating 400 mg/kg tocols subcutaneously 24 h before whole-body irradiation at a dose of 3 and 7 Gy. Among all the tocols studied, tocopherol succinate was most effective in stimulating granulocyte colony stimulating factor (G-CSF) and IL-6. Since G-CSF and IL-6 play an important role in hematopoietic injury, the study indicates that tocopherol succinate's radio protective activity is mediated by cytokines [8]. When tocopherol succinate injected mice were administered a neutralizing antibody to G-CSF, the protective effect of tocopherol succinate was significantly abrogated [9]. A study by Singh et al. [10] showed that tocopherol succinate protects mice against lethal doses of ionizing radiation by inhibiting radiation-induced apoptosis and DNA damage as well as by increasing cell proliferation. In a study by Singh et al. [37], the dose reduction factor of tocopherol succinate was determined to be 1.28 in mice, administered subcutaneously with 400 mg/kg of tocopherol succinate, 24 h before total body irradiation at 9, 9.5, 10, 10.5, 10.75, and 11 Gy. This study showed that tocopherol succinate stimulated high levels of G-CSF with a peak at 24 h, moderate levels of IL-6 between 24 and 48 h after treatment, and protected myeloid components from radiation injury at 3 and 7 Gy. A similar study [38] suggests that tocopherol succinate protects mice from radiation-induced gastrointestinal damage by promoting the generation of crypt cells and inhibiting apoptosis and translocation of gut bacteria to the heart, spleen, and liver in irradiated mice. Tocopherol succinate has also demonstrated radioprotection from total body irradiation by decreasing the number of CD68-positive cells, reducing DNA damage, and apoptotic cells and by increasing proliferating cells in irradiated mice [10]. Tocopherol succinate also modulates the expression of antioxidant enzymes and inhibits expression of oncogenes in irradiated mice, according to a study by Singh et al. [39].

3.2. Tocotrienols

Multiple studies have reported the antioxidant, anti-inflammatory, anticancer, hypocholesterolemic, and neuroprotective properties of tocotrienols in different cell lines, animal models, and in humans. This review will discuss their radioprotective activity studied in different animal models and in humans.

A number of studies have shown that tocotrienols are superior antioxidants compared to tocopherols [28,29,40–43]. Studies [24,44] have demonstrated that γ-tocotrienol (GT3) protects against radiation injury by increasing hematopoietic progenitors, neutrophils, platelets, white blood cells, and reticulocytes. Singh et al. [45] evaluated the protective effects of GT3 in nonhuman primates treated with 5.8, 6.5, and 7.2 Gy doses of cobalt-60 gamma radiation (0.6 Gy/min). This study reports the pharmacokinetic (PK) parameters (at 9.375, 18.75 and 37.5 mg/kg doses) and efficacy of

GT3 (37.5 mg/kg and 75 mg/kg). Their PK analysis showed increased area under the curve with increasing drug dose and half-life of GT3. Unexpectedly, t_{max} increased in a dose-dependent manner. This could be due to the slow release of GT3 from the site of injection (sub-cutaneous). The study also demonstrated that GT3's efficacy in reducing the severity of neutropenia and thrombocytopenia is dose-dependent, and 75 mg/kg treatment is more effective than 37.5 mg/kg treatment after a 5.8 Gy dose of ionizing radiation. However, there was no significant difference in animal survival at 60 days between the vehicle group and the GT3 treated groups.

The study by Li et al. [46] demonstrated that a single injection of δ-tocotrienol (DT3), given to mice 24 h before a total body irradiation, presented 100% survival, measured by 30-day post-irradiated survival, by increasing cell survival and regeneration of hematopoietic microfoci. Singh et al. [43] showed evidence that DT3 mediates its radioprotection by inducing G-CSF in irradiated mice and also showed that DT3 induces high levels of several cytokines, comparable to other tocols in mice. A study by Loose et al. [47] suggested that GT3 is more efficacious than the tocopherols in terms of radiation protection because of its greater potency to induce gene expression in human endothelial cells. This could be due to the low cellular uptake of α-tocopherol compared to GT3. When GT3 was administered s.c. at 200 mg/kg in combination with pentoxifylline, showed synergistic radioprotection activity in mice exposed to 11.5 Gy total body irradiation, and this radioprotective activity of GT3 was shown to be mediated through induction of G-CSF [48].

Studies by Satyamitra et al. [23] showed that DT3 has radiation protection and mitigation effects. DT3, when given s.c. at 150 mg/kg or 300 mg/kg 24 h before total body irradiation, showed effective radioprotection in mice. In addition, DT3 showed reduced lethality when administered at 150 mg/kg in mice 2, 6, or 12 h after irradiation. Another study by Kumar et al. [49] indicated that a GT3 and DT3 combination at 800 mg/kg given orally twice a day for six months to patients who had radiotherapy for head and neck cancer had significantly improved mouth opening and subjective symptoms due to radiation-induced fibrosis. Studies also suggested that tocols exert their biological effects not only by their antioxidant properties but also by inhibiting HMG-CoA reductase [49]. Tocotrienols accumulate in the small intestine as well as in the colon to a greater level than tocopherols, and this may aid with their ability to reduce GI injury [50]. A study by Naito et al. [51] demonstrated that GT3 concentrations in endothelial cells were 30–50 times greater than those of α-tocopherol. The effect of GT3 on tetrahydrobiopterin (BH4) bioavailability was studied by Berbee et al. [52], where GT3 counteracted the decrease in BH4. GT3 protected hematopoietic tissue by preserving the hematopoietic stem cells (HSCs) and hematopoietic progenitor cells (HPCs). The HPC numbers in GT3 treated mice recovered 90% at day seven after total body irradiation [44]. Modulation of sphingolipids leads to cellular stress and upregulation of A20, a well-established NF-kB negative regulator. It has been shown that the mechanism of GT3 radioprotection may involve the inhibition of NF-κB activation by induction of A20 [53,54]. It also has been shown that the ability of GT3 to protect against vascular injury is related to its ability to inhibit HMG-CoA reductase [55].

4. Vitamin E Tocols

Vitamin E in the diet passes through the gastrointestinal tract and gets absorbed in the small intestine. It is emulsified by bile and absorbed in the form of micelles [56]. Yap et al. [57] have reported that the dietary fat consumption plays an important role in the absorption of tocols. The administration route of vitamin E also influences its absorption [58,59].

4.1. α-Tocopherol Transfer Protein

The circulating levels of vitamin E in the body are maintained by α-tocopherol transfer protein (ATTP), which is abundantly found in the liver. This hepatic protein is a member of a lipid-binding protein family and plays a major discriminating role in the plasma and tissue retention of dietary tocols. This protein is regulated by α-tocopherol transfer gene present on chromosome 8q13 [60]. ATTP has two different conformations, closed and open [61]. The structure of ATTP has a hinge, which flips to a closed conformation after incorporating AT in the binding pocket. The fate of the tocol depends on the preferential binding of ATTP in the liver, and those that are not selected by ATTP are excreted via bile or renal excretion (Figure 2) [25,61]. ATTP has a much greater affinity AT than for all other tocols, and this would explain why the other tocols exhibit lower plasma levels over time [62–64]. Vitamin E supplements are commonly formulated with AT, which is often present as a synthetic racemic mixture. However, only the naturally occurring RRR isomer of AT has a high affinity for ATTP, causing the other isomers to be much less bioavailable [65]. Studies [25,66] have proposed that unsaturation in the side chain of tocotrienols accounts for their lower affinity for ATTP by making it impossible for the tocotrienol bend inside the ligand-binding pocket of ATTP and hindering the protein's ability to attain the closed conformation. Thus, there is a significant difference in the distribution and metabolism of tocols among various tissues [67–70].

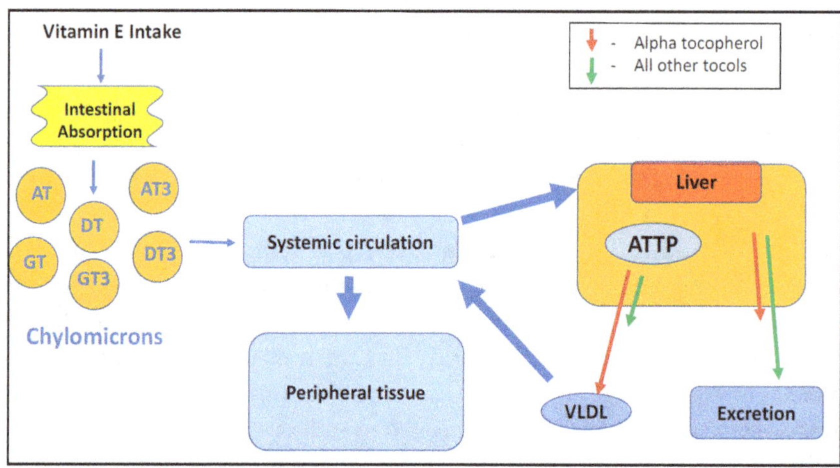

Figure 2. Major pathway for vitamin E absorption and metabolism.

There is a population, with a neurodegenerative disease known as ataxia, with vitamin E deficiency (AVED) [71]. Patients diagnosed with AVED have three frame shift mutations in the α-tocopherol transfer gene present on chromosome 8q13. AVED is an autosomal recessive defect in which the patient is not able to absorb vitamin E into the systemic circulation and becomes deficient [71]. Without a regular supply of this key antioxidant, the body becomes susceptible to damage by free radicals. The coordination of movement becomes uncontrolled and the patient experiences a loss of sensation [71]. Individuals suffering from AVED have normal intestinal absorption of vitamin E, but they are unable to maintain normal levels of vitamin E in systemic circulation. The reason for this is that AVED patients lack functional ATTP, thus the recirculation of α-tocopherol is inhibited. To maintain a normal blood concentration of vitamin E, patients suffering from AVED require very high doses of oral vitamin E throughout their lives [71]. AVED exemplifies the importance of the presence of functional ATTP. However, the fact that ATTP has a much greater affinity for α-tocopherol than for other tocols results in a much faster elimination rate and lower plasma levels over time for all the other tocopherols and for tocotrienols.

4.2. Absorption and Distribution

It is likely that the inconclusive outcomes of various vitamin E clinical trials may be due to limited understanding of the pharmacokinetics of tocols. The bioavailability of vitamin E in humans is dependent on many factors. Studies have shown that vitamin E bioavailability is greater when administered with food, particularly fat [57,58]. Reboul et al. [72] studied the role of the SR-B1 receptor in the intestinal absorption of vitamin E and showed that the expression of the SR-B1 receptor may be responsible for the inter-individual variability in vitamin E absorption and that this receptor mediates the intestinal vitamin E absorption.

Though there are several studies showing tocotrienol's radioprotective activity, their dosing, efficacy, and therapeutic concentrations still remain controversial. This is partially due to the lack of sufficient data explaining their absorption, distribution, and elimination. There is a large variability in the rate and extent of absorption of tocotrienols in different populations from healthy subjects to smokers and diseased patients. The route of administration can also play an important role in the plasma concentrations of tocotrienols [45,57,58].

The absorption of tocotrienols was negligible when administered via intraperitoneal and intramuscular route, whereas the absorption was incomplete when given orally [58]. Several studies have focused on developing a water-soluble delivery system to increase the solubility of the lipophilic tocols. The use of cyclodextrin and self-emulsifying formulations showed improved absorption and higher plasma levels in rats. The peak plasma concentration (C_{max}) and the area under the curve (AUC) of tocotrienols administered with self-emulsifying systems were increased 2–4-fold compared to non-emulsified formulations [73,74]. In a study by Yap et al. [57], comparisons were made between eight healthy male volunteers given 300 mg mixed tocotrienols (87 mg α-tocotrienol, 166 mg GT3, and 43 mg DT3) under a fasted state or after a fatty meal. The 24 h AUC of tocotrienols was increased by at least 2-fold in the fed state. The maximum plasma concentrations for α, γ, and δ tocotrienols were found to be 1.83, 2.13, and 0.34 μg/mL, respectively. While in another study, where tocotrienols were given at higher doses of 296 mg α-tocotrienol, 284 mg GT3, and 83 mg DT3, the maximum plasma concentrations were 1.55, 2.79, and 0.44 μg/mL, respectively [75]. The discrepancies in the plasma levels observed may be an indication that levels may depend on the ratios of the analogs [76]. It has been reported that tocotrienols were transported in triacylglycerol-rich fractions after administration of tocotrienol-rich fraction (TRF) at 1011 mg in healthy subjects, and tocotrienols were found in significant amounts in the plasma and lipoproteins [75]. This study [75], as well as other studies [77–79], indicate that high TRF doses from 200 to 3200 mg/d are safe for healthy human consumption. However, it was also mentioned in a review by Ju et al. [80] that the therapeutic efficacy of tocotrienols depends on dose, formulation, route of administration, and study population. Several studies [81–84] investigated the changes in lipid profile at different doses of tocotrienols.

In spite of all these studies, the dose dependent effect of TRF on the lipid profile is still inconclusive, and further studies are needed to identify the factors responsible for this disparity. For example, it was reported that reduced DNA damage was observed in people over the age of 50 years who were given tocotrienols [85]. This was supported by a later study by Chen et al. [86] who compared the absorption of tocotrienols in different age groups of subjects who were given TRF supplementations for six months. They observed that the plasma tocotrienol levels increased significantly in participants aged over 50 years but not in younger people between the ages of 35–49 years. In contrast to these studies, a study by Heng et al. [87] reported higher plasma concentrations of tocotrienols in younger people 30–34 years old, compared to people 50–54 years old after receiving TRF supplementations for six months. In study by Qureshi et al. [77], TRF doses at 125 mg/d, 250 mg/d, and 500 mg/d were given orally to healthy fed subjects (n = 11/dose), and dose-dependent increases in AUC and C_{max} were found. In a later study by Qureshi et al. [78], the safety and bioavailability of higher oral doses of 750 mg/d and 1000 mg/d of annatto-based tocotrienols in healthy fed subjects (n = 3/dose) were analyzed. This study showed a dose-dependent increase in plasma concentration (ng/mL) and plasma t_{max} of 3.33 and 4 h; elimination half-lives of 2.74 and 2.68 h for δ-tocotrienol. Similar results were reported for all other tocols, except for α-tocopherol. It was reported that a dose of δ-tocotrienol lower than 500 mg/d decreased the levels of serum total cholesterol, LDL-cholesterol, and triglycerides in a dose-dependent manner, but a higher dose of 750 mg/d increased the levels of these lipid parameters, compared to 250 mg/d [88]. Studies suggest that δ-tocotrienol has the unique dual biological property of inhibition (anti-inflammatory) and activation (pro-inflammatory), depending on its concentration [78,79,88–90]. The bioavailability of a mixture of α-tocotrienol, GT3, and DT3 was studied after administering a 300 mg capsule to fasted and fed healthy subjects (n = 8) and found the plasma t_{max} to be between 3 and 5 h for both fasted and fed subjects [57]. In another study, plasma t_{max}

after administering two 300 mg/capsules of a mixture of γ-tocotrienol and δ-tocotrienol was found to be 5.64 ± 1.50 h and 4.73 ± 0.90 h, respectively [91]. When a dose of 450 mg of a rich fraction of barley oil versus a rich fraction of palm oil was administered to healthy subjects ($n = 7$), the area under the curve (0–24 h) of total (α-, β-, γ-, δ-) tocotrienols was significantly (2.6-fold) higher in the barley oil than in the palm oil [92].

A study by Abuasal et al. [93] compared the intestinal absorption kinetics and the bioavailability of GT3 and AT administered to rats. The oral bioavailability of AT (36%) was significantly higher than GT3 (9%), and AT showed higher intestinal permeability than GT3. These results indicate that the intestinal permeability could be a contributing factor for the higher bioavailability of α-tocopherol and suggests that enhancing the permeability of γ-tocotrienol would increase its oral bioavailability. There are findings suggesting that increasing the permeability of GT3 via new approaches, like solid lipid nanoparticles, leads to an increase in its bioavailability [94]. It was reported that co-administration of tocotrienols with lipids causes a delay in the rate of gastric emptying and this leads to an increase in tocotrienol's solubility by stimulating the secretion of bile salts and phospholipids into the GI tract and therefore increasing the absorption and bioavailability of tocotrienols [95,96].

A self-emulsifying drug delivery system (SEDDS) has been used to achieve increased bioavailability of tocotrienols. GT3 dissolved in SEDDS versus commercial Tocovid was studied in vitro and in vivo in rats [97]. There was a 2-fold increase in the solubilization, higher cellular uptake in vitro, and a 2-fold increase in oral bioavailability for the SEDDS formulation [97]. Alqahtani et al. [98] also reported the bioavailability of γ and δ tocotrienols, administered to rats as SEDDS compared to commercially available UNIQUE E® tocotrienol capsules, and the results showed that SEDDS increased the bioavailability. However, bioavailability showed a progressive decrease with increased treatment dose due to nonlinear absorption kinetics [98].

Collectively these studies show that tocotrienols respond differently at different doses in different populations. The major determinant for the limited bioavailability of the tocotrienols could be their limited binding to the transporter, ATTP, which is responsible for transporting the tocols out of the liver into the systemic circulation [99]. The key role of ATTP in regulating the pharmacokinetics of vitamin E has been elegantly demonstrated in several studies [61,99–105]. Previous studies have shown that there is a good linear relationship between relative affinity of tocols to ATTP and their biological activity [106]. These studies also demonstrate the need to conduct more randomized controlled trials with large sample sizes to better understand the bioavailability mechanisms and the therapeutic window of tocotrienols. Thus, it is highly desirable to develop a new vitamin E analog with an increased half-life and improved pharmacokinetic properties. This can be achieved by increasing the affinity of the analogs to ATTP, which may be responsible for maintaining the plasma levels of these compounds and also by increasing their permeability. Multiple studies [25,63,66] have recently reported the development of such analogs, the tocoflexols (Figure 3). The tocoflexols were designed, using computer aided techniques, to behave like tocopherols in terms of their bioavailability and like tocotrienols in terms of their biological activity. To that effect, tocoflexol has been shown to have an antioxidant activity and rate of cell uptake on a par with DT3 and GT3, but it has a greater ability to bind to ATTP than the tocotrienols and thus has the potential for improved bioavailability.

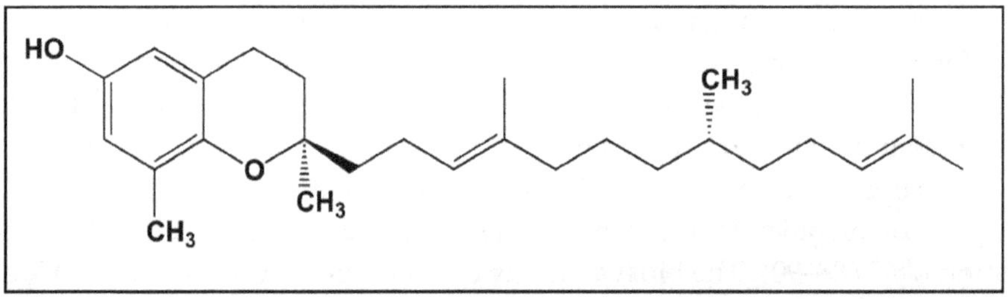

HO

CH_3

O

CH_3

CH_3

Figure 3. Chemical structure of δ-tocoflexol.

5. Conclusions and Future Directions

Given the increasing use of radioactive materials in healthcare as well as the number of nuclear reactors and the amplified nuclear terrorism risk, development of effective radioprotectors and radiomitigators that can be deployed immediately is the key to have a successful contingency strategy in case of unwanted/unexpected radiation exposures. Multiple studies have reported the mechanisms by which tocols exert their radioprotection. It has been suggested that tocols' mechanism of protection from radiation-induced hematopoietic death involves cytokines and chemokines [8]. The importance of G-CSF induction on the mechanism of radioprotection of tocotrienols was demonstrated when the protective effects of GT3 were abrogated in irradiated mice treated with G-CSF antibodies [9,40,48]. It has also been shown that tocols reduce post-irradiation GI syndrome by decreasing IL-1β and IL-6 [107]. Some studies have shown that tocotrienols have a greater radioprotective effect than tocopherols because of their ability to inhibit HMG-CoA reductase [55]. The radioprotective effects of GT3 depend not only on its antioxidant properties but also on its ability to concentrate in endothelial cells [51]. A study by Loose et al. [47] investigated the gene expression profile in human epithelial cells after treatment with GT3, γ-tocopherol (GT), and AT for 24 h. GT3 was found to be more effective in modulating changes in gene expression than GT and AT, when a genome wide analysis was performed. Several genes were affected, including those responsible for cell cycle, cell proliferation, cell death, hematopoiesis, angiogenesis, and DNA damage. The poor bioavailability of the tocotrienols is a major limiting factor for their clinical use as radioprotectants and radiomitigators [66]. In this regard, the development of the tocoflexols represents a promising approach [25].

Low doses of ionizing radiation in medical treatments and occupational exposure results in high risk for cardiovascular diseases [108]. Long distance space missions are associated with exposure to galactic cosmic rays and solar particle events that can increase the risk for cataract, cancers, and cardiovascular diseases [109–111]. Because of their effectiveness and low toxicity, the tocols may prove to be effective to protect against low-dose radiation, but further research is required to establish their potential.

Acknowledgments: This work was supported in part by the National Institutes of Health (P01AG012411-18; P20, GM109005; R15, ES022781, and P20 GM103429), the Arkansas Biosciences Institute FY13, and the Arkansas Science and Technology Authority 15-B-19.

Conflicts of Interest: The University of Arkansas has applied for patent protection on the tocoflexols and other tocotrienol containing products. A potential royalty stream to Shraddha Thakkar, Philip J. Breen, Cesar M. Compadre and Nukhet Aykin-Burns, may occur consistent with the University of Arkansas policy.

Disclaimer: The views presented in this article do not necessarily reflect current or future opinion or policy of the U.S. Food and Drug Administration. Any mention of commercial products is for clarification and not intended as an endorsement.

References

1. Singh, P.K.; Krishnan, S. Vitamin E analogs as radiation response modifiers. *Evid.-Based Complement. Altern. Med.* **2015**, *2015*, 741301. [CrossRef] [PubMed]
2. Lacroix, M.; Ouattara, B. Combined industrial processes with irradiation to assure innocuity and preservation of food products—A review. *Food Res. Int.* **2000**, *33*, 719–724. [CrossRef]
3. Pereira, E.; Antonio, A.L.; Barreira, J.C.; Barros, L.; Bento, A.; Ferreira, I.C. Gamma irradiation as a practical alternative to preserve the chemical and bioactive wholesomeness of widely used aromatic plants. *Food Res. Int.* **2015**, *67*, 338–348. [CrossRef]
4. Kobashigawa, S.; Kashino, G.; Suzuki, K.; Yamashita, S.; Mori, H. Ionizing radiation-induced cell death is partly caused by increase of mitochondrial reactive oxygen species in normal human fibroblast cells. *Radiat. Res.* **2015**, *183*, 455–464. [CrossRef] [PubMed]
5. Redza-Dutordoir, M.; Averill-Bates, D.A. Activation of apoptosis signalling pathways by reactive oxygen species. *Biochim. Biophys. Acta (BBA)-Mol. Cell Res.* **2016**, *1863*, 2977–2992. [CrossRef] [PubMed]

6. Chen, Q.; Chai, Y.C.; Mazumder, S.; Jiang, C.; Macklis, R.M.; Chisolm, G.M.; Almasan, A. The late increase in intracellular free radical oxygen species during apoptosis is associated with cytochrome c release, caspase activation, and mitochondrial dysfunction. *Cell Death Differ.* **2003**, *10*, 323–334. [CrossRef] [PubMed]
7. Singh, V.K.; Beattie, L.A.; Seed, T.M. Vitamin E: Tocopherols and tocotrienols as potential radiation countermeasures. *J. Radiat. Res.* **2013**, *54*, 973–988. [CrossRef] [PubMed]
8. Singh, V.K.; Shafran, R.L.; Jackson, W.E.; Seed, T.M.; Kumar, K.S. Induction of cytokines by radio protective tocopherol analogs. *Exp. Mol. Pathol.* **2006**, *81*, 55–61. [CrossRef] [PubMed]
9. Singh, P.K.; Wise, S.Y.; Ducey, E.J.; Brown, D.S.; Singh, V.K. Radioprotective efficacy of tocopherol succinate is mediated through granulocyte-colony stimulating factor. *Cytokine* **2011**, *56*, 411–421. [CrossRef] [PubMed]
10. Singh, V.K.; Singh, P.K.; Wise, S.Y.; Posarac, A.; Fatanmi, O.O. Radioprotective properties of tocopherol succinate against ionizing radiation in mice. *J. Radiat. Res.* **2012**, *54*, 210–220. [CrossRef] [PubMed]
11. Chitra, S.; Devi, C.S. Effect of alpha-tocopherol on pro-oxidant and antioxidant enzyme status in radiation-treated oral squamous cell carcinoma. *Indian J. Med. Sci.* **2008**, *62*, 141. [CrossRef] [PubMed]
12. Gomes, C.C.; Ramos-Perez, F.M.; Perez, D.E.; Novaes, P.D.; Boscolo, F.N.; Almeida, S.M. Radioprotective effect of vitamin E in parotid glands: A morphometric analysis in rats. *Braz. Dent. J.* **2013**, *24*, 183–187. [CrossRef] [PubMed]
13. Laurent, C.; Pouget, J.P.; Voisin, P. Modulation of DNA damage by pentoxifylline and α-tocopherol in skin fibroblasts exposed to gamma rays. *Radiat. Res.* **2005**, *164*, 63–72. [CrossRef] [PubMed]
14. Ferreira, P.R.; Fleck, J.F.; Diehl, A.; Barletta, D.; Braga-Filho, A.; Barletta, A.; Ilha, L. Protective effect of alpha-tocopherol in head and neck cancer radiation-induced mucositis: A double-blind randomized trial. *Head Neck* **2004**, *26*, 313–321. [CrossRef] [PubMed]
15. Sridharan, V.; Tripathi, P.; Sharma, S.; Corry, P.M.; Moros, E.G.; Singh, A.; Compadre, C.M.; Hauer-Jensen, M.; Boerma, M. Effects of late administration of pentoxifylline and tocotrienols in an image-guided rat model of localized heart irradiation. *PLoS ONE* **2013**, *8*, e68762. [CrossRef] [PubMed]
16. Misirlioglu, C.H.; Demirkasimoglu, T.; Kucukplakci, B.; Sanri, E.; Altundag, K. Pentoxifylline and alpha-tocopherol in prevention of radiation-induced lung toxicity in patients with lung cancer. *Med. Oncol.* **2007**, *24*, 308–311. [CrossRef] [PubMed]
17. Center for Disease Control. Acute Radiation Syndrome: A Brochure for Physicians. U.S. Department of Health and Human Services. Available online: https://emergency.cdc.gov/radiation/pdf/ars.pdf (accessed on 5 January 2018).
18. Singh, V.K.; Ducey, E.J.; Brown, D.S.; Whitnall, M.H. A review of radiation countermeasure works ongoing at the Armed Forces Radiobiology Research Institute. *Int. J. Radiat. Boil.* **2012**, *88*, 296–310. [CrossRef] [PubMed]
19. Weiss, J.F.; Landauer, M.R. History and development of radiation-protective agents. *Int. J. Radiat. Boil.* **2009**, *85*, 539–573. [CrossRef] [PubMed]
20. Dumont, F.; Roux, A.L.; Bischoff, P. Radiation countermeasure agents: An update. *Expert Opin. Ther. Pat.* **2010**, *20*, 73–101. [CrossRef] [PubMed]
21. Weiss, J.F.; Landauer, M.R. Protection against ionizing radiation by antioxidant nutrients and phytochemicals. *Toxicology* **2003**, *189*, 1–20. [CrossRef]
22. Agarwal, S.S.; Singh, V.K. Immunomodulators: A review of studies on Indian medicinal plants and synthetic peptides. Part I: Medicinal plants. *Proc. Ind. Nat. Sci. Acad. B* **1999**, *65*, 179–204.
23. Satyamitra, M.M.; Kulkarni, S.; Ghosh, S.P.; Mullaney, C.P.; Condliffe, D.; Srinivasan, V. Hematopoietic recovery and amelioration of radiation-induced lethality by the vitamin E isoform δ-tocotrienol. *Radiat. Res.* **2011**, *175*, 736–745. [CrossRef] [PubMed]
24. Ghosh, S.P.; Kulkarni, S.; Hieber, K.; Toles, R.; Romanyukha, L.; Kao, T.C.; Hauer-Jensen, M.; Kumar, K.S. Gamma-tocotrienol, a tocol antioxidant as a potent radioprotector. *Int. J. Radiat. Boil.* **2009**, *85*, 598–606. [CrossRef] [PubMed]
25. Compadre, C.M.; Singh, A.; Thakkar, S.; Zheng, G.; Breen, P.J.; Ghosh, S.; Kiaei, M.; Boerma, M.; Varughese, K.I.; Hauer-Jensen, M. Molecular dynamics guided design of tocoflexol: A new radio protectant tocotrienol with enhanced bioavailability. *Drug Dev. Res.* **2014**, *75*, 10–22. [CrossRef] [PubMed]
26. Felemovicius, I.; Bonsack, M.E.; Baptista, M.L.; Delaney, J.P. Intestinal radioprotection by vitamin E (alpha-tocopherol). *Ann. Surg.* **1995**, *222*, 504. [CrossRef] [PubMed]
27. Tsuzuki, W.; Yunoki, R.; Yoshimura, H. Intestinal epithelial cells absorb γ-tocotrienol faster than α-tocopherol. *Lipids* **2007**, *42*, 163. [CrossRef] [PubMed]

28. Serbinova, E.; Kagan, V.; Han, D.; Packer, L. Free radical recycling and intramembrane mobility in the antioxidant properties of alpha-tocopherol and alpha-tocotrienol. *Free Radic. Biol. Med.* **1991**, *10*, 263–275. [CrossRef]
29. Pearce, B.C.; Parker, R.A.; Deason, M.E.; Qureshi, A.A.; Wright, J.K. Hypocholesterolemic activity of synthetic and natural tocotrienols. *J. Med. Chem.* **1992**, *35*, 3595–3606. [CrossRef] [PubMed]
30. Qureshi, A.A.; Pearce, B.C.; Nor, R.M.; Gapor, A. Dietary alpha-tocopherol attenuates the impact of gamma-tocotrienol on hepatic 3-hydroxy-3-methylglutaryl coenzyme A reductase activity in chickens. *J. Nutr.* **1996**, *126*, 389. [CrossRef] [PubMed]
31. Srinivasan, V.; Weiss, J.F. Radioprotection by vitamin E: Injectable vitamin E administered alone or with WR-3689 enhances survival of irradiated mice. *Int. J. Radiat. Oncol. Biol. Phys.* **1992**, *23*, 841–845. [CrossRef]
32. Sarma, L.; Kesavan, P.C. Protective effects of vitamins C and E against γ-ray-induced chromosomal damage in mouse. *Int. J. Radiat. Boil.* **1993**, *63*, 759–764. [CrossRef]
33. Kumar, K.S. Nutritional approaches to radioprotection: Vitamin, E. *Mil. Med.* **2002**, *167*, 57. [PubMed]
34. Boerma, M.; Roberto, K.A.; Hauer-Jensen, M. Prevention and treatment of functional and structural radiation injury in the rat heart by pentoxifylline and alpha-tocopherol. *Int. J. Radiat. Oncol. Biol. Phys.* **2008**, *72*, 170–177. [CrossRef] [PubMed]
35. Empey, L.R.; Papp, J.D.; Jewell, L.D.; Fedorak, R.N. Mucosal protective effects of vitamin E and misoprostol during acute radiation-induced enteritis in rats. *Dig. Dis. Sci.* **1992**, *37*, 205–214. [CrossRef] [PubMed]
36. Roy, R.M.; Petrella, M.; Shateri, H. Effects of administering tocopherol after irradiation on survival and proliferation of murine lymphocytes. *Pharmacol. Ther.* **1988**, *39*, 393–395. [CrossRef]
37. Singh, V.K.; Brown, D.S.; Kao, T.C. Tocopherol succinate: A promising radiation countermeasure. *Int. Immunopharmacol.* **2009**, *9*, 1423–1430. [CrossRef] [PubMed]
38. Singh, P.K.; Wise, S.Y.; Ducey, E.J.; Fatanmi, O.O.; Elliott, T.B.; Singh, V.K. α-Tocopherol succinate protects mice against radiation-induced gastrointestinal injury. *Radiat. Res.* **2011**, *177*, 133–145. [CrossRef] [PubMed]
39. Singh, V.K.; Parekh, V.I.; Brown, D.S.; Kao, T.C.; Mog, S.R. Tocopherol succinate: Modulation of antioxidant enzymes and oncogene expression, and hematopoietic recovery. *Int. J. Radiat. Oncol. Biol. Phys.* **2011**, *79*, 571–578. [CrossRef] [PubMed]
40. Singh, V.K.; Newman, V.L.; Romaine, P.L.; Wise, S.Y.; Seed, T.M. Radiation countermeasure agents: An update (2011–2014). *Expert Opin. Ther. Pat.* **2014**, *24*, 1229–1255. [CrossRef] [PubMed]
41. Kamal-Eldin, A.; Appelqvist, L.Å. The chemistry and antioxidant properties of tocopherols and tocotrienols. *Lipids* **1996**, *31*, 671–701. [CrossRef] [PubMed]
42. Pearce, B.C.; Parker, R.A.; Deason, M.E.; Dischino, D.D.; Gillespie, E.; Qureshi, A.A.; Wright, J.K.; Volk, K. Inhibitors of cholesterol biosynthesis. 2. hypocholesterolemic and antioxidant activities of benzopyran and tetrahydronaphthalene analogs of the tocotrienols. *J. Med. Chem.* **1994**, *37*, 526–541. [CrossRef] [PubMed]
43. Singh, V.K.; Wise, S.Y.; Scott, J.R.; Romaine, P.L.; Newman, V.L.; Fatanmi, O.O. Radioprotective efficacy of delta-tocotrienol, a vitamin E isoform, is mediated through granulocyte colony-stimulating factor. *Life Sci.* **2014**, *98*, 113–122. [CrossRef] [PubMed]
44. Kulkarni, S.; Ghosh, S.P.; Satyamitra, M.; Mog, S.; Hieber, K.; Romanyukha, L.; Gambles, K.; Toles, R.; Kao, T.C.; Hauer-Jensen, M.; Kumar, K.S. Gamma-tocotrienol protects hematopoietic stem and progenitor cells in mice after total-body irradiation. *Radiat. Res.* **2010**, *173*, 738–747. [CrossRef] [PubMed]
45. Singh, V.K.; Kulkarni, S.; Fatanmi, O.O.; Wise, S.Y.; Newman, V.L.; Romaine, P.L.; Hendrickson, H.; Gulani, J.; Ghosh, S.P.; Kumar, K.S.; et al. Radio protective efficacy of gamma-tocotrienol in nonhuman primates. *Radiat. Res.* **2016**, *185*, 285–298. [CrossRef] [PubMed]
46. Li, X.H.; Fu, D.; Latif, N.H.; Mullaney, C.P.; Ney, P.H.; Mog, S.R.; Whitnall, M.H.; Srinivasan, V.; Xiao, M. δ-tocotrienol protects mouse and human hematopoietic progenitors from γ-irradiation through extracellular signal-regulated kinase/mammalian target of rapamycin signaling. *Haematologica* **2010**, *95*, 1996–2004. [CrossRef] [PubMed]
47. Loose, D.S.; Kumar, K.S.; Berbée, M.; Boerma, M.; Hauer-Jensen, M.; Fu, Q. Mechanisms underlying the radioprotective properties of γ-tocotrienol: Comparative gene expression profiling in tocol-treated endothelial cells. *Genes Nutr.* **2012**, *7*, 75.
48. Kulkarni, S.; Singh, P.K.; Ghosh, S.P.; Posarac, A.; Singh, V.K. Granulocyte colony-stimulating factor antibody abrogates radioprotective efficacy of gamma-tocotrienol, a promising radiation countermeasure. *Cytokine* **2013**, *62*, 278–285. [CrossRef] [PubMed]

49. Kumar, D.; Aggarwal, A.K.; Shukla, D.K.; Thimothy, G.; Rani, S. To study and evaluation of role of gamma and delta tocotrienol in radiation induced fibrosis. *Pharma Innov.* **2017**, *6 Pt B*, 91.
50. Yang, C.S.; Lee, M.J.; Zhao, Y.; Yang, Z. Metabolism of tocotrienols in animals and synergistic inhibitory actions of tocotrienols with atorvastatin in cancer cells. *Genes Nutr.* **2012**, *7*, 11. [CrossRef] [PubMed]
51. Naito, Y.; Shimozawa, M.; Kuroda, M.; Nakabe, N.; Manabe, H.; Katada, K.; Kokura, S.; Ichikawa, H.; Yoshida, N.; Noguchi, N.; et al. Tocotrienols reduce 25-hydroxycholesterol-induced monocyte-endothelial cell interaction by inhibiting the surface expression of adhesion molecules. *Atherosclerosis* **2005**, *180*, 19–25. [CrossRef] [PubMed]
52. Berbee, M.; Fu, Q.; Boerma, M.; Pathak, R.; Zhou, D.; Kumar, K.S.; Hauer-Jensen, M. Reduction of radiation-induced vascular nitrosative stress by the vitamin E analog γ-tocotrienol: Evidence of a role for tetrahydrobiopterin. *Int. J. Radiat. Oncol. Biol. Phys.* **2011**, *79*, 884–891. [CrossRef] [PubMed]
53. Bai, M.; Ma, X.; Li, X.; Wang, X.; Mei, Q.; Li, X.; Wu, Z.; Han, W. The accomplices of NF-κB lead to radioresistance. *Curr. Protein Pept. Sci.* **2015**, *16*, 279–294. [CrossRef] [PubMed]
54. Wang, Y.; Park, N.Y.; Jang, Y.; Ma, A.; Jiang, Q. Vitamin E γ-tocotrienol inhibits cytokine-stimulated NF-κB activation by induction of anti-inflammatory A20 via stress adaptive response due to modulation of sphingolipids. *J. Immunol.* **2015**, *195*, 126–133. [CrossRef] [PubMed]
55. Berbée, M.; Fu, Q.; Boerma, M.; Wang, J.; Kumar, K.S.; Hauer-Jensen, M. γ-Tocotrienol ameliorates intestinal radiation injury and reduces vascular oxidative stress after total-body irradiation by an HMG-CoA Reductase-dependent mechanism. *Radiat. Res.* **2009**, *171*, 596–605. [CrossRef] [PubMed]
56. Bjørneboe, A.; Bjørneboe, G.E.; Drevon, C.A. Absorption, transport and distribution of vitamin, E. *J. Nutr.* **1990**, *120*, 233–242. [CrossRef] [PubMed]
57. Yap, S.P.; Yuen, K.H.; Wong, J.W. Pharmacokinetics and bioavailability of α-, γ-and δ-tocotrienols under different food status. *J. Pharm. Pharmacol.* **2001**, *53*, 67–71. [CrossRef] [PubMed]
58. Yap, S.P.; Yuen, K.H.; Lim, A.B. Influence of route of administration on the absorption and disposition of α, γ-and δ-tocotrienols in rats. *J. Pharm. Pharmacol.* **2003**, *55*, 53–58. [CrossRef] [PubMed]
59. Abuasal, B.; Sylvester, P.W.; Kaddoumi, A. Intestinal absorption of γ-tocotrienol is mediated by Niemann-Pick C1-Like 1: In situ rat intestinal perfusion studies. *Drug Metab. Dispos.* **2010**, *38*, 939–945. [CrossRef] [PubMed]
60. Ouahchi, K.; Arita, M.; Kayden, H.; Hentati, F.; Hamida, M.B.; Sokol, R.; Arai, H.; Inoue, K.; Mandel, J.L.; Koenig, M. Ataxia with isolated vitamin E deficiency is caused by mutations in the α–tocopherol transfer protein. *Nat. Genet.* **1995**, *9*, 141–145. [CrossRef] [PubMed]
61. Meier, R.; Tomizaki, T.; Schulze-Briese, C.; Baumann, U.; Stocker, A. The molecular basis of vitamin E retention: Structure of human α-tocopherol transfer protein. *J. Mol. Biol.* **2003**, *331*, 725–734. [CrossRef]
62. Traber, M.G. Vitamin E bioavailability. In *The Encyclopedia of Vitamin E*; Preedy, V.R., Watson, R.R., Eds.; CABI: Oxon, UK, 2007; pp. 221–230.
63. Liu, X.; Gujarathi, S.; Zhang, X.; Shao, L.; Boerma, M.; Compadre, C.M.; Crooks, P.A.; Hauer-Jensen, M.; Zhou, D.; Zheng, G. Synthesis of (2R,8′S,3′E)-δ-tocodienol, a tocoflexol family member designed to have a superior pharmacokinetic profile compared to δ-tocotrienol. *Tetrahedron* **2106**, *72*, 4001–4006. [CrossRef] [PubMed]
64. Stocker, A.; Azzi, A. Tocopherol-binding proteins: Their function and physiological significance. *Antioxid. Redox Signal.* **2000**, *2*, 397–404. [CrossRef] [PubMed]
65. Traber, M.G.; Ramakrishnan, R.; Kayden, H.J. Human plasma vitamin E kinetics demonstrate rapid recycling of plasma RRR-alpha-tocopherol. *Proc. Natl. Acad. Sci. USA.* **1994**, *91*, 10005–10008. [CrossRef] [PubMed]
66. Singh, A.; Breen, P.J.; Ghosh, S.; Kumar, S.K.; Varughese, K.I.; Crooks, P.A.; Hauer-Jensen, M.; Compadre, C.M. Structural modification of tocotrienols to improve bioavailability. In *Tocotrienols: Vitamin E Beyond Tocopherols*, 2nd ed.; Tan, B., Watson, R.R., Preedy, V.R., Eds.; American Oil Chemists Society and Taylor & Francis: Urbana, IL, USA, 2012; pp. 359–370.
67. Kawakami, Y.; Tsuzuki, T.; Nakagawa, K.; Miyazawa, T. Distribution of tocotrienols in rats fed a rice bran tocotrienol concentrate. *Biosci. Biotechnol. Biochem.* **2007**, *71*, 464–471. [CrossRef] [PubMed]
68. Hayes, K.C.; Pronczuk, A.; Liang, J.S. Differences in the plasma transport and tissue concentrations of tocopherols and tocotrienols: Observations in humans and hamsters. *Proc. Soc. Exp. Biol. Med.* **1993**, *202*, 353–359. [CrossRef] [PubMed]

69. Ikeda, S.; Toyoshima, K.; Yamashita, K. Dietary sesame seeds elevate α-and γ-tocotrienol concentrations in skin and adipose tissue of rats fed the tocotrienol-rich fraction extracted from palm oil. *J. Nutr.* **2001**, *131*, 2892–2897. [CrossRef] [PubMed]
70. Okabe, Y.; Watanabe, A.; Shingu, H.; Kushibiki, S.; Hodate, K.; Ishida, M.; Ikeda, S.; Takeda, T. Effects of α-tocopherol level in raw venison on lipid oxidation and volatiles during storage. *Meat Sci.* **2002**, *62*, 457–462. [CrossRef]
71. Min, K.C.; Kovall, R.A.; Hendrickson, W.A. Crystal structure of human α-tocopherol transfer protein bound to its ligand: Implications for ataxia with vitamin E deficiency. *Proc. Natl. Acad. Sci. USA* **2003**, *100*, 14713–14718. [CrossRef] [PubMed]
72. Reboul, E.; Klein, A.; Bietrix, F.; Gleize, B.; Malezet-Desmoulins, C.; Schneider, M.; Margotat, A.; Lagrost, L.; Collet, X.; Borel, P. Scavenger receptor class B type I (SR-BI) is involved in vitamin E transport across the enterocyte. *J. Biol. Chem.* **2006**, *281*, 4739–4745. [CrossRef] [PubMed]
73. Miyoshi, N.; Wakao, Y.; Tomono, S.; Tatemichi, M.; Yano, T.; Ohshima, H. The enhancement of the oral bioavailability of γ-tocotrienol in mice by γ-cyclodextrin inclusion. *J. Nutr. Biochem.* **2011**, *22*, 1121–1126. [CrossRef] [PubMed]
74. Yap, S.P.; Yuen, K.H. Influence of lipolysis and droplet size on tocotrienol absorption from self-emulsifying formulations. *Int. J. Pharm.* **2004**, *281*, 67–78. [CrossRef] [PubMed]
75. Fairus, S.; Nor, R.M.; Cheng, H.M.; Sundram, K. Postprandial metabolic fate of tocotrienol-rich vitamin E differs significantly from that of α-tocopherol. *Am. J. Clin. Nutr.* **2006**, *84*, 835–842. [CrossRef] [PubMed]
76. Fairus, S.; Nor, R.M.; Cheng, H.M.; Sundram, K. Alpha-tocotrienol is the most abundant tocotrienol isomer circulated in plasma and lipoproteins after postprandial tocotrienol-rich vitamin E supplementation. *Nutr. J.* **2012**, *11*, 5. [CrossRef] [PubMed]
77. Qureshi, A.A.; Khan, D.A.; Saleem, S.; Silswal, N.; Trias, A.M. Pharmacokinetics and bioavailability of annatto δ-tocotrienol in healthy fed subjects. *J. Clin. Exp. Cardiol.* **2015**, *6*. [CrossRef]
78. Qureshi, A.A.; Khan, D.A.; Silswal, N.; Saleem, S.; Qureshi, N. Evaluation of Pharmacokinetics, and Bioavailability of Higher Doses of Tocotrienols in Healthy Fed Humans. *J. Clin. Exp. Cardiol.* **2016**, *7*, 434. [CrossRef] [PubMed]
79. Springett, G.M.; Husain, K.; Neuger, A.; Centeno, B.; Chen, D.T.; Hutchinson, T.Z.; Lush, R.M.; Sebti, S.; Malafa, M.P. A Phase I Safety, Pharmacokinetic, and Pharmacodynamic Presurgical Trial of Vitamin E δ-tocotrienol in Patients with Pancreatic Ductal Neoplasia. *eBioMedicine* **2015**, *2*, 1987–1995. [CrossRef] [PubMed]
80. Fu, J.Y.; Che, H.L.; Tan, D.M.; Teng, K.T. Bioavailability of tocotrienols: Evidence in human studies. *Nutr. Metab.* **2014**, *11*, 5. [CrossRef] [PubMed]
81. Wahlqvist, M.L.; Krivokuca-Bogetic, Z.; Lo, C.S.; Hage, B.; Smith, R.; Lukito, W. Differential serum responses of tocopherols and tocotrienols during vitamin supplementation in hypercholesterolaemic individuals without change in coronary risk factors. *Nutr. Res.* **1992**, *12*, S181–S201. [CrossRef]
82. Rasool, A.H.; Yuen, K.H.; Yusoff, K.; Wong, A.R.; Rahman, A.R. Dose dependent elevation of plasma tocotrienol levels and its effect on arterial compliance, plasma total antioxidant status, and lipid profile in healthy humans supplemented with tocotrienol rich vitamin, E. *J. Nutr. Sci. Vitaminol.* **2006**, *52*, 473–478. [CrossRef] [PubMed]
83. Rasool, A.H.; Rahman, A.R.; Yuen, K.H.; Wong, A.R. Arterial compliance and vitamin E blood levels with a self-emulsifying preparation of tocotrienol rich vitamin, E. *Arch. Pharm. Res.* **2008**, *31*, 1212–1217. [CrossRef] [PubMed]
84. Qureshi, A.A.; Sami, S.A.; Salser, W.A.; Khan, F.A. Dose-dependent suppression of serum cholesterol by tocotrienol-rich fraction (TRF 25) of rice bran in hypercholesterolemic humans. *Atherosclerosis* **2002**, *161*, 199–207. [CrossRef]
85. Chin, S.F.; Hamid, N.A.; Latiff, A.A.; Zakaria, Z.; Mazlan, M.; Yusof, Y.A.; Karim, A.A.; Ibahim, J.; Hamid, Z.; Ngah, W.Z. Reduction of DNA damage in older healthy adults by Tri E® Tocotrienol supplementation. *Nutrition* **2008**, *24*, 1–10. [CrossRef] [PubMed]
86. Chin, S.F.; Ibahim, J.; Makpol, S.; Hamid, N.A.; Latiff, A.A.; Zakaria, Z.; Mazlan, M.; Yusof, Y.A.; Karim, A.A.; Ngah, W.Z. Tocotrienol rich fraction supplementation improved lipid profile and oxidative status in healthy older adults: A randomized controlled study. *Nutr. Metab.* **2011**, *8*, 42. [CrossRef] [PubMed]

87. Heng, E.C.; Karsani, S.A.; Rahman, M.A.; Hamid, N.A.; Hamid, Z.; Ngah, W.Z. Supplementation with tocotrienol-rich fraction alters the plasma levels of Apolipoprotein AI precursor, Apolipoprotein E precursor, and C-reactive protein precursor from young and old individuals. *Eur. J. Nutr.* **2013**, *52*, 1811–1820. [CrossRef] [PubMed]
88. Qureshi, A.A.; Khan, D.A.; Mahjabeen, W.; Qureshi, N. Dose-dependent Modulation of Lipid Parameters, Cytokines and RNA by [delta]-tocotrienol in Hypercholesterolemic Subjects Restricted to AHA Step-1 Diet. *Br. J. Med. Med. Res.* **2015**, *6*, 351. [CrossRef]
89. Khor, H.T.; Chieng, D.Y.; Ong, K.K. Tocotrienols inhibit liver HMG CoA reductase activity in the guinea pig. *Nutr. Res.* **1995**, *15*, 537–544. [CrossRef]
90. Husain, K.; Francois, R.A.; Yamauchi, T.; Perez, M.; Sebti, S.M.; Malafa, M.P. Vitamin E δ-Tocotrienol Augments the Anti-tumor Activity of Gemcitabine and Suppresses Constitutive NF-κB Activation in Pancreatic Cancer. *Mol. Cancer Ther.* **2011**. [CrossRef] [PubMed]
91. Meganathan, P.; Jabir, R.S.; Fuang, H.G.; Bhoo-Pathy, N.; Choudhury, R.B.; Taib, N.A.; Nesaretnam, K.; Chik, Z. A new formulation of Gamma Delta Tocotrienol has superior bioavailability compared to existing Tocotrienol-Rich Fraction in healthy human subjects. *Sci. Rep.* **2015**, *5*. [CrossRef] [PubMed]
92. Drotleff, A.M.; Bohnsack, C.; Schneider, I.; Hahn, A.; Ternes, W. Human oral bioavailability and pharmacokinetics of tocotrienols from tocotrienol-rich (tocopherol-low) barley oil and palm oil formulations. *J. Funct. Foods* **2014**, *7*, 150–160. [CrossRef]
93. Abuasal, B.S.; Qosa, H.; Sylvester, P.W.; Kaddoumi, A. Comparison of the intestinal absorption and bioavailability of γ-tocotrienol and α-tocopherol: In vitro, in situ and in vivo studies. *Biopharm. Drug Dispos.* **2012**, *33*, 246–256. [CrossRef] [PubMed]
94. Abuasal, B.S.; Lucas, C.; Peyton, B.; Alayoubi, A.; Nazzal, S.; Sylvester, P.W.; Kaddoumi, A. Enhancement of intestinal permeability utilizing solid lipid nanoparticles increases γ-tocotrienol oral bioavailability. *Lipids* **2012**, *47*, 461–469. [CrossRef] [PubMed]
95. Pouton, C.W. Formulation of poorly water-soluble drugs for oral administration: Physicochemical and physiological issues and the lipid formulation classification system. *Eur. J. Pharm. Sci.* **2006**, *29*, 278–287. [CrossRef] [PubMed]
96. Charman, S.A.; Charman, W.N.; Rogge, M.C.; Wilson, T.D.; Dutko, F.J.; Pouton, C.W. Self-emulsifying drug delivery systems: Formulation and biopharmaceutic evaluation of an investigational lipophilic compound. *Pharm. Res.* **1992**, *9*, 87–93. [CrossRef] [PubMed]
97. Alqahtani, S.; Alayoubi, A.; Nazzal, S.; Sylvester, P.W.; Kaddoumi, A. Enhanced solubility and oral bioavailability of γ-Tocotrienol using a self-emulsifying drug delivery system (SEDDS). *Lipids* **2014**, *49*, 819–829. [CrossRef] [PubMed]
98. Alqahtani, S.; Alayoubi, A.; Nazzal, S.; Sylvester, P.W.; Kaddoumi, A. Nonlinear absorption kinetics of self-emulsifying drug delivery systems (SEDDS) containing tocotrienols as lipophilic molecules: In vivo and in vitro studies. *AAPS J.* **2013**, *15*, 684–695. [CrossRef] [PubMed]
99. Lim, Y.; Traber, M.G. Alpha-tocopherol transfer protein (α-TTP): Insights from alpha-tocopherol transfer protein knockout mice. *Nutr. Res. Pract.* **2007**, *1*, 247–253. [CrossRef] [PubMed]
100. Gohil, K.; Schock, B.C.; Chakraborty, A.A.; Terasawa, Y.; Raber, J.; Farese, R.V.; Packer, L.; Cross, C.E.; Traber, M.G. Gene expression profile of oxidant stress and neurodegeneration in transgenic mice deficient in α-tocopherol transfer protein. *Free Radic. Biol. Med.* **2003**, *35*, 1343–1354. [CrossRef]
101. Jishage, K.I.; Arita, M.; Igarashi, K.; Iwata, T.; Watanabe, M.; Ogawa, M.; Ueda, O.; Kamada, N.; Inoue, K.; Arai, H.; Suzuki, H. α-Tocopherol transfer protein is important for the normal development of placental labyrinthine trophoblasts in mice. *J. Biol. Chem.* **2001**, *276*, 1669–1672. [CrossRef] [PubMed]
102. Leonard, S.W.; Terasawa, Y.; Farese, R.V.; Traber, M.G. Incorporation of deuterated RRR-or all-rac-α-tocopherol in plasma and tissues of α-tocopherol transfer protein–null mice. *Am. J. Clin. Nutr.* **2002**, *75*, 555–560. [CrossRef] [PubMed]
103. Schock, B.C.; Van der Vliet, A.; Corbacho, A.M.; Leonard, S.W.; Finkelstein, E.; Valacchi, G.; Obermueller-Jevic, U.; Cross, C.E.; Traber, M.G. Enhanced inflammatory responses in α-tocopherol transfer protein null mice. *Arch. Biochem. Biophys.* **2004**, *423*, 162–169. [CrossRef] [PubMed]
104. Terasawa, Y.; Ladha, Z.; Leonard, S.W.; Morrow, J.D.; Newland, D.; Sanan, D.; Packer, L.; Traber, M.G.; Farese, R.V. Increased atherosclerosis in hyperlipidemic mice deficient in α-tocopherol transfer protein and vitamin, E. *Proc. Natl. Acad. Sci. USA* **2000**, *97*, 13830–13834. [CrossRef] [PubMed]

105. Yokota, T.; Igarashi, K.; Uchihara, T.; Jishage, K.I.; Tomita, H.; Inaba, A.; Li, Y.; Arita, M.; Suzuki, H.; Mizusawa, H.; et al. Delayed-onset ataxia in mice lacking α-tocopherol transfer protein: Model for neuronal degeneration caused by chronic oxidative stress. *Proc. Natl. Acad. Sci. USA* **2001**, *98*, 15185–15190. [CrossRef] [PubMed]

106. Hosomi, A.; Arita, M.; Sato, Y.; Kiyose, C.; Ueda, T.; Igarashi, O.; Arai, H.; Inoue, K. Affinity for α-tocopherol transfer protein as a determinant of the biological activities of vitamin E analogs. *FEBS Lett.* **1997**, *409*, 105–108. [CrossRef]

107. Li, X.H.; Ghosh, S.P.; Ha, C.T.; Fu, D.; Elliott, T.B.; Bolduc, D.L.; Villa, V.; Whitnall, M.H.; Landauer, M.R.; Xiao, M. Delta-tocotrienol protects mice from radiation-induced gastrointestinal injury. *Radiat. Res.* **2013**, *180*, 649–657. [CrossRef] [PubMed]

108. Little, M.P.; Tawn, E.J.; Tzoulaki, I.; Wakeford, R.; Hildebrandt, G.; Paris, F.; Tapio, S.; Elliott, P. A systematic review of epidemiological associations between low and moderate doses of ionizing radiation and late cardiovascular effects, and their possible mechanisms. *Radiat. Res.* **2008**, *169*, 99–109. [CrossRef] [PubMed]

109. Cucinotta, F.A.; Manuel, F.K.; Jones, J.; Iszard, G.; Murrey, J.; Djojonegro, B.; Wear, M. Space radiation and cataracts in astronauts. *Radiat. Res.* **2001**, *156*, 460–466. [CrossRef]

110. Cucinotta, F.A.; Schimmerling, W.; Wilson, J.W.; Peterson, L.E.; Badhwar, G.D.; Saganti, P.B.; Dicello, J.F. Space radiation cancer risks and uncertainties for Mars missions. *Radiat. Res.* **2001**, *156*, 682–688. [CrossRef]

111. Boerma, M.; Nelson, G.A.; Sridharan, V.; Mao, X.W.; Koturbash, I.; Hauer-Jensen, M. Space radiation and cardiovascular disease risk. *World J. Cardiol.* **2015**, *7*, 882. [CrossRef] [PubMed]

Superoxide Dismutase Mimetic GC4419 Enhances the Oxidation of Pharmacological Ascorbate and its Anticancer Effects in an H_2O_2-Dependent Manner

Collin D. Heer [1,*], Andrew B. Davis [1], David B. Riffe [1], Brett A. Wagner [1], Kelly C. Falls [1], Bryan G. Allen [1], Garry R. Buettner [1], Robert A. Beardsley [2], Dennis P. Riley [2] and Douglas R. Spitz [1,*]

1 Free Radical and Radiation Biology Program, Department of Radiation Oncology, Holden Comprehensive Cancer Center, The University of Iowa College of Medicine, Iowa City, IA 52242, USA; andrew-davis-2@uiowa.edu (A.B.D.); david-riffe@uiowa.edu (D.B.R.); brett-wagner@uiowa.edu (B.A.W.); kelly-falls@uiowa.edu (K.C.F.); bryan-allen@uiowa.edu (B.G.A.); garry-buettner@uiowa.edu (G.R.B.)

2 Galera Therapeutics, Malvern, PA 19355, USA; rbeardsley@galeratx.com (R.A.B.); driley@galeratx.com (D.P.R.)

* Correspondence: collin-heer@uiowa.edu (C.D.H.); douglas-spitz@uiowa.edu (D.R.S.)

Abstract: Lung cancer, together with head and neck cancer, accounts for more than one-fourth of cancer deaths worldwide. New, non-toxic therapeutic approaches are needed. High-dose IV vitamin C (aka, pharmacological ascorbate; P-$AscH^-$) represents a promising adjuvant to radiochemotherapy that exerts its anti-cancer effects via metal-catalyzed oxidation to form H_2O_2. Mn(III)-porphyrins possessing superoxide dismutase (SOD) mimetic activity have been shown to increase the rate of oxidation of $AscH^-$, enhancing the anti-tumor effects of $AscH^-$ in several cancer types. The current study demonstrates that the Mn(II)-containing pentaazamacrocyclic selective SOD mimetic GC4419 may serve as an $AscH^-/O_2^{\bullet-}$ oxidoreductase as evidenced by the increased rate of oxygen consumption, steady-state concentrations of ascorbate radical, and H_2O_2 production in complete cell culture media. GC4419, but not CuZnSOD, was shown to significantly enhance the toxicity of $AscH^-$ in H1299, SCC25, SQ20B, and Cal27 cancer cell lines. This enhanced cancer cell killing was dependent upon the catalytic activity of the SOD mimetic and the generation of H_2O_2, as determined using conditional overexpression of catalase in H1299T cells. GC4419 combined with $AscH^-$ was also capable of enhancing radiation-induced cancer cell killing. Currently, $AscH^-$ and GC4419 are each being tested separately in clinical trials in combination with radiation therapy. Data presented here support the hypothesis that the combination of GC4419 and $AscH^-$ may provide an effective means by which to further enhance radiation therapy responses.

Keywords: SOD mimetic; pharmacological ascorbate; vitamin C; head and neck cancer; lung cancer; radiation therapy; GC4419; oxidative stress; hydrogen peroxide

---

1. Introduction

Lung cancer, along with head and neck cancer, accounts for more than one-fourth of cancer deaths worldwide [1]. New, non-toxic therapeutic approaches are needed to improve survival outcomes. An emerging adjuvant therapy currently in clinical trials is high-dose IV vitamin C (aka, pharmacological ascorbate, P-$AscH^-$). Pharmacological ascorbate has shown promise when used in combination with radiation and chemotherapy in glioblastoma multiforme (NCT02344355), lung cancer (NCT02420314), and pancreatic cancer (NCT02905578) [2–5]. At physiological concentrations (40–80 μM in blood plasma), $AscH^-$ serves as a reducing agent and donor antioxidant [6]. However, at sufficiently high plasma concentrations (mM), $AscH^-$ can act as a selective pro-oxidant in cancer cells [2,5,7]. The pro-oxidant effects of $AscH^-$ are significantly increased in the presence of redox-active transition metals. With a metal catalyst, $AscH^-$ can rapidly transfer an electron to oxygen yielding $O_2^{\bullet-}$. The $O_2^{\bullet-}$ is then dismuted to H_2O_2 spontaneously or by the superoxide dismutase (SOD) family of enzymes [7,8]. The toxicity of $AscH^-$ to cancer cells can be inhibited by either catalase, which removes H_2O_2, or iron chelators that inhibit redox cycling. Thus, Fenton chemistry involving H_2O_2 and labile iron is thought to be responsible for the cancer-cell-specific cytotoxic effects of $AscH^-$ in vitro [5,9]. The role of transition metals in $AscH^-$ pro-oxidant chemistry has roused interest in combining $AscH^-$ with pharmaceutical agents containing redox-active transition metals. For example, the manganese–porphyrin [Mn(III)-porphyrin] class, which has SOD mimetic activity, has been shown to enhance $AscH^-$ toxicity toward cancer cells by increasing the generation of H_2O_2 in breast and pancreatic cancers [10–14].

A prominent class of SOD mimetics is the pentaazamacrocyclic Mn(II)-containing compounds, such as GC4419. GC4419 has exhibited therapeutic effects in several animal models and has recently completed a multi-site phase 2b clinical trial that investigated its ability to mitigate oral mucositis, a commonly experienced side effect of chemo-radiation and radiation therapy in head and neck cancer (NCT02508389) [15–17]. GC4419 is highly stable at pH 7.4 and selectively catalyzes the dismutation of $O_2^{\bullet-}$ with a rate constant at 2×10^7 M^{-1} s^{-1} [18]. GC4419 has been shown to selectively protect normal, but not malignant, human cells in culture and normal human tissue in a Phase 1b/2a clinical study, from radiation and chemotherapy [19,20].

While some Mn(III)-porphyrin SOD mimetics have been shown to augment the redox cycling and subsequent toxicity of $AscH^-$, the ability of Mn(II)-containing SOD mimetics to enhance the anticancer effects of $AscH^-$ has not been thoroughly investigated, primarily because the resting state of the pentaazamacrocyclic compounds is Mn(II) and is thus not amenable to reduction by $AscH^-$. However, it has been suggested that M40403 (aka, GC4403), a Mn(II)-pentaazamacrocyclic compound that is the mirror-image isomer of GC4419, may function as a $AscH^-/O_2^{\bullet-}$ oxidoreductase that catalyzes the transfer of an electron from $AscH^-$ to $O_2^{\bullet-}$, yielding H_2O_2 and $Asc^{\bullet-}$ [21]. Yet, the ability of GC4419 to enhance the anticancer effects of $AscH^-$ remains unknown. Here we present evidence that, when combined with pharmacological levels of $AscH^-$, GC4419 significantly increases cancer cell killing relative to $AscH^-$ alone. Our data suggest this cancer cell killing is dependent on H_2O_2 and is accompanied by increased rates of oxidation of $AscH^-$, oxygen consumption, and H_2O_2 production. In addition, GC4419 + $AscH^-$ (GC/$AscH^-$) sensitizes human lung and head and neck cancer cells to radiation. Both $AscH^-$ and GC4419 are currently being investigated individually in phase 2 clinical trials. Because both of these trials involve radiation therapy, the data presented here support the hypothesis that the combination of these agents may represent a viable approach to significantly improve patient outcomes in both head and neck and lung cancer.

2. Materials and Methods

2.1. Cell Lines and Media

H1299 lung cancer cells were obtained from ATCC and grown in RPMI 1640 media supplemented with 10% fetal bovine serum (FBS; Atlanta Biologicals, Flowery Brach, GA, USA). Cal27 and SCC25 head and neck cancer cells were obtained from ATCC. SQ20B cells were a gift from Andrean Simons-Burnett (Department of Pathology, University of Iowa, Iowa City, IA, USA). TSA201 cells were a gift from Dawn Quelle (Department of Pharmacology, University of Iowa, Iowa City, IA, USA). Cal27, SQ20B and TSA201 cells were maintained in DMEM (Gibco, Grand Island, NY, USA) media supplemented with 10% FBS. SCC25 cells were maintained in DMEM:F12 (Gibco) media containing 10% FBS, 1% HEPES and 400 ng mL^{-1} hydrocortisone. H1299T-CAT cells were derived from the H1299T cell line, as described below. All cultures were maintained in 5% CO_2, 20% O_2, and humidified in a 37 °C incubator.

2.2. Drug Treatment

Cells were treated with 5–20 μM GC4419 for 1 h or 24 h prior to and during treatment with $AscH^-$ (2.5–20 pmol $cell^{-1}$). L-Ascorbic acid stock solution (1.0 M) was prepared in Nanopure Type 1 water with the pH adjusted to 7.0 with NaOH. Concentration was determined spectrophotometrically, ε_{265} = 14,500 M^{-1} cm^{-1} [8]. $AscH^-$ was dosed per cell (pmol $cell^{-1}$), rather than by concentration, due to the dependence of $AscH^-$ and H_2O_2 toxicity on cell density [5,22–24]. All concentrations used in this study are relevant to in vivo measurements of $AscH^-$ in human plasma following IV infusion. GC4419 was dissolved in Nanopure water containing 5 mM sodium bicarbonate (Gibco). CuZnSOD (DDI Pharmaceuticals, Mountain View, CA, USA) was dissolved in Nanopure water. Cells were irradiated with a dose of 2 Gy (dose rate, 0.365 Gy min^{-1}) using a ^{37}Cs source (JL Shepherd, San Fernando, CA, USA).

2.3. Electron Paramagnetic Resonance (EPR) Spectroscopy

Spectra of the ascorbate free radical were collected with a Bruker EMX ESR spectrophotometer (Bruker BioSpin, Billerica, MA, USA) as previously described [10]. EPR instrument settings used to quantify [$Asc^{\bullet -}$] were center field, 3507.62 G; sweep width, 10.00 G; receiver gain, 5.02 × 10^4; modulation amplitude, 0.70 G; microwave frequency, 9.85 GHz; using an ER4119HS cavity with nominal microwave power of 10.0 mW. 3-Carboxyl-PROXYL (3-CxP, CAS: 2154-68-9; Sigma Aldrich, St. Louis, MO, USA) was used as the concentration standard taking into account potential saturation effects [25].

2.4. Oxygen Consumption by Clark Electrode

The rate of oxygen consumption was determined using a Clark electrode (YSI Inc., Yellow Springs, OH, USA). Data were collected using an ESA Biostat multielectrode system (ESA Dionex Corp, Chelmsford, MA, USA) and analyzed using Microsoft Excel (Microsoft, Redmond, WA, USA). Rates were determined from oxygen concentrations recorded every second over at least 60 s. Experiments were carried out in RPMI media containing 10% FBS.

2.5. H_2O_2 Quantification

Accumulation of H_2O_2 was determined using a Clark electrode (YSI Inc., Yellow Springs, OH, USA). $AscH^-$, GC4419 + $AscH^-$, or CuZnSOD + $AscH^-$ were added to RPMI media containing 10% FBS and O_2 concentrations were recorded every second. After 10 min, the concentration of H_2O_2 was determined based on the amount of O_2 generated following addition of 500 U mL^{-1} of catalase. The rate of production of H_2O_2 was then determined in units of nM H_2O_2 s^{-1}.

2.6. SOD Activity Assay

SOD activity was determined using the indirect competitive inhibition assay as described previously [26]. Briefly, the flux of superoxide generated by the metabolism of xanthine by xanthine oxidase was measured using nitroblue tetrazolium (NBT). The rate of NBT reduction can be measured spectrophotometrically at 560 nm and is inhibited by increasing concentrations of SOD or GC4419 that compete for the superoxide produced by xanthine oxidase. The rate of NBT reduction is calculated as percent inhibition relative to the NBT reduction in the absence of the native CuZnSOD or GC4419. The amount of CuZnSOD or GC4419 causing 50% maximum inhibition is defined as one unit of activity.

2.7. Clonogenic Assay

Cells (1.5–3.5 × 10^5) were plated in 60-mm dishes and allowed to grow for 48 h (SCC25) or 72 h (H1299, Cal27, SQ20B) prior to clonogenic assay. Cells were detached using 0.25% trypsin, combined with floating cells, and pelleted via centrifugation at 335× *g* for 5 min. Pellets were resuspended in fresh media and the total cell population was counted using a Beckman Coulter

Counter (Beckman Coulter Inc., Hialeaha, FL, USA). Cells were then plated in 60-mm dishes at a variety of densities ranging from 150–100,000 cells per dish. Clones were grown for 7–14 days in complete media with 0.1% gentamycin, fixed with 70% ethanol, stained with Coomassie blue, and colonies containing ≥50 cells were counted. The plating efficiencies of treatment groups for each cell line were normalized to the Control, GC4419, or GC4419/doxycycline (GC/Dox)-treated groups. The survival analysis was performed using a minimum of two cloning dishes per experimental condition, and the experiments were repeated a minimum of three times.

2.8. Lentivirus Production and Transduction

The doxycycline-inducible catalase overexpression plasmid was generated as previously described and obtained from Fenghuang Zahn's Lab (Department of Internal Medicine, University of Iowa, Iowa City, IA, USA) [27]. Lentivirus was produced in the TSA201 cell line using pCMV-VSV-G and psPAX2 helper vectors (Addgene, Caimbridge, MA, USA). H1299T cells (a clonal population derived from H1299 for aggressive growth in animals) were plated and allowed to grow for 48 h, and then virus was added to cells with 8 $\mu g\ mL^{-1}$ of polybrene every 24 h for two days. After transduction, cells were selected with 5 $\mu g\ mL^{-1}$ puromycin. Surviving cells were plated in 150-mm dishes with 1000 cells per dish. Clones were grown for 10 days, and then several colonies were picked and expanded. To test for maximal catalase overexpression, cells were treated with 1.5 $\mu g\ mL^{-1}$ of doxycycline for 48 h. Protein concentration was determined using the Lowry Assay. Increased catalase activity was verified by measuring the decomposition of H_2O_2 by cell lysates as previously described [28]. Maximal activity was found in clone 15. Optimal dose of doxycycline was determined by treating with 0.25–2 $\mu g\ mL^{-1}$ doxycycline for 24 or 48 h.

2.9. Statistical Analysis

Statistical analyses were performed using GraphPad Prism (Graphpad Software Inc., La Jolla, CA, USA) and an $\alpha = 0.05$. Two-way ANOVA analyses were performed with Tukey's multiple comparison post hoc test.

3. Results

3.1. GC4419 Increases the Rate of Oxygen Consumption and Ascorbate Radical Steady-State Concentration in Systems Containing AscH$^-$

To determine the effect of GC4419 on the rate of AscH$^-$ oxidation in complete RPMI media, we measured the steady-state concentration of ascorbate radical ($[Asc^{\bullet-}]_{ss}$) by EPR spectroscopy [29]. After adding AscH$^-$ or GC/AscH$^-$ to complete media, the solution was vortexed and immediately examined by EPR spectroscopy. When combined with 6 mM AscH$^-$, addition of 5 μM or 20 μM GC4419 resulted in a dose-dependent increase in $[Asc^{\bullet-}]_{ss}$ compared to AscH$^-$ alone (Figure 1A). When added to 6 mM AscH$^-$, 5 μM GC4419 increased the $[Asc^{\bullet-}]_{ss}$ by approximately 50%. When added to 3 mM or 6 mM AscH$^-$, 20 μM GC4419 roughly doubled the $[Asc^{\bullet-}]_{ss}$. These findings support the hypothesis that GC4419 catalyzes the oxidation of AscH$^-$.

To determine if the increase in $[Asc^{\bullet-}]_{ss}$ in the presence of GC4419 was accompanied by an increase in the production of reactive oxygen species (ROS), we evaluated the rate of oxygen consumption using a Clark Electrode. We observed that addition of 2 mM AscH$^-$ to complete RPMI media resulted in an increase in the rate of O_2 consumption from 15 to 35 nM s^{-1}. The addition of 20 μM GC4419 doubled the rate of O_2 consumption to 70 nM s^{-1} (Figure 1B). These findings support the hypothesis that the addition of GC4419 to solutions containing AscH$^-$ significantly increases the rate of oxygen consumption, which may indicate the production of ROS.

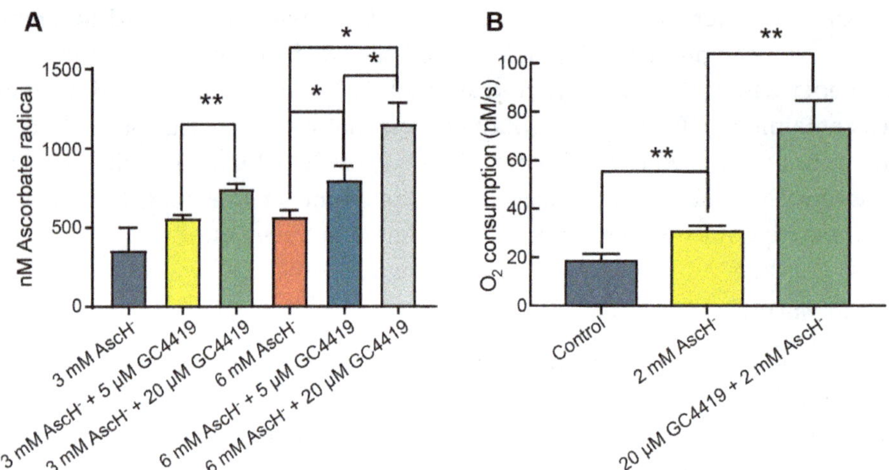

Figure 1. GC4419 increases the oxidative flux of systems containing $AscH^-$ (**A**) GC4419 increases $[Asc^{\bullet-}]_{ss}$ in complete media containing $AscH^-$. Ascorbate alone or GC/$AscH^-$ were added to complete RPMI media. Solutions were immediately examined by EPR and $[Asc^{\bullet-}]_{ss}$ was determined. 3-Carboxyl-PROXYL was used as a concentration standard [25]. Errors represent $\pm$ SEM, n = 3. * $p < 0.05$, ** $p < 0.01$ by unpaired t-test. (**B**) GC4419 increases oxygen consumption of complete media containing $AscH^-$. Ascorbate was added to complete RPMI media (Control) and the rate of oxygen consumption was measured. GC4419 was then added to the solution and oxygen consumption was measured. Errors represent $\pm$ SEM, n = 3. ** $p < 0.01$ by unpaired t-test.

3.2. GC4419, but Not CuZnSOD, Increases H_2O_2 Production and Cancer Cell Toxicity when Combined with $AscH^-$

To determine if the increased rate of oxygen consumption and higher $[Asc^{\bullet-}]_{ss}$ of systems containing GC4419 and $AscH^-$ translates to increased cancer cell killing, cancer cells were treated with 5–20 μM GC4419 for 24 h prior to and during the addition of $AscH^-$, then clonogenic survival was assessed. In multiple cancer cell lines, GC4419 significantly increased clonogenic cancer cell death in a manner that was dependent on the concentration of both GC4419 and $AscH^-$ (Figure 2A–D).

We next hypothesized that the increased oxygen consumption, $[Asc^{\bullet-}]_{ss}$, and cancer cell killing upon addition of GC4419 to systems containing $AscH^-$ may be due to the SOD activity of the mimetic. Specifically, GC4419 could enhance the rate of dismutation of $O_2^{\bullet-}$ produced by $AscH^-$, increasing the flux of H_2O_2 and resulting toxicity toward cancer cells. To test this hypothesis, H1299 lung cancer cells were treated with 0.1 or 1 μM CuZnSOD 24 h prior to and during a 1 h exposure to $AscH^-$. Concentrations of 0.1 and 1.0 μM CuZnSOD were chosen because these concentrations should be kinetically equivalent to 10 and 100 μM GC4419 based on rate constants for the dismutation reaction, 1.3×10^9 M^{-1} s^{-1} for CuZnSOD [30] and 2×10^7 M^{-1} s^{-1} for GC4419 [18]. The higher SOD activity of native CuZnSOD relative to GC4419 was confirmed using a NBT-reduction-based competitive inhibition assay where we found that the specific activity of CuZnSOD is approximately 240 times greater than that of GC4419 (Figure 2E, Inset). Interestingly, despite its higher SOD activity, no enhancement of cancer cell toxicity was observed upon addition of CuZnSOD to media containing $AscH^-$ (Figure 2E).

To determine if H_2O_2 production was increased upon the addition of GC4419, but not CuZnSOD, to systems containing $AscH^-$, we measured the generation of O_2 upon the addition of catalase to systems containing $AscH^-$ alone, GC4419 and $AscH^-$, or CuZnSOD and $AscH^-$. We found that GC4419, but not CuZnSOD, was able to significantly increase accumulation of H_2O_2 in systems containing $AscH^-$ (Figure 2F). These results suggest that increasing the SOD activity of the system does not affect H_2O_2 production or $AscH^-$ toxicity toward cancer cells. Similar results have been observed by other researchers combining PEG-SOD with $AscH^-$ [10]. These results also suggest that the SOD activity of GC4419 is not directly responsible for its ability to enhance $AscH^-$ toxicity, and support the hypothesis that GC4419 functions as an $AscH^-/O_2^{\bullet-}$ oxidoreductase that catalyzes the transfer of an electron from $AscH^-$ to $O_2^{\bullet-}$ to produce H_2O_2.

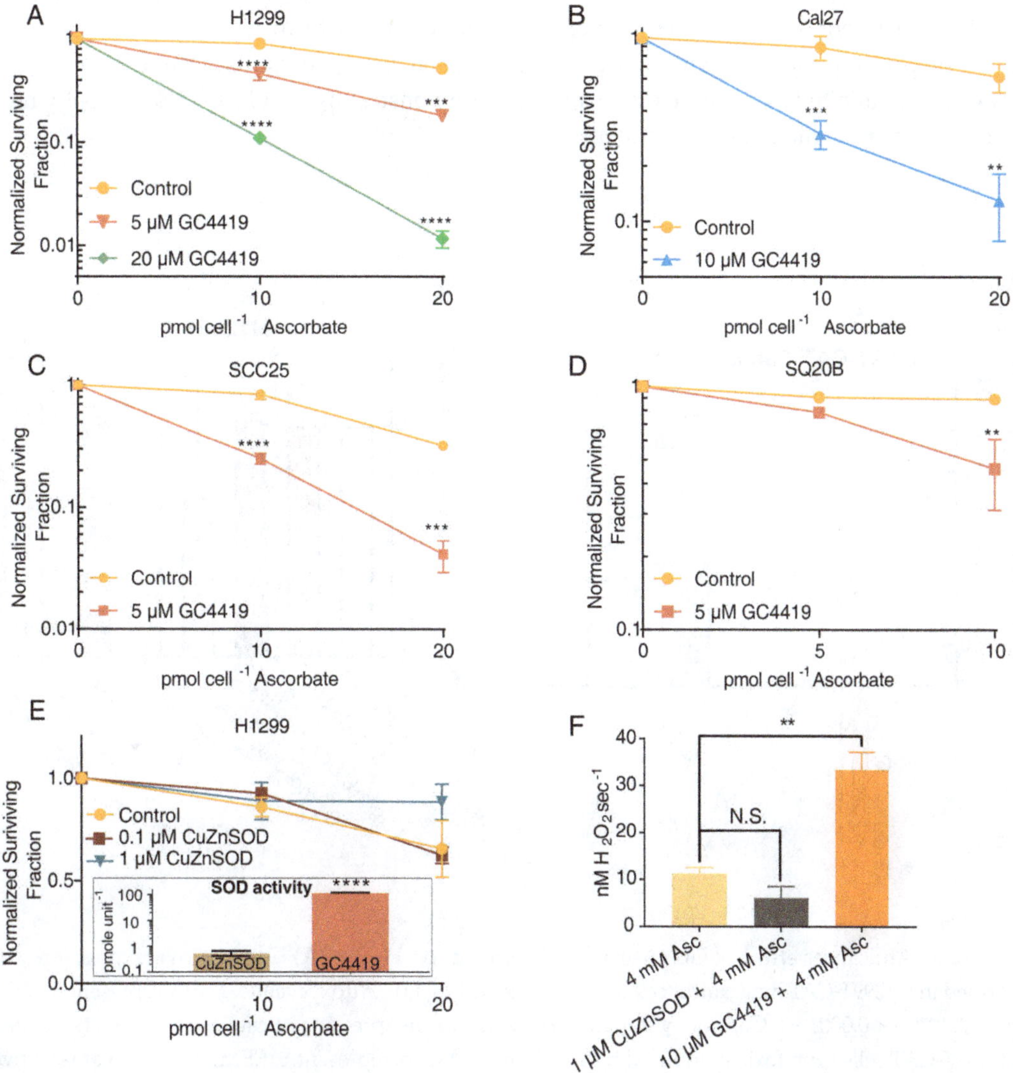

Figure 2. GC4419, but not CuZnSOD, increases cancer cell toxicity and H_2O_2 production when combined with $AscH^-$. (**A–D**) When added 24 h prior to and during 1 h $AscH^-$ treatment, GC4419 significantly increases the toxicity of $AscH^-$ in lung (H1299) and head-and-neck (Cal27, SQ20B, SCC25) cancer cell lines. Errors represent ± SEM, $n = 3$ with at least two cloning dishes per treatment. ** $p < 0.01$, *** $p < 0.001$, **** $p < 0.0001$ vs. Control by two-way ANOVA. Normalized to Control or GC4419-treated group. (**E**) Cells were treated with 0.1–10 µM CuZnSOD for 24 h prior to and during $AscH^-$ treatment. $n = 4$ with at least two cloning dishes per treatment. Normalized to Control or CuZnSOD groups. Inset: CuZnSOD exhibits approximately 240 times greater specific SOD activity relative to GC4419 as determined using a NBT-based competitive inhibition assay. Errors represent ± SEM, $n = 3$. **** $p < 0.0001$ vs. CuZnSOD by upaired *t*-test (**F**) Accumulation of H_2O_2 was determined using a Clark electrode (YSI Inc., Yellow Springs, OH, USA). $AscH^-$, GC4419 + $AscH^-$ or CuZnSOD + $AscH^-$ were added to RPMI media containing 10% FBS. The concentration of H_2O_2 was determined based on the amount of O_2 generated following addition of 500 U mL^{-1} of catalase. Errors represent ± SEM, $n = 3–4$. ** $p < 0.01$, vs. Control by unpaired *t*-test.

3.3. GC/AscH$^-$ Toxicity is Dependent on H_2O_2

To verify that the anti-cancer effect of GC/AscH$^-$ treatment is H_2O_2-dependent, we utilized an H1299T cell line that conditionally overexpresses catalase when exposed to doxycycline (H1299T-CAT). Cells were treated with 1 μg mL^{-1} of doxycycline 48 h prior to treatment with GC4419 and AscH$^-$. Doxycycline treatment was confirmed to increase catalase activity from 3.7 ± 1.5 m*k*U (mg protein)$^{-1}$ to 316 ± 9 m*k*U (mg protein)$^{-1}$ (Figure 3A). The cancer cell clonogenic killing capacity of GC/AscH$^-$ was completely inhibited by catalase overexpression, demonstrating that H_2O_2 was causally related to the cancer cell clonogenic killing (Figure 3B).

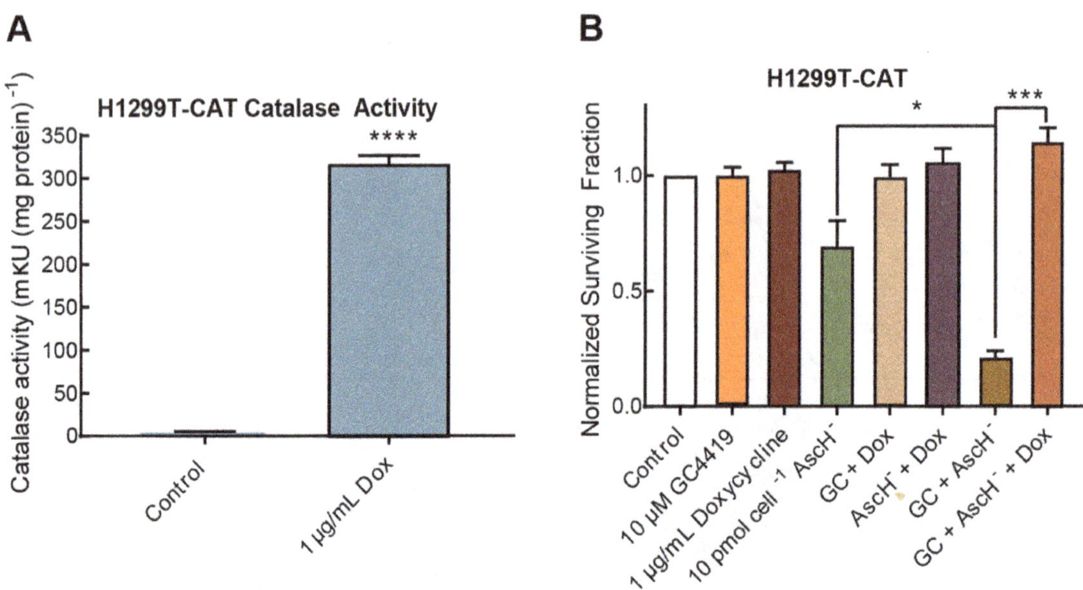

Figure 3. Anticancer effect of GC/AscH$^-$ is dependent on H_2O_2. (**A**) Catalase overexpression was verified in H1299T-CAT lung cancer cell lines exposed to 1 μg mL^{-1} doxycycline. Errors represent ± SEM, $n = 12$. **** $p < 0.0001$ vs. Control by unpaired *t*-test. (**B**) Overexpression of catalase completely rescued H1299T-CAT cells from toxicity induced by GC/AscH$^-$. Errors represent ± SEM, $n = 3$ with at least two cloning dishes per treatment. * $p < 0.05$, *** $p < 0.001$ by unpaired *t*-test. Normalized to Control.

3.4. Catalytic Activity of Mn(II)-Pentaazamacrocylces is Required for Enhancement of AscH− Toxicity

To determine if catalytic cycling of the pentaazamacrocycle is required for the enhancement of AscH$^-$ toxicity, we combined AscH$^-$ with GC4404, a Mn(II)-pentaazamacrocyclic derivative that is devoid of SOD activity. GC4404 does not form the Mn(III)-intermediate, which has been suggested to be reduced by AscH$^-$ [18,21]. Media were replaced, and H1299 lung cancer cells were treated with GC4419 or GC4404 for 1 h prior to and during the 1 h AscH$^-$ treatment. As predicted, GC4419 enhanced the toxicity of AscH$^-$ while GC4404 had no effect on AscH$^-$ toxicity (Figure 4). These results further support the hypothesis that catalytic cycling of the pentaazamacrocycle is required for the enhancement of AscH$^-$ toxicity.

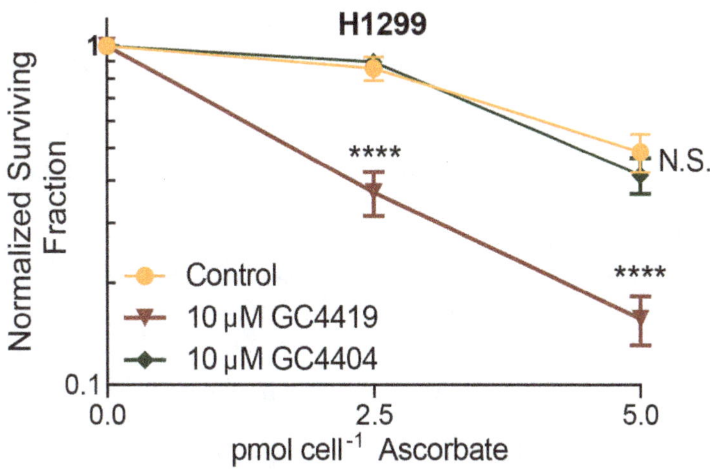

Figure 4. Catalytic activity of pentaazamacrocyclic mimetic is required to enhance $AscH^-$ toxicity as seen by clonogenic assay. Media were replaced and cells were treated with 10 μM of GC4419 or GC4404 (SOD inactive) for 1 h prior to 1 h $AscH^-$ treatment. Errors represent ± SEM, n = 4–7 with at least two cloning dishes per treatment. **** $p < 0.0001$, N.S. = no significance vs. Control by two-way ANOVA. Normalized to Control, GC4419, or GC4404 groups.

3.5. GC/AscH⁻ Treatment Increases Cancer Cell Response to Ionizing Radiation

Patients being treated with GC4419 in clinical trials to date (i.e., NCT02508389) all received radiation treatment; H_2O_2 is known to increase tumor response to radiation [5,31]. Thus, combining $AscH^-$ and GC4419 with radiation has the potential to improve tumor therapy outcomes. To investigate the ability of GC/$AscH^-$ to enhance the response of cancer cells to ionizing radiation (IR), cancer cells were exposed to GC4419 for 24 h and $AscH^-$ for 1 h prior to exposure to IR. Interestingly, the treatment with GC/$AscH^-$ prior to 2 Gy IR resulted in cancer cell killing that was at least additive and significantly exceeded that seen with either agent alone in two cell lines, with a third trending toward significance (Figure 5).

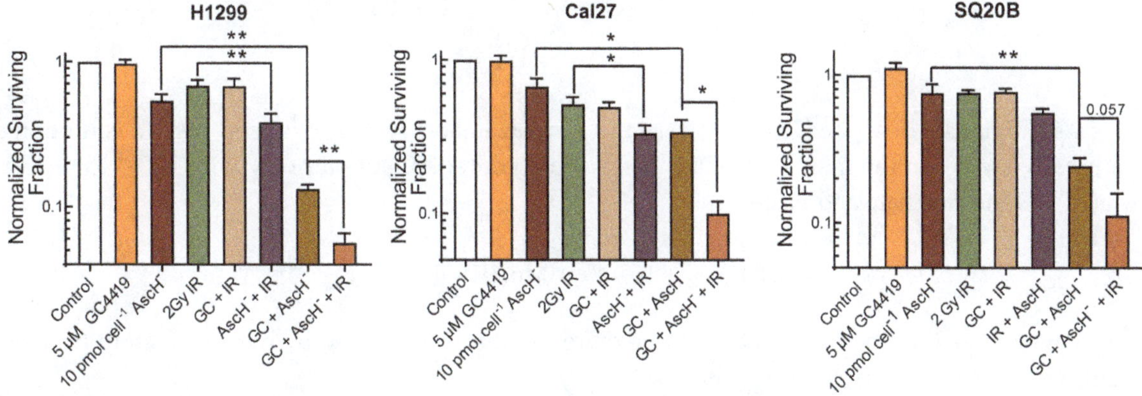

Figure 5. GC/$AscH^-$ treatment sensitizes cancer cells to IR as seen by clonogenic assay. H1299 lung cancer cells and Cal27 and SQ20B head and neck cancer cells were treated with GC4419 24 h before and $AscH^-$ 1 h before exposure to IR. Errors represent ± SEM, n = 3–4 with at least two cloning dishes per treatment. * $p < 0.05$, ** $p < 0.01$, by unpaired t-test. Normalized to Control.

4. Discussion

We have shown that the Mn(II)-pentaazamacrocyclic SOD mimetic GC4419 increases the rate of oxygen consumption, $[Asc^{\bullet -}]_{ss}$, and H_2O_2 production in complete media containing pharmacological levels of $AscH^-$. When applied to cells, the combination of GC4419/$AscH^-$ results in increased clonogenic cancer cell killing that is dependent on H_2O_2 and the catalytic activity of the pentaazamacrocycle. Another exciting finding is that the combination of GC4419 and $AscH^-$ sensitizes cancer cells to IR.

Understanding the similarities and differences of reaction mechanisms of various classes of SOD mimetics with $AscH^-$ is of potential importance for the clinical implementation of SOD mimetics in combination with $AscH^-$. In addition, this understanding will be critical for the development of novel or structurally-related compounds that combine with $AscH^-$ to enhance cancer cell toxicity. For the Mn(III)-porphyrins possessing SOD mimetic activity, it has been proposed that the Mn(III) is reduced by $AscH^-$, yielding Mn(II) and $Asc^{\bullet-}$. The Mn(II) then reduces O_2 to $O_2^{\bullet-}$ [11].

$$\mathrm{Mn(III)} + \mathrm{AscH^-} \rightarrow \mathrm{Mn(II)} + \mathrm{Asc^{\bullet-}}$$

$$\mathrm{Mn(II)} + \mathrm{O_2} \rightarrow \mathrm{Mn(III)} + \mathrm{O_2^{\bullet-}}$$

Because the Mn(III)-porphyrin simply serves as a catalyst, the net reaction is:

$$\mathrm{O_2} + \mathrm{AscH^-} \rightarrow \mathrm{O_2^{\bullet-}} + \mathrm{Asc^{\bullet-}}$$

The $O_2^{\bullet-}$ then dismutes spontaneously or through the action of the Mn(III)-porphyrin as an SOD mimetic to yield H_2O_2. Because catalase overexpression has been shown to completely inhibit killing, this H_2O_2 is principally responsible for the toxicity of $AscH^-$ [10,11].

$$\mathrm{O_2^{\bullet-}} + \mathrm{O_2^{\bullet-}} + 2\mathrm{H^+} \rightarrow \mathrm{H_2O_2} + \mathrm{O_2}$$

In the case of Mn(II)-pentaazamacrocyclic mimetics, we propose that the $O_2^{\bullet-}$ or $HO_2^{\bullet}$ necessary to initiate the oxidation of GC4419 is primarily produced by reactions between $AscH^-$ and redox-active transition metals in cell culture media [32,33]. For example,

$$\mathrm{AscH^-} + (\mathrm{Cu/Fe})^{n} \rightarrow \mathrm{Asc^{\bullet-}} + (\mathrm{Cu/Fe})^{n-1}$$

$$(\mathrm{Cu/Fe})^{n-1} + \mathrm{O_2} \rightarrow \mathrm{O_2^{\bullet-}} + (\mathrm{Cu/Fe})^{n}$$

$$\mathrm{O_2^{\bullet-}} + \mathrm{H^+} \leftrightarrow \mathrm{HO_2^{\bullet}}$$

As previously described, the Mn(II) of the pentaazamacrocycle is oxidized by two competing pathways [34,35]. In the first, $Mn(II)OH_2$ reacts via an outer-sphere pathway with $HO_2^{\bullet}$ to yield a Mn(III)OH intermediate and H_2O_2.

$$\mathrm{Mn(II)OH_2} + \mathrm{HO_2^{\bullet}} \rightarrow \mathrm{Mn(III)OH} + \mathrm{H_2O_2}$$

We propose that the Mn(III)OH intermediate can then be reduced by hydrogen atom transfer from $AscH^-$, yielding H_2O, Mn(II), and $Asc^{\bullet-}$.

$$\mathrm{Mn(III)OH} + \mathrm{AscH^-} \rightarrow \mathrm{Mn(II)} + \mathrm{H_2O} + \mathrm{Asc^{\bullet-}}$$

Removing the Mn(II)-pentaazamacrocycle from the equation, because it serves as a catalyst, the net reaction is:

$$\mathrm{HO_2^{\bullet}} + \mathrm{AscH^-} \rightarrow \mathrm{Asc^{\bullet-}} + \mathrm{H_2O_2}$$

The second mechanism is in-line with the conclusion that GC4419 can act as an $AscH^-/O_2^{\bullet-}$ oxidoreductase by catalyzing the transfer of an electron from $AscH^-$ to $O_2^{\bullet-}$, yielding H_2O_2 and

$Asc^{\bullet-}$ [21]. In this reaction, the Mn(II) intermediate is complexed by $O_2^{\bullet-}$ and oxidation is initiated following protonation of the bound $O_2^{\bullet-}$.

$$\mathrm{Mn(II)} + \mathrm{O_2}^{\bullet-} + \mathrm{H^+} \rightarrow \mathrm{Mn(III)O_2H}$$

We propose that the $Mn(III)O_2H$ intermediate is also then reduced by a hydrogen atom transfer from $AscH^-$, yielding H_2O_2 and $Asc^{\bullet-}$.

$$\mathrm{Mn(III)O_2H} + \mathrm{AscH^-} \rightarrow \mathrm{Mn(II)} + \mathrm{H_2O_2} + \mathrm{Asc}^{\bullet-}$$

Removing the Mn(II)-pentaazamacrocycle complex from the equation, because it serves as a catalyst, the net reaction is:

$$\mathrm{O_2}^{\bullet-} + \mathrm{H^+} + \mathrm{AscH^-} \rightarrow \mathrm{H_2O_2} + \mathrm{Asc}^{\bullet-}$$

Several findings in the present study support these conclusions:

(1) the reduction of the Mn(III) intermediate by $AscH^-$ is thermodynamically favorable, as the reduction potential of GC4419 Mn(III)/Mn(II) (+525 mV, acetonitrile) is considerably greater than $Asc^{\bullet-}/AscH^-$ (+282 mV, aqueous) [32,36];

(2) Native CuZnSOD does not enhance cancer cell toxicity or H_2O_2 production when combined with $AscH^-$, supporting the hypothesis that the SOD activity of GC4419 is not responsible for increased $AscH^-$ toxicity;

(3) Addition of GC4419 to solutions containing $AscH^-$ results in a significant increase in $[Asc^{\bullet-}]_{ss}$, supporting the hypothesis that addition of GC4419 increases the one-electron oxidation of $AscH^-$;

(4) The structurally-similar Mn(II)-pentaazamacrocycle complex, GC4404, which does not form the Mn(III)-intermediate which has been suggested to be reduced by $AscH^-$ [35], does not enhance $AscH^-$ cancer cell toxicity, strongly supporting the hypothesis that catalytic cycling of the pentaazamacrocycle is required for the enhancement of $AscH^-$ toxicity; and

(5) GC4419 enhances H_2O_2 production when combined with $AscH^-$, and the cancer cell toxicity of $GC/AscH^-$ is completely inhibited by catalase overexpression, demonstrating that H_2O_2 is responsible for the toxicity of $GC/AscH^-$.

5. Conclusions

Thus, our findings support the conclusion that, in the presence of mM levels of $AscH^-$ in complete media, GC4419 can function as an $AscH^-/O_2^{\bullet-}$ oxidoreductase catalyst [21], killing human lung and head and neck cancer cells by a mechanism involving the formation of H_2O_2. However, the role of the two competing pathways of oxidation and how this relates to the potential $AscH^-/O_2^{\bullet-}$ oxidoreductase activity of GC4419 requires further investigation. Future studies will also investigate the utility of $GC/AscH^-$ in enhancing the response of cancer cells and tumors to radiation and chemotherapy in vivo as well as examine the ability of other pentaazamacrocyclic compounds to enhance $AscH^-$ cancer cell toxicity.

6. Patents

Authors Collin D. Heer, Robert A. Beardsley, Dennis P. Riley, and Douglas R. Spitz and have submitted one or more patent applications covering some of the aspects of these discoveries.

Acknowledgments: The authors would like to thank the Radiation and Free Radical Research Core in the Holden Comprehensive Cancer Center. This work was supported by Galera Therapeutics Inc., as well as NIH grants T32 CA078586, T32 DC000040, R01CA182804, R01CA169046, P30CA086862, T35HL007485-34, F30 CA213817, 5T32 GM007337 and the Carver Research Program of Excellence in Redox Biology and Medicine and the Carver College of Medicine Medical Student Summer Research Program. The authors would also like to thank Gareth Smith for assistance in preparing the manuscript.

Author Contributions: Collin D. Heer and Douglas R. Spitz conceived and designed the experiments; Collin D. Heer, Andrew B. Davis, and David B. Riffe performed the experiments; Collin D. Heer, Bryan G. Allen, Robert A. Beardsley, Dennis P. Riley, and Douglas R. Spitz analyzed the data; Brett A. Wagner, Dennis P. Riley, Garry R. Buettner, and Kelly C. Falls contributed reagents/materials/analysis tools; Collin D. Heer and Douglas R. Spitz wrote the manuscript and all authors edited the manuscript.

Conflicts of Interest: Dennis P. Riley and Robert A. Beardsley are employed by and hold equity interests in Galera Therapeutics, Inc. which provided the pentaazamacrocyclic compounds used in this study. Douglas R. Spitz and Bryan G. Allen have Sponsored Research Agreements supported by Galera Therapeutics, Inc. to study GC4419 in preclinical and clinical studies of cancer therapy. No other author has competing financial interests in this work.

References

1. Siegel, R.L.; Miller, K.D.; Jemal, A. Cancer statistics, 2016. *CA Cancer J. Clin.* **2016**, *66*, 7–30. [CrossRef] [PubMed]
2. Welsh, J.L.; Wagner, B.A.; van't Erve, T.J.; Zehr, P.S.; Berg, D.J.; Halfdanarson, T.R.; Yee, N.S.; Bodeker, K.L.; Du, J.; Roberts, L.J.; et al. Pharmacological ascorbate with gemcitabine for the control of metastatic and node-positive pancreatic cancer (PACMAN): Results from a phase I clinical trial. *Cancer Chemother. Pharmacol.* **2013**, *71*, 765–775. [CrossRef] [PubMed]
3. Stephenson, C.M.; Levin, R.D.; Spector, T.; Lis, C.G. Phase I clinical trial to evaluate the safety, tolerability, and pharmacokinetics of high-dose intravenous ascorbic acid in patients with advanced cancer. *Cancer Chemother. Pharmacol.* **2013**, *72*, 139–146. [CrossRef] [PubMed]
4. Ma, Y.; Chapman, J.; Levine, M.; Polireddy, K.; Drisko, J.; Chen, Q. High-dose parenteral ascorbate enhanced chemosensitivity of ovarian cancer and reduced toxicity of chemotherapy. *Sci. Transl. Med.* **2014**, *6*, 222ra18. [CrossRef] [PubMed]
5. Schoenfeld, J.D.; Sibenaller, Z.A.; Mapuskar, K.A.; Wagner, B.A.; Cramer-Morales, K.L.; Furqan, M.; Sandhu, S.; Carlisle, T.L.; Smith, M.C.; Abu Hejleh, T.; et al. $O_2^{\bullet-}$ and H_2O_2-Mediated Disruption of Fe Metabolism Causes the Differential Susceptibility of NSCLC and GBM Cancer Cells to Pharmacological Ascorbate. *Cancer Cell* **2017**, *31*, 487–500.e8. [CrossRef] [PubMed]
6. Buettner, G.R. The pecking order of free radicals and antioxidants: Lipid peroxidation, alpha-tocopherol, and ascorbate. *Arch. Biochem. Biophys.* **1993**, *300*, 535–543. [CrossRef] [PubMed]
7. Du, J.; Martin, S.M.; Levine, M.; Wagner, B.A.; Buettner, G.R.; Wang, S.; Taghiyev, A.F.; Du, C.; Knudson, C.M.; Cullen, J.J. Mechanisms of ascorbate-induced cytotoxicity in pancreatic cancer. *Clin. Cancer Res.* **2010**, *16*, 509–520. [CrossRef] [PubMed]
8. Buettner, G.R. In the absence of catalytic metals ascorbate does not autoxidize at pH 7: Ascorbate as a test for catalytic metals. *J. Biochem. Biophys. Methods* **1988**, *16*, 27–40. [CrossRef]
9. Du, J.; Wagner, B.A.; Buettner, G.R.; Cullen, J.J. Role of labile iron in the toxicity of pharmacological ascorbate. *Free Radic. Biol. Med.* **2015**, *84*, 289–295. [CrossRef] [PubMed]
10. Rawal, M.; Schroeder, S.R.; Wagner, B.A.; Cushing, C.M.; Welsh, J.L.; Button, A.M.; Du, J.; Sibenaller, Z.A.; Buettner, G.R.; Cullen, J.J. Manganoporphyrins increase ascorbate-induced cytotoxicity by enhancing H_2O_2 generation. *Cancer Res.* **2013**, *73*, 5232–5241. [CrossRef] [PubMed]
11. Tovmasyan, A.; Sampaio, R.S.; Boss, M.-K.; Bueno-Janice, J.C.; Bader, B.H.; Thomas, M.; Reboucas, J.S.; Orr, M.; Chandler, J.D.; Go, Y.-M.; et al. Anticancer therapeutic potential of Mn porphyrin/ascorbate system. *Free Radic. Biol. Med.* **2015**, *89*, 1231–1247. [CrossRef] [PubMed]
12. Evans, M.K.; Tovmasyan, A.; Batinic-Haberle, I.; Devi, G.R. Mn porphyrin in combination with ascorbate acts as a pro-oxidant and mediates caspase-independent cancer cell death. *Free Radic. Biol. Med.* **2014**, *68*, 302–314. [CrossRef] [PubMed]
13. Cieslak, J.A.; Strother, R.K.; Rawal, M.; Du, J.; Doskey, C.M.; Schroeder, S.R.; Button, A.; Wagner, B.A.; Buettner, G.R.; Cullen, J.J. Manganoporphyrins and ascorbate enhance gemcitabine cytotoxicity in pancreatic cancer. *Free Radic. Biol. Med.* **2015**, *83*, 227–237. [CrossRef] [PubMed]
14. Batinić-Haberle, I.; Rajić, Z.; Benov, L. A Combination of Two Antioxidants (An SOD Mimic and Ascorbate) Produces a Pro-Oxidative Effect Forcing Escherichia coli to Adapt via Induction of oxyR Regulon. *Anticancer Agents Med. Chem.* **2011**, *11*, 329–340. [CrossRef] [PubMed]

15. Salvemini, D.; Mazzon, E.; Dugo, L.; Riley, D.P.; Serraino, I.; Caputi, A.P.; Cuzzocrea, S. Pharmacological manipulation of the inflammatory cascade by the superoxide dismutase mimetic, M40403. *Br. J. Pharmacol.* **2001**, *132*, 815–827. [CrossRef] [PubMed]
16. Salvemini, D.; Mazzon, E.; Dugo, L.; Serraino, I.; De Sarro, A.; Caputi, A.P.; Cuzzocrea, S. Amelioration of joint disease in a rat model of collagen-induced arthritis by M40403, a superoxide dismutase mimetic. *Arthritis Rheum.* **2001**, *44*, 2909–2921. [CrossRef]
17. Masini, E.; Cuzzocrea, S.; Mazzon, E.; Marzocca, C.; Mannaioni, P.F.; Salvemini, D. Protective effects of M40403, a selective superoxide dismutase mimetic, in myocardial ischaemia and reperfusion injury in vivo. *Br. J. Pharmacol.* **2002**, *136*, 905–917. [CrossRef] [PubMed]
18. Aston, K.; Rath, N.; Naik, A.; Slomczynska, U.; Schall, O.F.; Riley, D.P. Computer-Aided Design (CAD) of Mn(II) Complexes: Superoxide Dismutase Mimetics with Catalytic Activity Exceeding the Native Enzyme. *Inorg. Chem.* **2001**, *40*, 1779–1789. [CrossRef] [PubMed]
19. Mapuskar, K.A.; Flippo, K.H.; Schoenfeld, J.D.; Riley, D.P.; Strack, S.; Abu-Hejleh, T.; Furqan, M.; Monga, V.; Domann, F.E.; Buatti, J.M.; et al. Mitochondrial superoxide increases age-associated susceptibility of human dermal fibroblasts to radiation and chemotherapy. *Cancer Res.* 2017. [CrossRef] [PubMed]
20. Anderson, C.M.; Sonis, S.T.; Lee, C.M.; Adkins, D.; Allen, B.G.; Sun, W.; Agarwala, S.S.; Venigalla, M.L.; Chen, Y.; Zhen, W.; et al. Phase 1b/2a Trial of The Superoxide Dismutase Mimetic GC4419 to Reduce Chemoradiotherapy-induced Oral Mucositis in Patients with Oral Cavity or Oropharyngeal Carcinoma. *Int. J. Radiat. Oncol. Biol. Phys.* 2017. [CrossRef] [PubMed]
21. Kelso, G.F.; Maroz, A.; Cochemé, H.M.; Logan, A.; Prime, T.A.; Peskin, A.V.; Winterbourn, C.C.; James, A.M.; Ross, M.F.; Brooker, S.; et al. A Mitochondria-Targeted Macrocyclic Mn(II) Superoxide Dismutase Mimetic. *Chem. Biol.* **2012**, *19*, 1237–1246. [CrossRef] [PubMed]
22. Doskey, C.M.; van't Erve, T.J.; Wagner, B.A.; Buettner, G.R. Moles of a Substance per Cell Is a Highly Informative Dosing Metric in Cell Culture. *PLoS ONE* **2015**, *10*, e0132572. [CrossRef] [PubMed]
23. Spitz, D.R.; Dewey, W.C.; Li, G.C. Hydrogen peroxide or heat shock induces resistance to hydrogen peroxide in Chinese hamster fibroblasts. *J. Cell. Physiol.* **1987**, *131*, 364–373. [CrossRef] [PubMed]
24. Doskey, C.M.; Buranasudja, V.; Wagner, B.A.; Wilkes, J.G.; Du, J.; Cullen, J.J.; Buettner, G.R. Tumor cells have decreased ability to metabolize H_2O_2: Implications for pharmacological ascorbate in cancer therapy. *Redox Biol.* **2016**, *10*, 274–284. [CrossRef] [PubMed]
25. Buettner, G.R.; Kiminyo, K.P. Optimal EPR detection of weak nitroxide spin adduct and ascorbyl free radical signals. *J. Biochem. Biophys. Methods* **1992**, *24*, 147–151. [CrossRef]
26. Spitz, D.R.; Oberley, L.W. An assay for superoxide dismutase activity in mammalian tissue homogenates. *Anal. Biochem.* **1989**, *179*, 8–18. [CrossRef]
27. Brandt, K.E.; Falls, K.C.; Schoenfeld, J.D.; Rodman, S.N.; Gu, Z.; Zhan, F.; Cullen, J.J.; Wagner, B.A.; Buettner, G.R.; Allen, B.G.; et al. Augmentation of intracellular iron using iron sucrose enhances the toxicity of pharmacological ascorbate in colon cancer cells. *Redox Biol.* **2018**, *14*, 82–87. [CrossRef] [PubMed]
28. Spitz, D.R.; Elwell, J.H.; Sun, Y.; Oberley, L.W.; Oberley, T.D.; Sullivan, S.J.; Roberts, R.J. Oxygen toxicity in control and H_2O_2-resistant Chinese hamster fibroblast cell lines. *Arch. Biochem. Biophys.* **1990**, *279*, 249–260. [CrossRef]
29. Buettner, G.R.; Jurkiewicz, B.A. Ascorbate free radical as a marker of oxidative stress: An EPR study. *Free Radic. Biol. Med.* **1993**, *14*, 49–55. [CrossRef]
30. Goldstein, S.; Fridovich, I.; Czapski, G. Kinetic properties of Cu,Zn-superoxide dismutase as a function of metal content—order restored. *Free Radic. Biol. Med.* **2006**, *41*, 937–941. [CrossRef] [PubMed]
31. Spitz, D.R.; Azzam, E.I.; Li, J.J.; Gius, D. Metabolic oxidation/reduction reactions and cellular responses to ionizing radiation: A unifying concept in stress response biology. *Cancer Metastasis Rev.* **2004**, *23*, 311–322. [CrossRef] [PubMed]
32. Du, J.; Cullen, J.J.; Buettner, G.R. Ascorbic acid: Chemistry, biology and the treatment of cancer. *Biochim. Biophys. Acta* **2012**, *1826*, 443–457. [CrossRef] [PubMed]
33. Buettner, G.R.; Jurkiewicz, B.A. Catalytic metals, ascorbate and free radicals: Combinations to avoid. *Radiat. Res.* **1996**, *145*, 532–541. [CrossRef] [PubMed]
34. Riley, D.P.; Lennon, P.J.; Neumann, W.L.; Weiss, R.H. Toward the rational design of superoxide dismutase mimics: Mechanistic studies for the elucidation of substituent effects on the catalytic activity of macrocyclic manganese(ii) complexes. *J. Am. Chem. Soc.* **1997**, *119*, 6522–6528. [CrossRef]

35. Riley, D.P.; Schall, O.F. Structure—Activity Studies and the Design of Synthetic Superoxide Dismutase (SOD) Mimetics as Therapeutics. In *Advances in Inorganic Chemistry: Template Effects and Molecular Organization*; van Eldik, R., Bowman-James, K., Eds.; Academic Press: Cambridge, MA, USA, 2006; Volume 59, pp. 233–263.
36. Maroz, A.; Kelso, G.F.; Smith, R.A.J.; Ware, D.C.; Anderson, R.F. Pulse radiolysis investigation on the mechanism of the catalytic action of Mn(II)−pentaazamacrocycle compounds as superoxide dismutase mimetics. *J. Phys. Chem. A* **2008**, *112*, 4929–4935. [CrossRef] [PubMed]

Permissions

All chapters in this book were first published in ANTIOXIDANTS, by MDPI; hereby published with permission under the Creative Commons Attribution License or equivalent. Every chapter published in this book has been scrutinized by our experts. Their significance has been extensively debated. The topics covered herein carry significant findings which will fuel the growth of the discipline. They may even be implemented as practical applications or may be referred to as a beginning point for another development.

The contributors of this book come from diverse backgrounds, making this book a truly international effort. This book will bring forth new frontiers with its revolutionizing research information and detailed analysis of the nascent developments around the world.

We would like to thank all the contributing authors for lending their expertise to make the book truly unique. They have played a crucial role in the development of this book. Without their invaluable contributions this book wouldn't have been possible. They have made vital efforts to compile up to date information on the varied aspects of this subject to make this book a valuable addition to the collection of many professionals and students.

This book was conceptualized with the vision of imparting up-to-date information and advanced data in this field. To ensure the same, a matchless editorial board was set up. Every individual on the board went through rigorous rounds of assessment to prove their worth. After which they invested a large part of their time researching and compiling the most relevant data for our readers.

The editorial board has been involved in producing this book since its inception. They have spent rigorous hours researching and exploring the diverse topics which have resulted in the successful publishing of this book. They have passed on their knowledge of decades through this book. To expedite this challenging task, the publisher supported the team at every step. A small team of assistant editors was also appointed to further simplify the editing procedure and attain best results for the readers.

Apart from the editorial board, the designing team has also invested a significant amount of their time in understanding the subject and creating the most relevant covers. They scrutinized every image to scout for the most suitable representation of the subject and create an appropriate cover for the book.

The publishing team has been an ardent support to the editorial, designing and production team. Their endless efforts to recruit the best for this project, has resulted in the accomplishment of this book. They are a veteran in the field of academics and their pool of knowledge is as vast as their experience in printing. Their expertise and guidance has proved useful at every step. Their uncompromising quality standards have made this book an exceptional effort. Their encouragement from time to time has been an inspiration for everyone.

The publisher and the editorial board hope that this book will prove to be a valuable piece of knowledge for researchers, students, practitioners and scholars across the globe.

List of Contributors

Giuseppina Barrera, Stefania Pizzimenti, Martina Daga and Marie Angele Cucci
Dipartimento di Scienze Cliniche e Biologiche, Università di Torino, 10124 Turin, Italy

Chiara Dianzani
Dipartimento di Scienze e Tecnologia del Farmaco, Università di Torino, 10124 Turin, Italy

Alessia Arcaro, Giovanni Paolo Cetrangolo and Fabrizio Gentile
Dipartimento di Medicina e Scienze della Salute "V. Tiberio", Università del Molise, 86100 Campobasso, Italy

Giulio Giordano and Maria Graf
Presidio Ospedaliero "A. Cardarelli", Azienda Sanitaria Regione Molise, 86100 Campobasso, Italy

Abbey Symes, Amin Shavandi, Hongxia Zhang and Alaa El-Din Ahmed Bekhit
Department of Food Science, University of Otago, Dunedin 9054, New Zealand

Isam A. Mohamed Ahmed and Fahad Y. Al-Juhaimi
Department of Food Science and Nutrition, College of Food and Agricultural Sciences, King Saud University, Riyadh 11451, Saudi Arabia

Arpita Chatterjee, Yuxiang Zhu, Elizabeth A. Kosmacek, Eliezer Z. Lichter and Rebecca E. Oberley-Deegan
Department of Biochemistry and Molecular Biology, University of Nebraska Medical Center, Omaha, NE 68198, USA

Qiang Tong
Department of Biochemistry and Molecular Biology, University of Nebraska Medical Center, Omaha, NE 68198, USA
Department of Gastrointestinal Surgery, Union Hospital, Tongji Medical College, Huazhong University of Science and Technology, Wuhan 430022, China

Julio César Camarena-Tello
Programa Institucional de Doctorado en Ciencias Biológicas, Universidad Michoacana de San Nicolás de Hidalgo, Morelia 58240, Mich., Mexico

Héctor Eduardo Martínez-Flores, María Carmen Bartolomé-Camacho and José Octavio Rodiles-López
Facultad de Químico Farmacobiología, Universidad Michoacana de San Nicolás de Hidalgo, Morelia 58240, Mich., Mexico

Ma. Guadalupe Garnica-Romo
Facultad de Ingeniería Civil, Universidad Michoacana de San Nicolás de Hidalgo, Morelia 58240, Mich., Mexico

José Saúl Padilla-Ramírez
Instituto Nacional de Investigaciones Forestales, Agrícolas y Pecuarias, Centro de Investigación Regional Norte-Centro, Campo Experimental Pabellón, Pabellón de Arteaga 20660, Aguascalientes, Mexico

Alfredo Saavedra-Molina
Instituto de Investigaciones Químico Biológicas, Universidad Michoacana de San Nicolás de Hidalgo, Morelia 58030, Mich., Mexico

Osvaldo Alvarez-Cortes
Departamento de Bioquímica, Instituto Tecnológico de Morelia, Morelia 58120, Mich., Mexico

Jean-Claude Lavoie
Department of Nutrition, Faculty of Medicine, Université de Montréal, Sainte-Justine Hospital, Montréal, QC H3T 1C5, Canada

André Tremblay
Department Obstetrics & Gynecology, and department of Biochemistry and Molecular Medicine, Faculty of Medicine, University of Montreal, Sainte-Justine Hospital, Montréal, QC H3T 1C5, Canada

Muhammad Jawad Nasim, Muhammad Sarfraz and Claus Jacob
Division of Bioorganic Chemistry, School of Pharmacy, Saarland University, D-66123 Saarbruecken, Germany

Sharoon Griffin
Division of Bioorganic Chemistry, School of Pharmacy, Saarland University, D-66123 Saarbruecken, Germany
Institute of Pharmaceutics and Biopharmaceutics, Philipps University of Marburg, 35037 Marburg, Germany

Cornelia M. Keck
Institute of Pharmaceutics and Biopharmaceutics, Philipps University of Marburg, 35037 Marburg, Germany

Muhammad Irfan Masood
Division of Bioorganic Chemistry, School of Pharmacy, Saarland University, D-66123 Saarbruecken, Germany
Department of Biotechnology, University of Applied Sciences Kaiserslautern, 66482 Zweibruecken, Germany

Karl-Herbert Schäfer
Department of Biotechnology, University of Applied Sciences Kaiserslautern, 66482 Zweibruecken, Germany

Azubuike Peter Ebokaiwe
Department of Chemistry/Biochemistry and Molecular Biology, Federal University, Ndufu-Alike Ikwo, 482131 Ndufu-Alike, Nigeria

Juliet M. Pullar, Anitra C. Carr, Stephanie M. Bozonet and Margreet C. M. Vissers
Centre for Free Radical Research, Department of Pathology and Biomedical Science, University of Otago, Christchurch, Christchurch 8140, New Zealand

Gwendolyn N. Y. van Gorkom, Roel G. J. Klein Wolterink, Catharina H. M. J. Van Elssen, Wilfred T. V. Germeraad and Gerard M. J. Bos
Division of Hematology, Department of Internal Medicine, GROW-School for Oncology and Developmental Biology, Maastricht University Medical Center, 6202AZ Maastricht, The Netherlands

Lotte Wieten
Department of Transplantation Immunology, Maastricht University Medical Center, 6202 AZ Maastricht, The Netherlands

Kin Sum Leung and Jetty Chung-Yung Lee
School of Biological Sciences, The University of Hong Kong, Pokfulam Road, Hong Kong, China

Jean-Marie Galano and Thierry Durand
Institut des Biomolécules Max Mousseron (IBMM), UMR 5247, CNRS Université de Montpellier, ENSCM, F-34093 Montpellier, France

Giovanna Fia, Ginevra Bucalossi and Bruno Zanoni
Dipartimento di Gestione dei Sistemi Agrari, Alimentari e Forestali, University of Florence, Via Donizetti, 6, 50144 Firenze, Italy

Claudio Gori
Vino Vigna, Via Claudio Monteverdi, 9, 50053 Empoli, Italy

Francesca Borghini
ISVEA Srl, Servizi Analitici di Eccellenza per i Settori Enologico, Viticolo e il Comparto Alimentare, Via Basilicata 1/3, Poggibonsi, 53036 Siena, Italy

Sara Rocha
i3S—Instituto de Investigação e Inovação em Saúde, Universidade do Porto, 4200-135 Porto, Portugal
IBMC—Instituto de Biologia Molecular e Celular, Universidade do Porto, 4200-135 Porto, Portugal

Ana Freitas
i3S—Instituto de Investigação e Inovação em Saúde, Universidade do Porto, 4200-135 Porto, Portugal
INEB—Instituto de Engenharia Biomédica, Universidade do Porto, 4200-135 Porto, Portugal
FMUP—Faculdade de Medicina da Universidade do Porto, 4200-319 Porto, Portugal

Sofia C. Guimaraes, Miguel Aroso and Maria Gomez-Lazaro
i3S—Instituto de Investigação e Inovação em Saúde, Universidade do Porto, 4200-135 Porto, Portugal
INEB—Instituto de Engenharia Biomédica, Universidade do Porto, 4200-135 Porto, Portugal

Rui Vitorino
iBiMED, Department of Medical Sciences, University of Aveiro, 3810-193 Aveiro, Portugal
Unidade de Investigação Cardiovascular, Departamento de Cirurgia e Fisiologia, Universidade do Porto, 4200-319 Porto, Portugal

Mariola Cano Sanchez
Laboratory of Cardiovascular Physiology, Antilles University, P-97200 Fort de France, France
Tissue Repair and Regeneration Laboratory (TR2Lab), University of Vic-UCC, Vic P-08500 Barcelone, Spain

Steve Lancel
INSERM U1011-EGID, Institut Pasteur de Lille, Université Lille, CHU Lille, F-59000 Lille, France

Eric Boulanger
INSERM U995-LIRIC Inflammation Research International Centre, Université Lille, F-59000 Lille, France
Département de Gériatrie, CHU Lille, F-59000 Lille, France

Remi Neviere
Laboratory of Cardiovascular Physiology, Antilles University, P-97200 Fort de France, France
INSERM U995-LIRIC Inflammation Research International Centre, Université Lille, F-59000 Lille, France

Département de Physiologie, CHU Lille, F-59000 Lille, France

Kimberly J. Krager
Department of Pharmaceutical Sciences, College of Pharmacy, University of Arkansas for Medical Sciences, Little Rock, AR 72205, USA

Ujwani Nukala
Department of Pharmaceutical Sciences, College of Pharmacy, University of Arkansas for Medical Sciences, Little Rock, AR 72205, USA
Joint Bioinformatics Graduate Program, University of Arkansas at Little Rock, Little Rock, AR 72204, USA

Shraddha Thakkar
Division of Bioinformatics and Biostatistics, National Center for Toxicological Research, US Food and Drug Administration, Jefferson, AR 72079, USA

Philip J. Breen, Cesar M. Compadre and Nukhet Aykin-Burns
Department of Pharmaceutical Sciences, College of Pharmacy, University of Arkansas for Medical Sciences, Little Rock, AR 72205, USA
Tocol Pharmaceuticals, LLC, Little Rock, AR 77205, USA

Collin D. Heer, Andrew B. Davis, David B. Riffe, Brett A. Wagner, Kelly C. Falls, Bryan G. Allen, Garry R. Buettner and Douglas R. Spitz
Free Radical and Radiation Biology Program, Department of Radiation Oncology, Holden Comprehensive Cancer Center, The University of Iowa College of Medicine, Iowa City, IA 52242, USA

Robert A. Beardsley and Dennis P. Riley
Galera Therapeutics, Malvern, PA 19355, USA

Index

R

S

T

V